Respiratory Medicine

Series Editor:
Sharon I.S. Rounds

Stephanie D. Davis • Ernst Eber
Anastassios C. Koumbourlis

Editors

Diagnostic Tests in Pediatric Pulmonology

Applications and Interpretation

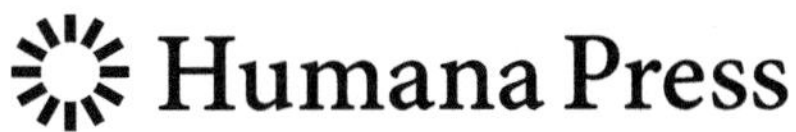

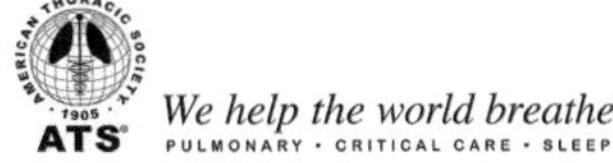

Editors
Stephanie D. Davis, M.D.
Section of Pediatric Pulmonology
  Allergy and Sleep Medicine
Riley Hospital for Children
Indiana University School of Medicine
Indianapolis, IN, USA

Ernst Eber, M.D.
Respiratory and Allergic Disease Division
Department of Paediatrics
  and Adolescent Medicine
Medical University of Graz
Graz, Austria

Anastassios C. Koumbourlis, M.D., M.P.H.
Division of Pulmonary and Sleep Medicine
Children's National Medical
  Center/George Washington University
School of Medicine and Health Sciences
Washington, DC, USA

ISSN 2197-7372
ISBN 978-1-4939-4400-2
DOI 10.1007/978-1-4939-1801-0
Springer New York Heidelberg Dordrecht London

ISSN 2197-7380 (electronic)
ISBN 978-1-4939-1801-0 (eBook)

Preface

Over the past 20 years, diagnostic tests for pediatric pulmonologists have revolutionized care of children afflicted with respiratory disorders. These tests have been used to help not only in diagnosis but also in the management and treatment of these children. Bronchoscopic, imaging, and physiologic advances have improved clinical care and have also been used as outcome measures in research trials.

The aims of this book are to (1) describe the various diagnostic modalities (especially the newer ones) that are available for the evaluation of pediatric respiratory disorders; (2) understand the advantages and limitations of each test so that the clinician may choose the most appropriate modality; and (3) describe how best to interpret the key findings in a variety of tests as well as the possible pitfalls in interpretation.

The book focuses on the main diagnostic modalities used in the evaluation of pediatric patients with respiratory disorders and presents up-to-date information on a number of tests that are used for a variety of conditions encountered in the practice of pediatric pulmonology. The clinical applications of the tests are highlighted within each chapter.

The book contains 14 chapters written by 30 authors; the authors are both young pediatric pulmonologists who are emerging as leaders in our field as well as well-known international experts.

Target readers are practicing clinicians including pediatric pulmonologists, intensivists, pediatricians, and primary care practitioners. Other readers may include trainees, respiratory therapists, nurses, radiologists, and clinical researchers.

We would like to thank the staff at Springer, especially Maureen Alexander and Amanda Quinn, for endorsing and editing the book. We especially would like to thank our expert authors for writing such detailed and outstanding chapters. Finally, we would like to thank our families for their continual love, support, and encouragement during this endeavor.

Indianapolis, IN, USA	Stephanie D. Davis
Graz, Austria	Ernst Eber
Washington, DC, USA	Anastassios C. Koumbourlis

Contents

Contributors

Alan S. Brody, M.D. Cincinnati Children's Hospital and the University of Cincinnati College of Medicine, Cincinnati, OH, USA

Department of Radiology, Cincinnati Children's Medical Center, Cincinnati, OH, USA

Mark A. Chilvers, M.D. Division of Pediatric Respiratory Medicine, British Columbia's Children's Hospital, University of British Columbia, Vancouver, BC, Canada

Andrew A. Colin, M.D. Division of Pediatric Pulmonology, Miller School of Medicine, Batchelor Children's Research Institute, University of Miami, Miami, FL, USA

Daniel P. Credeur, Ph.D. Department of Medical Pharmacology and Physiology, University of Missouri, Columbia, MO, USA

Stephanie D. Davis, M.D. Section of Pediatric Pulmonology, Allergy and Sleep Medicine, Riley Children Hospital, Indiana University School of Medicine, Indianapolis, IN, USA

Ernst Eber, M.D. Respiratory and Allergic Disease Division, Department of Paediatrics and Adolescent Medicine, Medical University of Graz, Graz, Austria

Graham L. Hall, Ph.D., F.R.A.N.Z.S.R.S. Telethon Kids Institute, University of Western Australia, West Perth, WA, Australia

Respiratory Medicine, Princess Margaret Hospital for Children, Perth, WA, Australia

Carolyn M. Kercsmar, M.S., M.D. Pediatrics, Asthma Center, Cincinnati Children's Hospital Medical Center, Cincinnati, OH, USA

Young-Jee Kim, M.D. Section of Pediatric Pulmonology, Allergy and Sleep Medicine, Indiana University School of Medicine, Riley Hospital for Children, Indianapolis, IN, USA

Anastassios C. Koumbourlis, M.D., M.P.H. Division of Pulmonary and Sleep Medicine, Children's National Medical Center/George Washington University, School of Medicine and Health Sciences, Washington, DC, USA

Margaret W. Leigh, M.D. Pediatric Pulmonology Division, Department of Pediatrics, UNC Hospitals, University of North Carolina, Chapel Hill, NC, USA

Carolina Z. Marcus, M.D. Department of Pediatrics, University of Rochester Medical Center, Rochester, NY, USA

Fabio Midulla, M.D. Department of Paediatrics, "Sapienza" University of Rome, Rome, Italy

Raffaella Nenna, M.D. Department of Paediatrics, "Sapienza" University of Rome, Rome, Italy

Judith A. Owens, M.D., D,A.B.S.M. Division of Pulmonary and Sleep Medicine, Children's National Health System, Washington, DC, USA

Annabelle Quizon, M.D. Section of Pediatric Pulmonology, Baystate Medical Center, Springfield, MA, USA

Mantosh S. Rattan, M.D. Cincinnati Children's Hospital and the University of Cincinnati College of Medicine, Cincinnati, OH, USA

Department of Radiology, Cincinnati Children's Medical Center, Cincinnati, OH, USA

Joel Reiter, M.D. Division of Pediatric Pulmonology, Miller School of Medicine, Batchelor Children's Research Institute, University of Miami, Miami, FL, USA

Clement L. Ren, M.D. Department of Pediatrics, Golisano Children's Hospital at Strong, University of Rochester, Rochester, NY, USA

Paul D. Robinson, M.B.Ch.B., M.R.C.P.C.H., F.R.A.C.P., Ph.D. Respiratory Medicine, The Children's Hospital at Westmead, Sydney, NSW, Australia

Margaret Rosenfeld, M.D., M.P.H. Division of Pulmonary Medicine, Seattle Children's Hospital, Seattle, WA, USA

Giovanni A. Rossi, M.D. Pediatric Pulmonology and Allergy Unit, Istituto Giannina Gaslini, Largo Gaslini, Genoa, Italy

Steven M. Rowe, M.D., M.S.P.H. Division of Pulmonary Allergy and Critical Care Medicine, Department of Medicine, University of Alabama at Birmingham, Birmingham, AL, USA

Iman R. Sami, M.D., M.R.C.P. Division of Pulmonary and Sleep Medicine, Children's National Health System, Washington, DC, USA

Adam J. Shapiro, M.D. Pediatric Respiratory Medicine, Montreal Children's Hospital, McGill University, Montreal, QC, Canada

George M. Solomon, M.D. Division of Pulmonary Allergy and Critical Care Medicine, Department of Medicine, University of Alabama at Birmingham, Birmingham, AL, USA

Sanja Stanojevic, Ph.D. Division of Respiratory Medicine, The Hospital for Sick Children, Toronto, ON, Canada

Janet Stocks, Ph.D. Respiratory, Critical Care and Anaesthesia Section, UCL, Institute of Child Health, London, UK

David Thomas, M.D., Ph.D. Pediatric Center for Respiratory, Exercise and Sleep Medicine, Athletic Training Facility Football Operations, Louisiana State University, Baton Rouge, LA, USA

Louisiana Healthcare Connections, Baton Rouge, LA, USA

Robert E. Wood, Ph.D., M.D. Pulmonary Medicine and Otolaryngology, Cincinnati Children's Hospital, Cincinnati, OH, USA

Chapter 1
The Evaluation of the Upper and Lower Airways in Infants and Children: Principles and Pearls from Four Decades in the Trenches

Robert E. Wood

Abstract Diagnostic bronchoscopy is an often underutilized technique in pediatric patients. However, with proper equipment, appropriate technical and cognitive skills, and effective and careful attention to safety and comfort, bronchoscopy can be a powerful tool for the pediatric pulmonologist. This review is a distillation of the author's four decades of experience.

Keywords Flexible bronchoscopy • Airway dynamics • Sedation/anesthesia for pediatric bronchoscopy • Airway management for pediatric flexible bronchoscopy • Indications for pediatric flexible bronchoscopy • Complications of pediatric flexible bronchoscopy • Techniques for pediatric flexible bronchoscopy • Clinical utility of pediatric flexible bronchoscopy

Bronchoscopy is a powerful diagnostic and therapeutic tool for the evaluation and management of children with pulmonary or airway issues. During the 1970s, dramatic progress was made in the development of instrumentation suitable for pediatric bronchoscopy, including the glass rod telescope for rigid instruments and a flexible bronchoscope small enough to be safely used in children. Over the ensuing nearly four decades, further progress has been made in instrumentation as well as experience in the utilization of these instruments.

R.E. Wood, Ph.D., M.D. (✉)
Pulmonary Medicine and Otolaryngology, Cincinnati Children's Hospital,
3333 Burnet Ave MLC 2021, Cincinnati, OH 45229-3039, USA
e-mail: rewood@cchmc.org

© Springer Science+Business Media New York 2015
S.D. Davis et al. (eds.), *Diagnostic Tests in Pediatric Pulmonology*,
Respiratory Medicine, DOI 10.1007/978-1-4939-1801-0_1

The discussion in this chapter is predicated on the assumption that the operator will be equipped with the proper equipment (which is properly cleaned and prepared for use in the patient), trained assistants, a proper venue, appropriate provision for sedation/anesthesia and monitoring of the patient's physiologic status, and a plan for safe recovery from the sedation, and that the parents/guardians have provided appropriate informed consent.

This chapter is primarily a distillation of my personal experience over the past four decades of spelunking in the pediatric airways. The views expressed are mine, and are based on more than 20,000 procedures. I have made (and learned from) many mistakes … my practices and perspective have evolved over this time.

Principles

There are four criteria for successful bronchoscopy: (1) safety, (2) safety, (3) comfort, and (4) achieving the correct diagnosis or result.

Other than death of the patient, the most serious complication of a bronchoscopy is to have done the procedure but obtained the wrong diagnostic or therapeutic result.

Match the instrument(s) to the patient and purpose of the procedure.

Be aware of the effect of sedation level and body position as well as the effect of the instrument itself and techniques utilized for airway management on the visualized anatomy and airway dynamics.

The airways begin at the nostril ….

Children often have more than one significant airway abnormality—examine the entire airway unless contraindicated.

"WNL" too often really means, "We Never Looked."

The endoscopic findings must be interpreted *in the context of the patient's history*—some things that look bad may not be physiologically important and may be the result of the sedation or conditions under which the examination is performed. Or vice versa ….

Stridor is always visible.

Every bronchoscopic procedure performed in children should be recorded so that the video record can be examined again when necessary.

Indications for Procedures

There are only two indications for bronchoscopy in children, diagnostic and therapeutic. Diagnostic bronchoscopy is indicated when there is information in the lungs or airways of the child, necessary for the care of the child, that is best obtained with a bronchoscope. Similarly, therapeutic bronchoscopy is indicated when it is the best way to achieve the necessary therapeutic goals. The specific indications for bronchoscopy will vary considerably among different institutions, as there will inevitably be wide variation in the patient populations.

A Basic Philosophy of Bronchoscopy

No one knows what lurks in the airways of a child, and surprises abound. The bronchoscopist must be careful to examine the entire airway in each patient, unless there is a very good reason not to do so. For example, an intubated immunosuppressed patient who is thrombocytopenic does not need to have a scope passed through the nose unless in search of specific pathology, as there is more risk than benefit involved.

The bronchoscopist must adopt a surgical mentality—you are sent to drain the swamp, not merely to survey and report back—i.e., take care of things that can be taken care of …. Discovering and then simply reporting the finding of a mucus plug is not enough—remove the mucus plug if it is possible/reasonable to do so. Every diagnostic bronchoscopy has the potential to also be a therapeutic procedure. Likewise, every therapeutic bronchoscopy includes a diagnostic component. When a flexible bronchoscope is employed to facilitate a difficult intubation, for example, the operator should recognize and report the abnormal anatomy or other factors that make the intubation difficult; otherwise, a golden opportunity may be missed, and the patient may be forced to undergo yet another procedure.

The goals of bronchoscopy are to evaluate the airway anatomy, dynamics, and contents, to obtain appropriate specimens for further analysis (as indicated), to relate the findings to the patient's history and clinical context, and to improve the patient's clinical status when feasible. When contemplating a bronchoscopy, the assessment of risk must also include the risk of *not* doing the bronchoscopy.

Bronchoscopy is a visual procedure—the work product is primarily *images*. Every procedure should be recorded for review at some later point in time—this will improve the quality of patient care, facilitate teaching (parents, patients, and medical trainees), and reduce the potential for medicolegal liability. Written documentation is also important, and should include enough descriptive language to enable the reader to develop a reasonably accurate picture of what was actually seen and done.

Instruments

Diagnostic and/or therapeutic bronchoscopy may be done with either rigid or flexible instruments, and in many cases, either instrument will suffice for the patient's immediate need. However, there are clearly indications for which a rigid instrument is much more suitable, and some for which a flexible instrument is more suitable. Additionally, for the adequate evaluation of some pediatric patients, utilization of *both* rigid and flexible instruments may be necessary.

A bronchoscope must be small enough to safely traverse the airway of the patient. The most common flexible instrument utilized in pediatric patients today has an outer diameter of 2.8 mm, and this instrument can be safely used in children as small as approximately 600 g (although in children smaller than about 1,200 g, great care must be taken to ensure adequate ventilation or very rapid completion of the procedure). This instrument (and its predecessor, which is approximately 3.7 mm) has a 1.2 mm suction channel; this limits the devices that can be passed through the channel. Instruments with a larger suction channel can be used in older children, and may be necessary when airway secretions are extremely thick or instrumentation is necessary.

Rigid instruments utilize a glass rod telescope, which produces an image with extremely high resolution. Rigid bronchoscopes and telescopes are available in a variety of sizes. A major limitation of rigid instrumentation is that it is necessary to pass the instrument through the mouth, extending the neck and elevating the mandible. This may not be possible in all patients, and, in any event, will distort the anatomy and airway dynamics.

The traditional techniques for flexible bronchoscopy involve transnasal passage, thus enabling examination of the entire airway, and placing minimal traction on airway structures, giving the most effective visualization of airway dynamics. However, transnasal passage means that the tip of the instrument must be flexed forward to view and enter the larynx (Fig. 1.1), making evaluation of the posterior aspects of the larynx much more difficult. It can be virtually impossible to diagnose a laryngoesophageal cleft, for example, with a flexible bronchoscope. A rigid bronchoscope, on the other hand, approaches the larynx from a very different angle (Fig. 1.1), and is the instrument of choice for evaluation of the anatomic details of the larynx, and especially the posterior commissure. Children suspected of aspiration should in most cases be evaluated with both rigid and flexible instruments in order to definitively ensure that there is no laryngoesophageal cleft or "H-type" TE fistula.

Sedation, Anesthesia, and Airway Management for Flexible Bronchoscopy in Children

It is possible to examine a child's airway without sedation. The most common setting for this approach is a simple evaluation of the nasopharyngeal airway and larynx in an office setting, including the endoscopic assessment of swallowing. Most children do not like this, and it may be difficult for the operator as well. However, full assessment of vocal cord function may require this approach. When the bronchoscope needs to be passed beyond the glottis, it is much wiser and safer to provide sedation for pediatric patients.

In the early days of pediatric flexible bronchoscopy, most procedures were done with sedation provided by the bronchoscopist. Today, most procedures are performed with the aid of an anesthesiologist, and this is very appropriate, in order to enhance safety; it also enables the use of agents that are generally restricted to use by anesthesiologists and can provide a more smooth and comfortable evaluation. However, choice of the wrong technique for sedation is one of the easiest ways to achieve the wrong diagnosis. Sedation that is too deep may mask dynamic pathology, and sedation that is not sufficiently deep may increase the risk of complications and possibly lead to termination of the procedure before the answer has been obtained. It is vitally important that the bronchoscopist and the person responsible

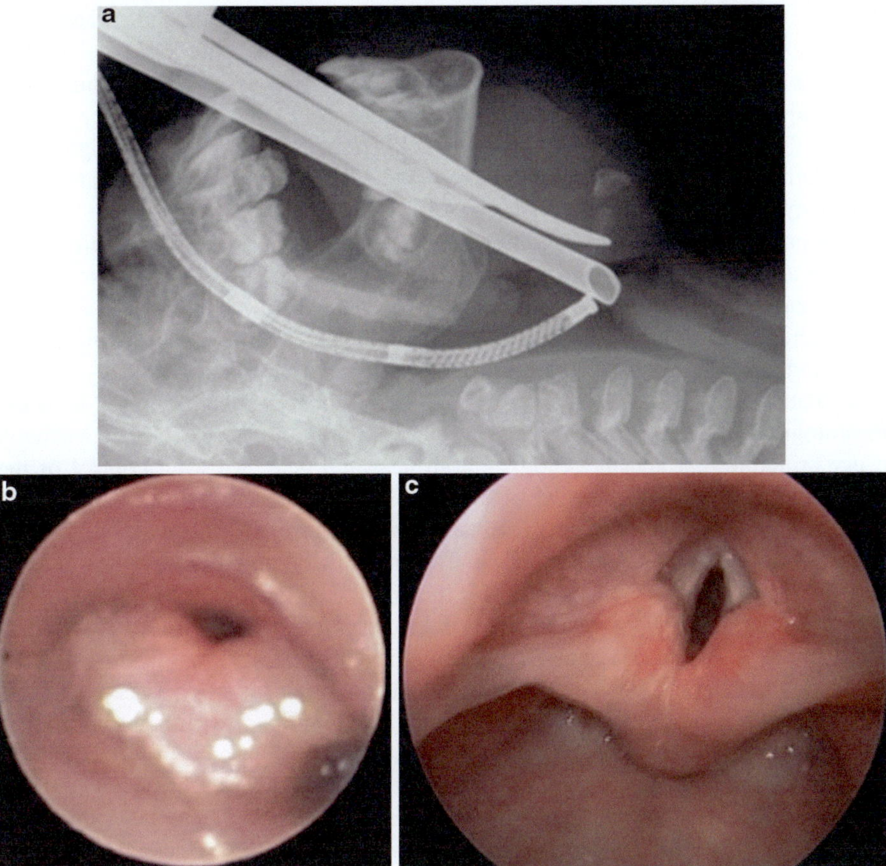

Fig. 1.1 Flexible and rigid instruments approach the larynx from very different perspectives. A rigid instrument necessarily elevates the hyoid and tongue base, lifting and distorting the larynx, while at the same time allowing more detailed anatomic evaluation as well as manipulation of the tissues under direct vision. The flexible instrument, on the other hand, approaches from behind, and is much more suitable for evaluation of laryngeal dynamics. When there is any suspicion of posterior laryngeal pathology (laryngoesophageal cleft, for example) both instruments may need to be employed in order to obtain a full understanding of the laryngeal anatomy and dynamics. (**a**) Lateral radiograph showing the path taken by rigid and flexible instruments. Note the elevation of the hyoid and tongue base by the rigid instrument and the angle of approach to the larynx by both instruments (this is not the same patient as in **b** and **c**). (**b**) The larynx of a child with a history of inspiratory stridor, seen by a flexible instrument. There is no traction on the larynx, and in this view, the mucosa overlying the arytenoid cartilages completely obscures the view of the glottis, and produces significant inspiratory obstruction. (**c**) The same larynx as seen by a rigid instrument. The larynx is being elevated by a rigid laryngoscope. The mucosa, which through the flexible instrument looked redundant and possibly edematous, now looks anatomically normal, and there is no obvious obstruction

for the sedation and monitoring of the child both have an adequate understanding of the purpose of the procedure and that they communicate effectively before, during, and after the procedure. It is often useful to change the level of sedation during the course of an examination. For example, a deeper level of sedation at the beginning may facilitate the anatomic evaluation and collection of specimens, while lightening the sedation near the end of the procedure may facilitate documentation of abnormal airway dynamics.

The precise techniques utilized for sedation of children for bronchoscopic procedures is as much a matter of personal preference as anything, as long as the patient is safe and the goals of the procedure are adequately met. Mask induction followed by establishment of intravenous access and maintenance with a short-acting parenteral drug can be a very effective technique.

Pediatric bronchoscopy is certainly among the most challenging tasks an anesthesiologist is called upon to perform. As bronchoscopists, we violate virtually every principle that anesthesiologists hold near and dear: we want control of the airway, we want to see the airway obstruct (at least, long enough for us to be able to understand why the child's airway is obstructing), and we often want to see the child cough (so that we can see lower airway dynamics). Modern bronchoscopes employ digital display, and it is very helpful for the anesthesiologist to be able to visualize what the bronchoscopist is seeing. This does not in itself suffice for effective communication between the bronchoscopist and the anesthesiologist.

Airway management can be one of the most contentious issues between the anesthesiologist and the bronchoscopist. Typically, the child is placed under light anesthesia so that spontaneous ventilation is maintained, and an oral airway is placed. The bronchoscope is then inserted through one nostril. However, the presence of the oral airway distorts the anatomy, and it often needs to be removed, at least temporarily, while the upper airway anatomy and dynamics are assessed. Once this is accomplished, the oral airway can be reinserted and the bronchoscope directed into the lower airways. The bronchoscopist should evaluate the position of the oral airway (in many cases, the oral airway may actually push the posterior tongue over the larynx, obstructing, rather than opening, the airway). It is quite effective (so long as the patient is breathing spontaneously) to insert an endotracheal tube into the oral airway to provide for delivery of oxygen and anesthetic gas directly to the larynx (Fig. 1.2).

Many bronchoscopists and anesthesiologists routinely perform their procedures through a laryngeal mask airway (LMA). While this is easy, and allows positive pressure ventilation from start to finish, there are many reasons to condemn this as a routine practice. An LMA completely bypasses the nasopharyngeal airway, and many diagnoses will be missed. The LMA also presses against the post-cricoid region of the larynx, and can interfere with vocal cord motion; it also can put downward traction on the post-cricoid mucosa, making it impossible to adequately diagnose some forms of laryngomalacia (see Figs. 1.3 and 1.4). An LMA does not prevent laryngospasm or even, necessarily, aspiration of oral secretions. When positive pressure support is given through the LMA, it can be impossible to adequately evaluate tracheomalacia or bronchomalacia. On the other hand, there are clearly some circumstances where the use of an LMA may be appropriate and effective;

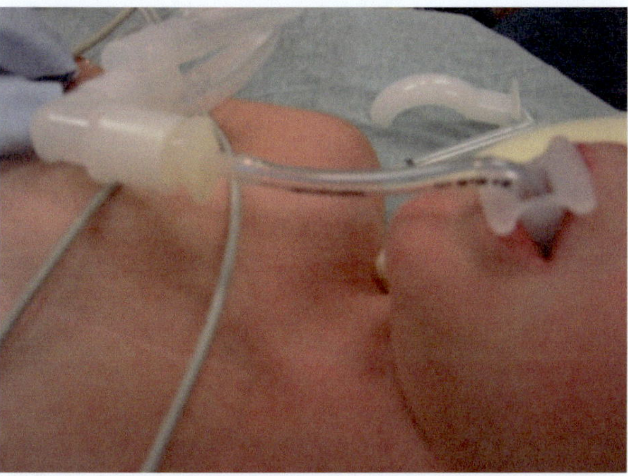

Fig. 1.2 Placement of a shortened RAE tube into the oral airway allows insufflation of oxygen and anesthetic gas and does not obstruct the space above the patient's face (which can interfere with manipulation of the flexible bronchoscope)

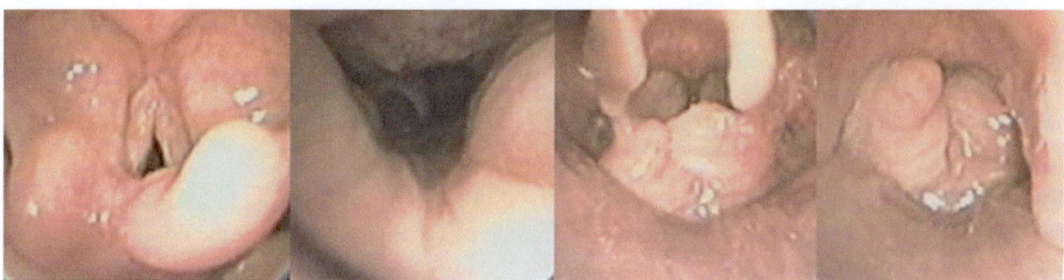

Fig. 1.3 How an LMA can lead to erroneous diagnoses. The *first panel* shows the larynx of a child with MPS II with an LMA in place. The patient has a history of significant stridor, but through the LMA, the larynx does not look too abnormal (and no stridor could be heard). The LMA was removed; the *second panel* shows hypopharyngeal collapse (this photo does not show the full extent of the collapse, which was complete). The *third panel* shows the larynx with mandibular lift; the mucosa overlying the post-cricoid area is redundant, and the arytenoids are large. The *final panel* shows the dramatic inspiratory prolapse of the arytenoid mucosa when mandibular lift was relaxed. The LMA did not allow evaluation of the supraglottic airway, and the traction on the post-cricoid mucosa created by the tip of the LMA in the upper esophagus made it impossible to appreciate the laryngomalacia

these primarily involve situations in which there is no clinical concern about the upper airway anatomy or dynamics, and the child may be too small to utilize an endotracheal tube with the flexible bronchoscope. However, as the 2.8 mm flexible bronchoscope can readily and safely be used through a 3.5 mm endotracheal tube, there are relatively few situations in which this may be the technique of choice. If the bronchoscopist feels strongly that an LMA is essential to safe and effective

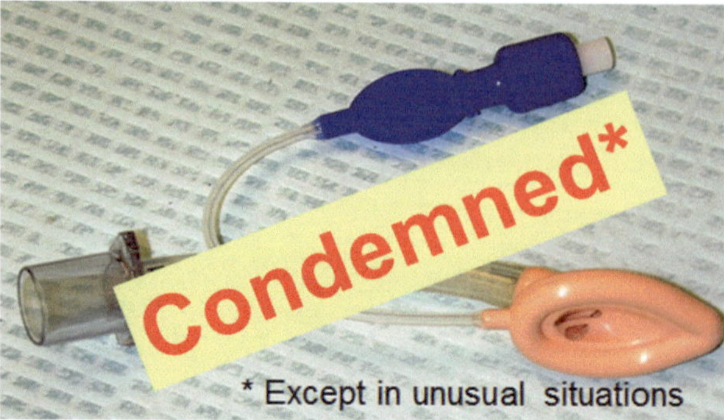

Fig. 1.4 The laryngeal mask airway can be useful, but it is inappropriate to employ the device for every procedure as the primary technique for airway management

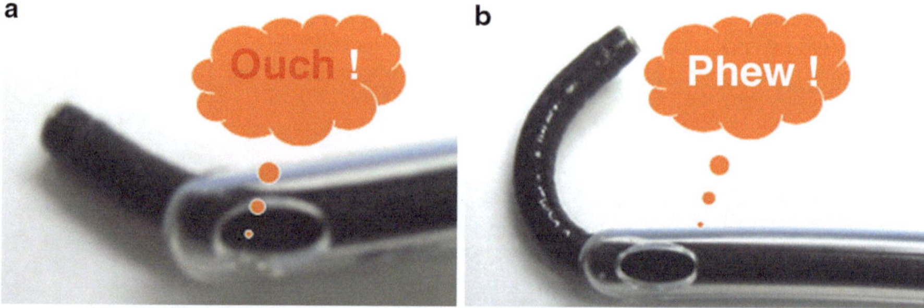

Fig. 1.5 Care must be taken when passing a flexible bronchoscope through an artificial airway (endotracheal or tracheostomy tube) to not flex the tip of the instrument until the bending segment has passed beyond the end of the tube. Otherwise, the bronchoscope can be damaged

evaluation of the *lower* airways, then very serious consideration should be given to an evaluation of the *upper* airways without the presence of the LMA. If this is done as the last step in the global procedure, then there will be less chance for contamination of the BAL specimens with upper airway secretions, and can be done as the patient recovers from the sedation.

It is often necessary or desirable to perform a flexible bronchoscopy through an endotracheal tube. Care must be taken to ensure that the tube is adequately lubricated (otherwise, manipulation of the bronchoscope may be difficult, or the bronchoscope may be physically damaged). Care must also be taken to ensure that the tip of the flexible bronchoscope extends far enough beyond the end of the endotracheal (or tracheostomy) tube before the tip is flexed; attempting to flex the tip of the scope while the bending segment of the instrument is still within the confines of the tube can result in breaking the control wires (Fig. 1.5).

A 2.8 mm bronchoscope can be safely utilized through a tube that is only 3.5 mm in diameter. However, this will result in a high level of obstruction to airflow through the tube. It is much easier to force air through the tube and into the lung than for the air to passively escape, and if there is not a sufficient leak around the outside of the tube, a very high level of airway pressure ("inadvertent PEEP") can develop, even leading to a tension pneumothorax. Conversely, excessive suctioning when the instrument is passed through a relatively small tube can result in a dramatic decrease in the patient's functional residual capacity and rather impressive oxygen desaturation can result. This is generally easily managed, however, by removing the bronchoscope and applying positive pressure ventilation through the endotracheal or tracheostomy tube (an alveolar recruitment maneuver is often most beneficial).

Techniques for Flexible Bronchoscopy

In the majority of diagnostic flexible bronchoscopies, it is desirable to obtain a specimen (bronchoalveolar lavage "BAL") for cytologic and microbiologic analysis. This specimen should be representative of the state of the lungs prior to the procedure—it is therefore important to minimize the risk of aspiration of oral secretions before the specimen can be obtained. The nose and hypopharynx should be gently suctioned prior to inserting the bronchoscope. Continuous insufflation of oxygen (~2 L/min) through the suction channel of the bronchoscope during passage through the nose and to the larynx can minimize contamination of the suction channel. Application of topical lidocaine to the larynx, while essential, also immediately leads to the risk of aspiration. Employing a small volume (0.5 mL) can help minimize this. However, when a patient is lying supine, the carina is at an approximately 30° downhill position from the larynx, and it is very common to visualize secretions draining from the mouth towards the carina as the bronchoscope is initially inserted. Suctioning of these secretions will of course contaminate the instrument and therefore the subsequent specimen, as will delay in obtaining the BAL specimen (Fig. 1.6)

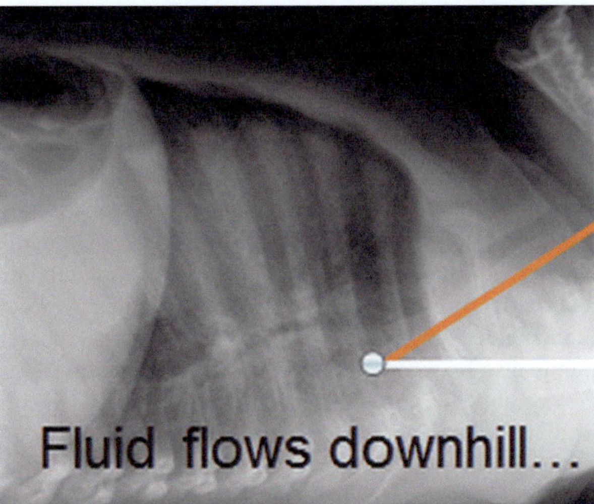

Fig. 1.6 Secretions readily drain from the larynx to the carina when the patient is supine. This often results in contamination of BAL specimens by oral secretions

If the proposed site for BAL specimen collection can be determined beforehand, it can be very helpful to immediately go to this site and perform the BAL; after the specimen has been obtained, one can aspirate secretions, either endogenous or aspirated, in order to evaluate the remaining airway anatomy, etc. Sometimes, however, there will be no clue in advance, and a very quick inspection of the bronchial anatomy (which should take no more than ~10 s once the tip of the bronchoscope reaches the carina, assuming that there are minimal secretions present, so that the anatomy can be clearly seen) can inform the site selection.

When it is important to obtain a BAL specimen with absolutely minimal risk of contamination by upper airway secretions, the most effective technique is to electively intubate the patient without placing any topical anesthetic on the larynx and then pass the bronchoscope through the clean endotracheal tube. After obtaining the BAL specimen, the endotracheal tube can be removed (if desired) and the anatomic (and dynamic) evaluation can then be completed. When I utilize this technique, in patients in whom I expect a sterile BAL specimen, the culture is indeed sterile more often than not.

When there is diffuse lung disease, the precise location from which a BAL specimen is obtained may be relatively unimportant. However, site selection can be a serious concern. For example, if there is a peripheral lesion seen on chest radiography, one may wish to sample that specific area. It is easy to sample a different area than the one intended, by simply passing the bronchoscope too far distally, and missing the bronchus leading to the intended target. This is an especially insidious problem when one is utilizing a smaller diameter instrument in a larger patient. Even one bronchial generation, which can be only 2–3 mm, can make a difference (Fig. 1.7).

There have been attempts to "standardize" BAL technique, with the goal of achieving a consistent dilution of alveolar lining fluid (ALF) components in the specimen obtained. However, it makes no rational sense to specify the aliquot volume (for example, xx mL/kg or xx ml/100 mL estimated FRC) unless the size of the bronchoscope and the bronchial generation number into which the tip of the instrument will be gently wedged are also specified (see Fig. 1.7). Almost by definition, each bronchial generation reduces the volume of lung being sampled beyond the tip of the bronchoscope by half, thereby potentially doubling the concentration of ALF constituents in the resulting specimen.

When airway dynamics are an important part of the evaluation, it may be necessary to lighten the level of sedation (this may be most effectively done after the anatomic evaluation has been completed). Bronchoscopy performed under deep anesthesia or with neuromuscular paralysis is almost guaranteed to prevent the accurate diagnosis of dynamic airway problems. It is not at all uncommon for the anatomy to look perfectly normal until the patient coughs, at which time surprisingly dramatic bronchomalacia or tracheomalacia may become apparent (Fig. 1.8). For this reason, it may also be desirable not to routinely apply topical anesthetic agents to the distal airway until the airway dynamics have been adequately evaluated. When a more involved or prolonged procedure is needed, the sedation can be deepened (or the procedure may be temporarily interrupted while an endotracheal tube or LMA is placed to provide for positive pressure ventilation during the remainder of the procedure).

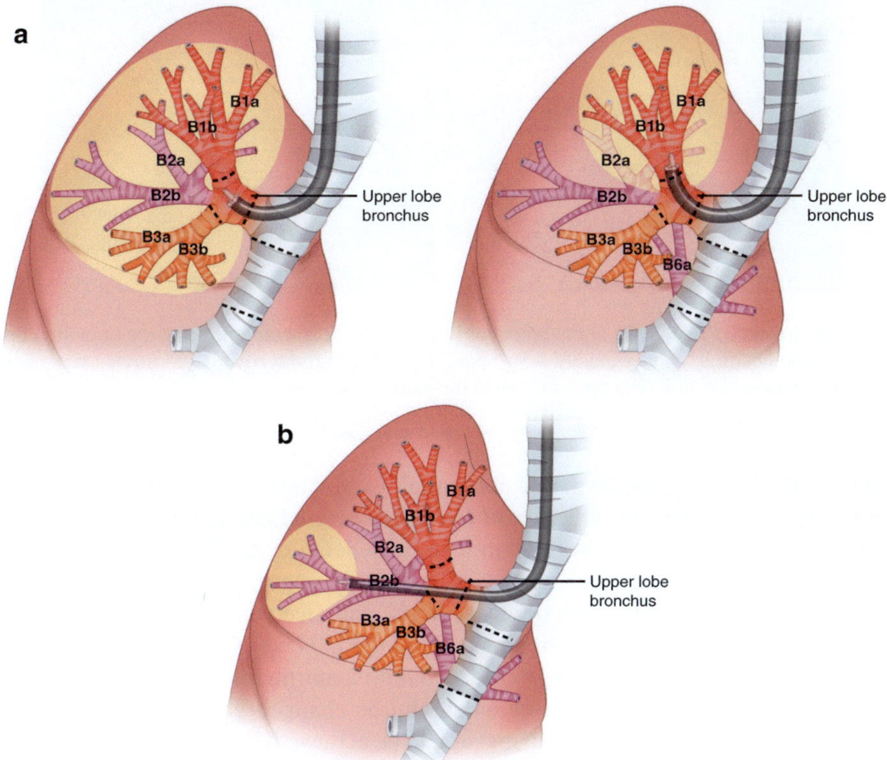

Fig. 1.7 The effect of scope size and position on BAL: Advancing the tip of the bronchoscope to a more peripheral position (which may be especially easy to do when a smaller diameter instrument is used) can result in sampling of a much smaller lung volume than may be intended (or recognized). This can, in some circumstances, produce erroneous results

This is often very useful when there is extensive mucus plugging or some other indication for a more prolonged procedure, especially a procedure that will require extensive suctioning.

The bronchoscopist should systematically evaluate the anatomy of the entire airway, beginning at the nostril. Generally, the easiest pathway through the nasal airway is through the middle meatus, and it is a smart idea to evaluate both sides of the nose, as unilateral obstruction is not rare. The presence of an oral airway can push the soft palate down, and make the adenoids appear to occupy much more of the airway than is the case under natural conditions. An oral airway can also push the tongue base down over the larynx, giving the appearance of glossoptosis. It is important to remove the oral airway, at least long enough to adequately evaluate the anatomy and dynamics of the upper airway. As the bronchoscope is advanced beyond the choana, the operator must also be alert to the changes that are produced by relatively small changes in the position of the head and neck. This is particularly

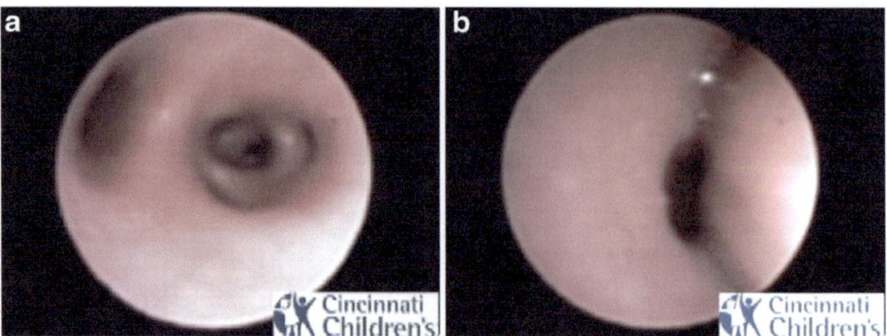

Fig. 1.8 (**a** and **b**) Two views of the bronchus intermedius, taken with the tip of the bronchoscope in the same position, approximately 0.5 s apart. The image on the *right* demonstrates significant bronchomalacia that was only apparent when the patient coughed

true for the tongue base. Dynamic abnormalities in the supraglottic region are also dependent on inspiratory effort (and the pressure gradient generated) as well as muscle tone, and this will vary significantly, depending on the level of sedation. Some children who have no history of stridor or upper airway obstruction can appear to have laryngomalacia or glossoptosis, and vice versa. The bronchoscopist must correlate the endoscopic findings within the context of the clinical history of the patient. If there is a history of stridor, but no abnormalities are apparent during the examination, the level of sedation should be changed until the symptoms are reproduced, so that an accurate diagnosis can be achieved. If there is audible stridor, the vibrating structures producing the sound must always be visualized; if not, the only explanation is that one is not looking in the right place. If there appears to be a significant dynamic abnormality but there is no history of upper airway obstruction or noisy breathing, this may be due to the effects of sedation, and not clinically relevant. In other cases, however, the history is incomplete or even wrong…

Because the tip of the flexible bronchoscope must be flexed anteriorly to view and then enter the larynx, it is much easier to obtain a view of the anterior commissure than of the posterior commissure. The posterior aspects of the larynx can often be more easily evaluated as the bronchoscope is being withdrawn than during insertion.

Complications of Bronchoscopy

All human activity involves risk. If the potential risk outweighs the potential benefit, then the activity should not be performed. This is also true of bronchoscopy. A complication may be defined as the occurrence of an event that is unexpected, and either causes harm to the patient or results in a significant change in the performance of the procedure. The most common "complication" listed in literature reviews is transient oxygen desaturation. Low oxygen saturation is often noted as a relative contraindication to doing a bronchoscopy. However, in many patients, the need for the procedure outweighs the potential risk of producing some hypoxemia (indeed, the low oxygen saturation is often the very *indication* for the procedure, with the anticipation that the result of the procedure will be an improvement in the hypoxemia). There is little evidence to suggest that transient oxygen desaturations result in harm to the patient, and I do not feel that they should be considered a true complication. The operator and anesthesiologist can do much to minimize the potential, and to respond appropriately when a desaturation event does occur, but procedures should not be terminated simply because there are some desaturation events that resolve promptly and with reasonable effort. If a patient is unable to ventilate adequately to maintain oxygenation, then the procedure can be continued after providing an artificial airway (endotracheal tube or LMA).

Mechanical complications can include mucosal edema or hemorrhage, and pneumothorax. Microbiological complications include introducing pathogens into a previously non-infected lung or spread from an infected to a non-infected portion of the lungs; this is most likely to occur when there has been failure to adequately clean and disinfect/sterilize the instrument between patients. The most serious complication, other than death of the patient, is cognitive: failure to obtain the correct diagnosis or therapeutic outcome. There are many paths that can lead to this unhappy state of affairs.

One subtle but potentially very serious complication is failure to do the procedure when it is truly needed. I have seen a number of children who have undergone major thoracic surgical procedures (repair of VSD, repair of pulmonary artery sling, as two examples) and despite difficult intubations, only after the chest was closed did someone think to do a bronchoscopy … which revealed potentially life-threatening airway anomalies (complete tracheal rings). The incidence of complete tracheal rings is on the order of 60 % in children with pulmonary artery slings ….

When discussing the risk of a proposed procedure with parents/guardians, it is important to place the potential risks in proper context. It is also important to recognize, and to point out to parents, that sometimes, the most valuable finding is the definitive exclusion of serious pathology that had been suspected (and worried/agonized about) prior to the procedure.

The Clinical Utility of Bronchoscopy

The specific indications for bronchoscopy, as well as the findings, will vary enormously from institution to institution, and depend on many factors, the most important of which is the referral practice in that institution. At Cincinnati Children's Hospital, we have a referral pattern that encompasses virtually the entire USA, and a very high number of children who are being referred for consideration for airway reconstructive surgery. This is a very different patient population from that which might be seen, for example, in a hospital that focuses on children's oncology. Because of the high percentage of our patients with structural airway problems, we perform ~50 % of our flexible bronchoscopies in conjunction with our otolaryngology colleagues, who perform rigid endoscopy. One might question the practice of doing both flexible and rigid bronchoscopy in the same patient by two different physicians, and that would be a legitimate question, if the only issue were the technical performance of the procedure. However, there is a world of difference between a flexible bronchoscopy performed by a pulmonologist and rigid bronchoscopy performed by a surgeon; we have very different perspectives, different instruments, and different procedural goals, we look at different aspects of the airway, and our follow-up is different. We believe that $1 + 1 = >2$. We also frequently engage our colleagues in gastroenterology and do a triple endoscopy; we attempt to make the most effective and efficient use of anesthesia events as possible.

When we perform multidisciplinary evaluations, we sequence the procedures so that the flexible bronchoscopy/BAL is performed first, the rigid laryngoscopy/bronchoscopy is performed second, and then the patient is electively intubated for the GI endoscopy. This maximizes the potential to obtain a valid BAL specimen without contamination from prior laryngeal anesthesia and manipulation.

The clinical utility of a bronchoscopy will depend on the indication for the procedure, the care and skill with which it is performed, and other factors. No listing of "diagnostic yield" will be applicable to other institutions. Surprise diagnoses are common; I found a clinically unsuspected foreign body in 1 % of the first 1,000 flexible bronchoscopies I did (excluding patients in whom the presence of a foreign body *was* suspected). We often evaluate patients prior to bone marrow ablation for a bone marrow transplant; it is not uncommon to find previously unsuspected problems, including occult infection, anatomic problems, evidence of ongoing aspiration, or significant amounts of retained secretions. In those patients in whom the findings are normal, we may, in retrospect, question why we did the procedure. However, in those patients in whom there are significant findings, their entire management may be changed. Since it can be extremely difficult to define in advance who may have an abnormality, an attitude of "guilty until proven innocent" is defensible, *within reason* (we are not excused from using common sense and careful clinical judgment). Our approach to patients referred for airway reconstruction is based on the recognition that lung disease (due to aspiration or anatomic abnormalities, for example) is a major risk factor in the potential success of the surgical procedures, and we aggressively manage such patients before clearing them for repair.

Simple factors can dramatically reduce the clinical value of a bronchoscopy. The value of a culture of a BAL specimen can be neutralized, for example, by antibiotic therapy prior to the bronchoscopy. Failure to obtain a specimen from the proper location or failure to perform the appropriate analyses on the specimen can also lead to erroneous diagnosis. It is not safe to assume that lung disease is uniformly distributed throughout the lungs; I have seen many patients in whom one part of the lung was heavily inflamed and infected, while a BAL from another part of the lung was sterile, and yielded no evidence of inflammation on cytologic examination. The operator must review all available information prior to performing the bronchoscopy, and must also examine all parts of the lung, unless there is a truly compelling reason not to do so.

The decision to perform a bronchoscopy is predicated on the clinical situation, the experience and skill of the bronchoscopist, and an (admittedly, subjective) assessment of the risk/benefit ratio. For what specific indications is flexible bronchoscopy most likely to be useful? As noted, this will depend in large degree on the patient population, so let us look at some principles …. The most profound statement of relevance here is, "statistics do not apply to individuals," and one truly never knows what may be found.

In the following discussion, I will focus on generalities rather than specifics; this is not an attempt to provide a comprehensive review of the literature … this is a distillation of my own four decades of experience with pediatric flexible bronchoscopy ….

A carefully performed flexible bronchoscopy with appropriate BAL can usually yield a definitive etiologic diagnosis of pneumonia. In the vast majority of patients with pneumonia, however, this is not an enormous diagnostic challenge, and bronchoscopy is not likely to be cost effective, nor is the benefit likely to exceed the risk (although minimal) and cost. However, in a patient who is at risk for unusual organisms, who is immunosuppressed, who has an unusual clinical presentation, or who does not respond to treatment with empirically chosen antibiotics, bronchoscopy becomes much more reasonable. One situation which frequently arises in busy pediatric hospitals is pneumonia in the immunocompromised host. There is often a clinical urgency to initiate therapy ASAP, and not wait for the patient to achieve a satisfactory NPO status and for a procedural time slot to become available. Such patients are often immediately begun on Thundercillin, Megastompamycin, Amphoterrible, and assorted other agents in a desperate attempt to get control of the putative infection before it gets out of hand, and this is often a life-saving maneuver. A subsequent bronchoscopy and BAL are therefore much less likely to yield a definitive diagnosis, and even when it does, many practitioners will not alter the antimicrobial treatment plan, fearing that the BAL might still have missed something. The pulmonologist usually hears about such patients after a week or two of unsuccessful therapy, and then it is challenging to decide whether a bronchoscopy can be justified, since the yield can be fully expected to be low. It has been my personal experience in many of these patients that we find something not infectious—pulmonary hemorrhage, for example, or a foreign body or an endobronchial lesion—that explains the clinical history. It is impossible to cite any meaningful statistics to help decide which patient in this situation can be anticipated to benefit from bronchoscopy ….

Recurrent or persistent pneumonia is a very valid indication for bronchoscopy. While the vast majority of pneumonias in children are viral, pneumonia that is recurrent in the same area of the lungs is often due to a specific anatomic problem (including occult foreign body aspiration). Some such patients are discovered to have recurrent pulmonary hemorrhage, which can occur without overt hemoptysis or other clinical manifestations.

Noisy breathing is another common indication for diagnostic bronchoscopy. Most patients with a history of recurrent wheezing have a form of asthma. These patients do not need bronchoscopy. However, I have seen many patients with "severe" asthma, not responsive or only very poorly responsive to conventional asthma treatment, who do not have asthma. Rather, they have anatomic abnormalities, occult foreign bodies, bronchomalacia, bronchial compression, etc. Some of these children have become Cushingoid due to escalating dosing with systemic steroids in an ill-fated attempt to gain control of their severe asthma symptoms .... Many physicians believe that poorly controlled asthma is a *contraindication* to bronchoscopy—in fact, it can be a highly productive *indication* for bronchoscopy.

Persistent stridor in an infant is a common cause of much anxiety on the part of parents, grandparents, and pediatricians. Most such children have laryngomalacia, and can be expected to "grow out of it"—it could be argued that bronchoscopy is unnecessary. However, any child with persistent stridor who is also failing to thrive, or who requires supplemental oxygen without an identifiable pulmonary cause, or whose parents cannot sleep at night due to the anxiety produced by their child's noisy breathing can be greatly benefitted by a diagnostic bronchoscopy. Knowledge is power, and if the parents can be assured, definitively, that there is no other lesion, they will sleep better, be more confident in their care of the child, and will be much less likely to go searching from doctor to doctor for CT scans, etc. There is great power in the definitive knowledge that your child's noisy breathing is truly benign. On the other hand, 15–20 % of patients whose airways I have examined for stridor, and in whom I find laryngomalacia, also have other significant airway abnormalities such as tracheomalacia, tracheal or bronchial compression, and complete tracheal rings. Other published reports have noted similar results. The great Godfather of bronchoscopy, Chevalier Jackson, said (in 1915) "If in doubt as to whether bronchoscopy should be performed, bronchoscopy should always be performed." I agree.

Children with obstructive sleep apnea most commonly have adenoidal or tonsillar hypertrophy, and can be treated with simple measures (T&A). However, if these measures do not relieve the obstruction, examination with a flexible instrument can be very helpful. Glossoptosis, laryngomalacia, and other problems can be identified. As discussed earlier, the bronchoscopist must pay close attention to the position of the head and neck, and to the level of sedation. If, during the examination, there is no noise, and no dynamic collapse is seen, the level of sedation should be altered so that the obstruction will occur and can be documented.

Chronic cough is a common indication for bronchoscopy. In this case, airway dynamics are often as important as the findings on BAL (microbiology, cytology). Patients with tracheomalacia or bronchomalacia may develop an intractable cough due to mechanical trauma to the mucosa produced by the cough. I have seen a number of patients previously diagnosed with "psychogenic cough" who actually had tracheomalacia or (central) bronchomalacia—understanding the nature of the problem can lead to resolution. I teach these patients to cough against pursed lips to maintain some back pressure and thus avoid making the "barking" sound with their cough, and this reduces the risk of mechanical irritation produced by the cough itself (which can then perpetuate the cough).

Not every child with atelectasis requires bronchoscopy, although the procedure can be both diagnostic and therapeutic. Most children with atelectasis resolve quickly on their own. However, if the atelectasis is functionally significant, or is recurrent, or is persistent, then bronchoscopy can be valuable. Mucus plugging, foreign bodies, bronchial compression or stenosis, and other diagnoses lurk, waiting to be discovered. In a significant percentage of patients with atelectasis, no anatomic abnormality will be discovered; in these patients, the cytology and microbiology of BAL specimens will be important, and the BAL may in itself be helpful to speed resolution of the atelectasis (by loosening mucus plugging beyond the visual range of the bronchoscope).

One area of confusion is the bronchoscopic diagnosis of aspiration. Ideally, aspiration could be defined by the discovery of a marker that can only get into the lungs by aspiration. Many surrogate markers have been evaluated, including lipid-laden macrophages (LLM) and gastric enzymes. Unfortunately, there is no marker that is both specific and sensitive, and the clinician must place everything into the proper context for interpretation. For example, while it is clear that aspiration of lipid-containing liquids or even solids can produce an elevated number of LLM in subsequent BAL specimens, a patient who is NPO and aspirates only oral secretions cannot be expected to produce lipid laden macrophages. Even a patient who is clearly aspirating may have a highly variable number of LLM, depending on the amount of material aspirated, the lipid content of the material, the physical state of the material (i.e., liquid vs. solid), and most importantly, the time between the aspiration event and the sampling. Sampling immediately after an aspiration event cannot be expected to yield LLM—the process takes time. It may also take weeks to clear LLM after a single aspiration event, but the factors influencing the rate of clearance are totally unknown and almost surely variable. Finally, processes other than aspiration can produce LLM, including bone marrow infarction (as in sickle cell anemia) and hemophagocytic lymphohistiocytosis. The presence of large numbers of dead or dying neutrophils could be expected to result in LLM, since alveolar macrophages readily ingest dead cells, but, perhaps surprisingly, many patients with chronic purulence (i.e., cystic fibrosis) do not have elevated LLM in their BAL specimens.

In the evaluation of a patient with suspected aspiration, I do look at the percentage of lipid laden macrophages. I also look for large numbers of squamous epithelial cells (assuming that the BAL specimen has not been contaminated with saliva during the procedure—see previous discussion), and large numbers of "oral flora" on culture. I place these findings in the context of the child's history and known anatomic/functional defects, and will report "findings consistent with aspiration" but almost never am willing to state that the BAL findings are "diagnostic of" aspiration.

Pediatric radiologists often tease their pulmonary colleagues that multi-detector CT techniques have made bronchoscopy obsolete. While it is true that imaging techniques can yield much important information about the lungs and airways, the truth is that bronchoscopy and radiologic techniques are complementary. Neither can give the entire picture, and both are often necessary for accurate and complete evaluation of patients. For example, while a CT scan can demonstrate extrinsic compression of central airways, and identify the offending structure, radiographic studies are often confused by the accumulation of airway secretions, and in any case, the radiographic studies do not provide microbiologic information nor therapeutic benefit. On the other hand, bronchoscopy can easily miss sampling a lesion that is beyond the visual range unless the bronchoscopy is guided by radiologic imaging.

Bronchoscopy can be a very important adjunct to surgical manipulation of the pediatric airway. Transillumination of the bronchi can assist the surgeon in the identification of specific regions of the lung. Direct observation of the trachea during an aortopexy, for example, can improve the likelihood that the surgical procedure will be effective.

The potential value of diagnostic bronchoscopy in children is perhaps best embodied in the statement of the indications for bronchoscopy: information in the lungs or airways of the child, necessary for the care of the child, and best obtained with the bronchoscope.

"Seek, and ye shall find." Matt 7:7

Chapter 2
Bronchoalveolar Lavage: Tests and Applications

Fabio Midulla, Raffaella Nenna, and Ernst Eber

Abstract Bronchoalveolar lavage (BAL) is a diagnostic procedure used for recovering cellular and non-cellular components of the epithelial lining fluid of the alveolar and bronchial airspaces. Non-bronchoscopic BAL involves the insertion of simple catheters or balloon-type devices through an endotracheal tube, while bronchoscopic BAL involves the instillation and immediate withdrawal of pre-warmed sterile 0.9 % saline solution through the working channel of a flexible bronchoscope, preferably in the middle lobe or the lingula. The parameters measured in BAL fluid (BALF) include the percentage of the instilled normal saline that is recovered as well as various BALF cellular and non-cellular components. BAL is performed for diagnostic, therapeutic, and research purposes. The most important indication for BAL in children is in the work up of infectious diseases. Other indications for BAL include non-specific chronic respiratory symptoms, non-specific radiological findings, and clinical symptoms suggestive of interstitial lung disease. BAL is still considered to be the gold standard for diagnosing chronic pulmonary aspiration. BAL is a well-tolerated and safe procedure; however, on occasion, fever, cough, transient wheezing, and pulmonary infiltrates have been observed, which usually resolve within 24 h.

Keywords Bronchoalveolar lavage • Bronchoscopy • Complications • Epithelial lining fluid • Indications • Reference values • Techniques • Therapeutic applications

Bronchoalveolar lavage (BAL) is a predominantly diagnostic procedure used for recovering cellular and non-cellular components of the epithelial lining fluid (ELF) of the alveolar and bronchial airspaces. The procedure usually consists of the instillation and immediate withdrawal of pre-warmed sterile 0.9 % (normal) saline solution (NSS) through the working channel of a flexible bronchoscope (FB), which has been wedged into a bronchus with a matching diameter.

F. Midulla, M.D. • R. Nenna, M.D.
Department of Paediatrics, "Sapienza" University of Rome,
V.le Regina Elena, 324, Rome 00161, Italy

E. Eber, M.D. (✉)
Respiratory and Allergic Disease Division, Department of Paediatrics and Adolescent Medicine, Medical University of Graz, Auenbruggerplatz 34/2, Graz 8036, Austria
e-mail: ernst.eber@medunigraz.at

© Springer Science+Business Media New York 2015
S.D. Davis et al. (eds.), *Diagnostic Tests in Pediatric Pulmonology*,
Respiratory Medicine, DOI 10.1007/978-1-4939-1801-0_2

Procedures

Current clinical practice utilises two techniques: non-bronchoscopic and broncho-scopic BAL. Non-bronchoscopic BAL involves the insertion of simple catheters or balloon-type devices (size 4–8 French) through an endotracheal tube [1].

Bronchoscopic BAL involves instillation and withdrawal of NSS through the working channel of a flexible bronchoscope. The preferred sites for BAL in diffuse lung diseases are the middle lobe and the lingula because, being the smallest lobes of each lung, they offer better fluid recovery. When lung disease is localised, BAL must target the radiologically or endoscopically identified involved lobe or segment. In patients with cystic fibrosis, samples from multiple sites should be obtained in order to avoid underestimation of the extent of infection [2]. To avoid contamination, BAL must precede any other planned bronchoscopic procedure.

In order to obtain the lavage specimen in the dedicated collection trap, gentle manual or mechanical suction (3.33–13.3 kPa, i.e. 25–100 mmHg) is applied, while maintaining the tip of the bronchoscope wedged into the selected site. The saline utilised for BAL is pre-warmed to body temperature (37 °C) in order to prevent the cough reflex. Flow from the distal tip of the bronchoscope can be observed during fluid instillation.

Three optional methods are currently used for calculating the total amount of sterile NSS for BAL to obtain samples that are representative of the alveolar com-partment [3]. Some authors choose to use 2–4 aliquots of equal volume (10 ml per aliquot for children less than 6 years, and 20 ml per aliquot for children over 6 years of age), irrespective of the patient's body weight [4]. Others suggest the use of three aliquots, each consisting of 1 ml/kg body weight for children weighing up to 20 kg, and three 20 ml aliquots for heavier children. Lastly, de Blic et al. [5] have recom-mended that the amount of instilled NSS be adjusted up to a maximum volume of 10 % of the child's functional residual capacity (FRC).

In general, BAL is considered technically acceptable if more than 40 % of the total NSS instilled is recovered, and the lavage fluid (except for the first sample) contains few epithelial cells.

Processing of Bronchoalveolar Lavage Fluid

To optimise cell viability, BAL fluid (BALF) must be kept at 4 °C until analysed. BALF specimens should be processed as soon as possible. The variables measured in the BALF include the percentage of fluid recovered (as compared to the amount of NSS instilled) as well as various cellular and non-cellular components. The first unfiltered BALF aliquot is usually processed separately for microbiological studies. While BALF is centrifuged for direct detection of bacteria, viruses, and fungi and to culture fungi, protozoa, and viruses, it is not centrifuged to culture bacteria. The rest of the aliquots are filtered through sterile gauze to remove mucus; then they are pooled and submitted for cytological studies and analysis of the BALF solutes.

BALF can be prepared in two ways: (a) by obtaining cytospin preparations of the whole BALF, and (b) by re-suspension of the specimen in a small amount of medium which is then centrifuged. At least four slides should be prepared for each patient and we recommend storing one or two slides for research purposes. The number of cells per ml in the recovered BALF is counted with a cytometer on whole BALF specimens stained with trypan blue, or with a cytoscan. Alternatively, the slides can be stained with May-Grünwald, Giemsa, or Diff-Quick stains for the evaluation of differential cell counts and cellular morphological features. In particular clinical settings, the slides can also be prepared with specific stains, e.g. Oil Red O stain to detect lipid-laden macrophages, iron stain to identify iron-positive macrophages in patients with alveolar haemorrhage, and periodic acid-Schiff (PAS) to identify glycogen.

Materials for the evaluation of non-cellular components must be obtained from the supernatant after centrifugation.

The composition of the BALF can be influenced by several technical factors including: site of lavage, fluid pH, temperature and volume of instilled NSS, number of aliquots, size of bronchoscope, dwell time, and suction pressure. Another important precautionary measure is to keep the samples in anaerobic transport media that contain reducing agents in order to avoid air exposure that destroys anaerobic bacteria.

Reference Values

Mean BALF total cell count ranges from 10.3 to 59.9×10^4 cells/ml, with a mean of 81.2–90 % for macrophages, 8.7–16.2 % for lymphocytes, 1.2–5.5 % for neutrophils, and 0.2–0.4 % for eosinophils, respectively [6]. The predominant cells, regardless of the child's age, are macrophages, followed by lymphocytes (Table 2.1).

Normal values of BALF lymphocyte subsets in children resemble those found in healthy adults, except for the CD4/CD8 ratio, which is often lower in children, possibly because children frequently suffer from viral infections [7, 8].

The concentration of serum-derived proteins is higher in children than in adults, whereas locally produced mediators do not differ (Tables 2.2 and 2.3). Surfactant phospholipid concentrations are higher in 3–8 year old than in older children, whereas surfactant protein concentrations are independent of the child's age.

Indications for Bronchoalveolar Lavage

BAL is performed for diagnostic, therapeutic and research applications. The most important indication for BAL in children is in the work-up of infectious diseases. BAL can be done in both immunocompromised (lung transplant, HIV infection, chemotherapy) and immunocompetent children (chronic pneumonia, tuberculosis, cystic fibrosis). Other indications for BAL include non-specific chronic respiratory symptoms, non-specific radiological findings, and clinical symptoms suggestive of chronic interstitial lung disease (CILD; diffuse parenchymal lung disease, DPLD).

Table 2.1 Total and differential cell counts in bronchoalveolar lavage fluid (BALF) from control children

		Midulla et al. [20]
Number of patients		16
Age range		2–32 m
Sedation		LA
Number of aliquots		2
Lavage volume		20 ml
BALF recovered %	Mean ± SD	43.1 ± 12.2
	Median	42.5
	Range	20–65
Cell count (10^4 cells·ml^{-1})	Mean ± SD	59.9 ± 8.2
	Median	51
	Range	20–130
AM %	Mean ± SD	86 ± 7.8
	Median	87
	Range	71–98
Lym %	Mean ± SD	8.7 ± 5.8
	Median	7
	Range	2–22
Neu %	Mean ± SD	5.5 ± 4.8
	Median	3.5
	Range	0–17
Eos %	Mean ± SD	0.2 ± 0.3
	Median	0
	Range	0–1

m months, *LA* local anaesthesia, *AM* alveolar macrophages, *Lym* lymphocytes, *Neu* neutrophils, *Eos* eosinophils

Table 2.2 Concentration (mg L^{-1}) of serum-derived proteins in bronchoalveolar lavage fluid (BALF) from control children

		Midulla et al. [20]
Number of patients		7
Age		1–3 y
Total protein	Mean ± SD	108 ± 39
	Median	67
	Range	44–336
Albumin	Mean ± SD	58 ± 26
	Median	29
	Range	14–210

y years

Table 2.3 Concentration (mg L^{-1}) of locally produced mediators in bronchoalveolar lavage fluid (BALF) from control children

		Midulla et al. [20]
Number of patients		7
	Age	1–3 y
Fibronectin	Mean ± SD	172 ± 83
	Median	80
	Range	25–640
Hyaluronic acid	Mean ± SD	26 ± 5
	Median	18
	Range	16–45

y years

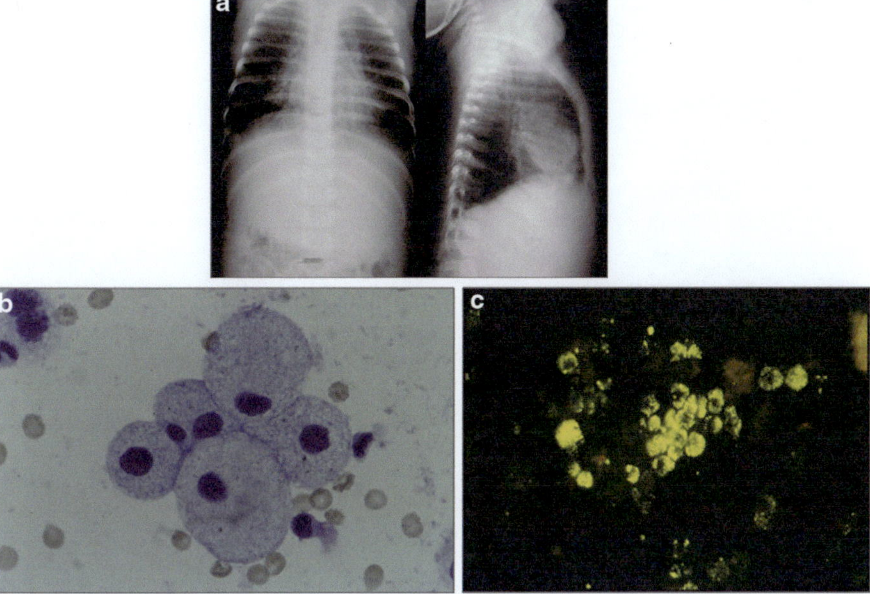

Fig. 2.1 A child with interstitial pneumonia. (**a**) chest X-ray, (**b**) bronchoalveolar lavage cytology showing several alveolar macrophages with foamy cytoplasm (May-Grünwald Giemsa stain, ×100), (**c**) positive direct immunofluorescence for cytomegalovirus antigens

BAL results should be analysed carefully; in fact, BAL is diagnostic only when pathogens not usually found in the lung are recovered, such as *Pneumocystis jirovecii*, *Toxoplasma gondii*, *Strongyloides stercoralis*, *Legionella pneumophila*, *Histoplasma capsulatum*, *Mycobacterium tuberculosis*, *Mycoplasma pneumoniae*, influenza virus, and respiratory syncytial virus. The isolation of herpes simplex virus, cytomegalovirus, Aspergillus, *Candida albicans*, Cryptococcus, and atypical mycobacteria from BALF is not diagnostic but may contribute to diagnosis and management of infectious diseases (Fig. 2.1). The presence of equal to or more than 10^4 colony-forming units/ml BALF will identify patients with bacterial pneumonia with reasonable accuracy. Hence, when evaluating the microbiological results, the physician must take into account the underlying disease and the overall clinical picture.

The role of BAL in the diagnosis of lung infection in immunocompetent children is controversial. Bronchoscopy including BAL as invasive procedure is hardly ever justified as a first step in the diagnosis of primary respiratory infection in otherwise healthy children, but should be reserved for patients with atypical manifestations. BAL may be a useful tool in patients with chronic pneumonia, tuberculosis, and cystic fibrosis. In the latter, BAL has an important role in detecting respiratory pathogens and inflammation, especially in young children who are unable to expectorate or in those who fail to improve after therapy [2].

CILD is a heterogeneous group of disorders characterised by typical radiological findings, restrictive lung disease, and inflammation of the pulmonary interstitium [9].

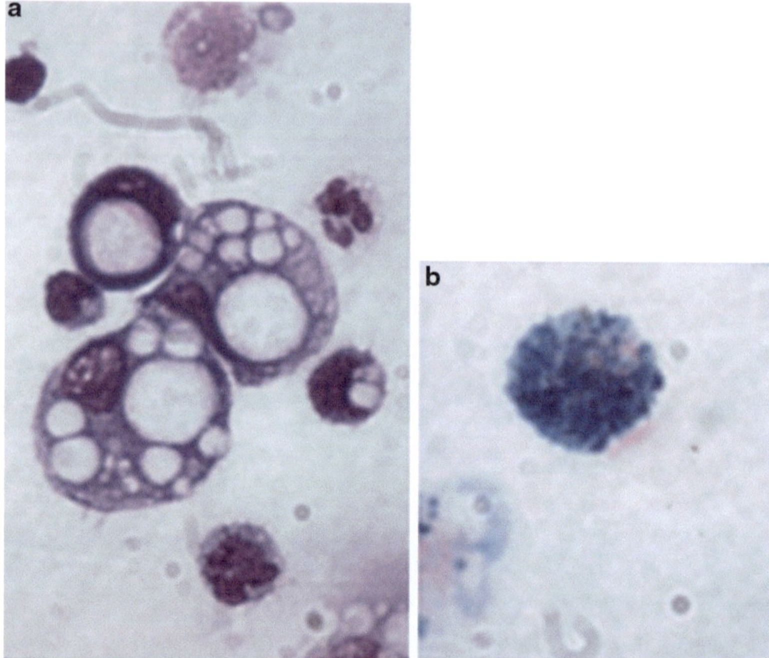

Fig. 2.2 (**a**) Lipoid pneumonia. Bronchoalveolar lavage fluid cytology showing vacuolated alveolar macrophages (May-Grünwald Giemsa stain, ×100). (**b**) Haemosiderin-laden alveolar macrophages in the bronchoalveolar lavage fluid of a patient with alveolar haemorrhage (Prussian blue staining, ×100)

In these patients, BAL may have an important role in reaching or confirming a specific diagnosis, in characterising the alveolitis, and in monitoring the patient during treatment and follow-up [10].

In addition, BALF findings usually provide a specific diagnosis in children with alveolar proteinosis, chronic lipoid pneumonia (Fig. 2.2a), pulmonary histiocytosis, pulmonary haemorrhage (Fig. 2.2b), and pulmonary microlithiasis.

With BALF analysis, three different forms of alveolitis can be identified: lymphocytic, neutrophilic, and eosinophilic (Fig. 2.3):

1. When patients present with clinical manifestations typical of sarcoidosis, a high percentage of lymphocytes (more than 30 %) with predominating CD4 T-cells in the BALF is strongly suggestive, although not definitively confirmatory, of the diagnosis [11].

   Hypersensitivity pneumonitis typically causes lymphocytic alveolitis with the BALF containing predominantly CD8 T-lymphocytes. Similarly, in children with histiocytosis X, or with interstitial lung disease related to collagen disease, or in cryptogenic organising pneumonia (COP; previously termed bronchiolitis obliterans and organising pneumonia—BOOP) the predominant cells are CD8 T-lymphocytes.

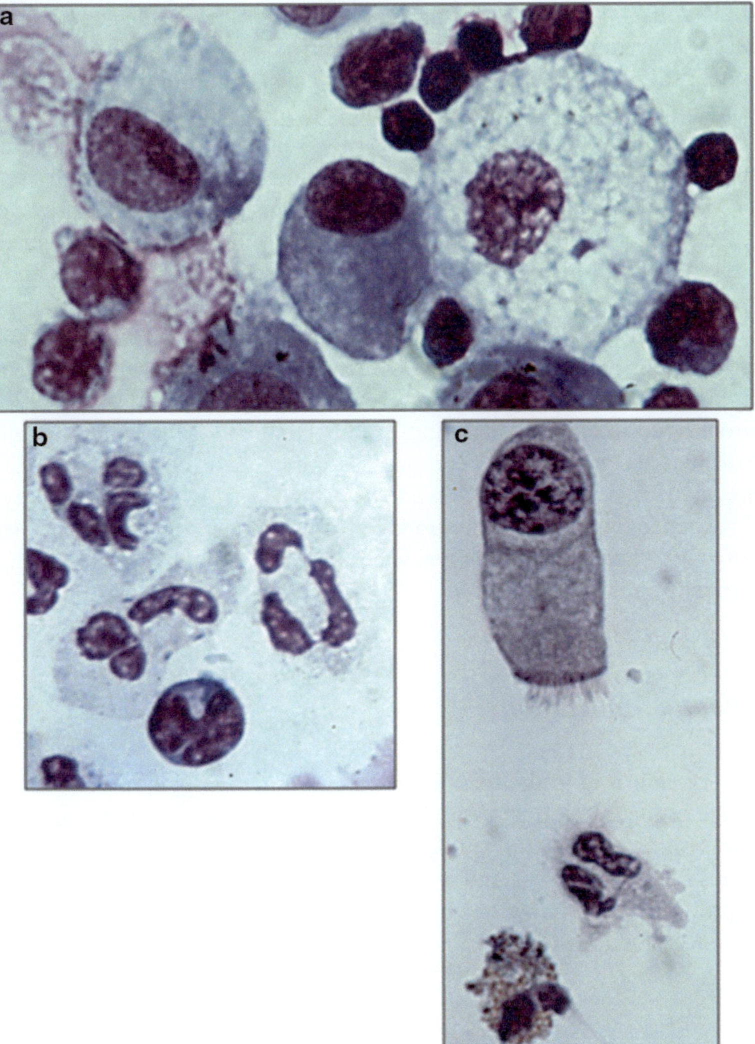

Fig. 2.3 Bronchoalveolar lavage fluid cytology features in (**a**) lymphocytic, (**b**) neutrophilic, and (**c**) eosinophilic alveolitis (May-Grünwald Giemsa stain, ×100)

2. A neutrophilic alveolitis is usually found in idiopathic pulmonary fibrosis and in COP. The histological features are accumulation of macrophages accompanied by mild chronic interstitial pneumonia and, at the worst, mild interstitial fibrosis.
3. Patients with eosinophilic alveolitis or interstitial lung disease always show a predominance of eosinophils in BALF with focal eosinophilic abscesses. The aetiology of this condition often remains elusive; a number of causes (e.g. drug reactions, fungi, parasites, and vapour inhalation) have been described.

BAL is still considered to be the gold standard for the diagnosis of chronic pulmonary aspiration (CPA), i.e. the repeated passage of food material, gastric refluxate, or saliva into the subglottic airways causing chronic or recurrent respiratory symptoms [12]. BAL remains the procedure of choice to diagnose CPA by determining the lipid-laden macrophage (LLM) index [13] and by measuring gastric pepsin concentrations [14, 15]. The LLM index can be calculated by assigning each LLM a score that ranges from 0 to 4 according to the amount of cytoplasmic lipid and scoring one hundred consecutive alveolar macrophages; thus, the highest possible score (LLM index) is 400. A LLM index of more than 100 is considered positive for aspiration [13]. However, the LLM index has certain limitations such as a lack of reproducibility, the inability to differentiate between exogenous and endogenous lipids, and the false-positive results that it may yield in patients with lung disease unrelated to aspiration or even in healthy children [16, 17]. LLM may also be observed in cases of fat embolism [18] and endogenous lipoid pneumonia [19]. Tracheal pepsin has also been used as a marker of reflux aspiration. Pepsin detection in the BALF has been shown to have high sensitivity and specificity values for reflux-related pulmonary aspiration. Unfortunately, pepsin detection is still possible only with "home-made" assays, and its use is strictly limited to the diagnosis of gastric reflux-related aspiration.

Therapeutic Applications

BAL has a major role in the therapy of certain lung diseases, in the form of total lung lavage or mucus plug removal. In particular, children with persistent and massive atelectasis can successfully undergo selective lavage, usually with sterile saline. Mucolytics including DNase and *N*-acetylcysteine as well as exogenous surfactant to help prevent reabsorption atelectasis have also been used, but efficacy has not been demonstrated for these.

Complications

BAL is a well-tolerated and safe procedure; however, on occasion, fever, cough, transient wheezing, and pulmonary infiltrates have been observed, which usually resolve within 24 h. The most frequent complication is fever; the only treatment needed is antipyretics. In immunocompromised patients antibiotic therapy must be performed for 48 h.

BAL may cause hypoxaemia, hypercapnia, or both. Severe bleeding, bronchial perforation, mediastinal emphysema, pneumothorax, and cardiac arrest are extremely rare. Contraindications to the procedure include bleeding disorders, severe hemoptysis, and severe hypoxemia that persists despite oxygen treatment.

References

1. Heaney LG, Stevenson EC, Turner G, Cadden IS, Taylor R, Shields MD, Ennis M. Investigating paediatrics airways by non-bronchoscopic lavage: normal cellular data. Clin Exp Allergy. 1996;26:799–806.
2. Gutierrez JP, Grimwood K, Armstrong DS, Carlin JB, Carzino R, Olinsky A, Robertson CF, Phelan PD. Interlobar differences in bronchoalveolar lavage fluid from children with cystic fibrosis. Eur Respir J. 2001;17:281–6.
3. Midulla F, Ratjen F. Special considerations for bronchoalveolar lavage in children. Eur Respir Rev. 1999;9:38–42.
4. Ratjen F, Bruch J. Adjustment of bronchoalveolar lavage volume to body weight in children. Pediatr Pulmonol. 1996;21:184–8.
5. de Blic J, Mc Kelvie P, Le Bourgeois M, Blanche S, Benoist MR, Scheinmann P. Value of bronchoalveolar lavage in the management of severe acute pneumonia and interstitial pneumonitis in the immunocompromised child. Thorax. 1987;42:759–65.
6. Eber E. Bronchoalveolar lavage in pediatric patients. J Bronchol. 1998;5:227–41.
7. Ratjen F, Bredendiek M, Bredel M, Meltzer J, Costabel U. Differential cytology of bronchoalveolar lavage fluid in normal children. Eur Respir J. 1994;7:1865–70.
8. Riedler J, Grigg J, Stone C, Tauro G, Robertson CF. Bronchoalveolar lavage cellularity in healthy children. Am J Respir Crit Care Med. 1995;152:163–8.
9. Fan LL, Langston C. Chronic interstitial lung disease in children. Pediatr Pulmonol. 1993; 16:184–96.
10. Ronchetti R, Midulla F, Sandstrom T, Bjermer L, Zabrak J, Pawlik J, Villa MP, Villani A. Bronchoalveolar lavage in children with chronic diffuse parenchymal lung disease. Pediatr Pulmonol. 1999;27:1–8.
11. Chadelat K, Baculard A, Grimfeld A, Tournier G, Boule M, Boccon-Gibod L, Clement A. Pulmonary sarcoidosis in children: serial evaluation of bronchoalveolar lavage cells during corticosteroid treatment. Pediatr Pulmonol. 1993;16:41–7.
12. Boesch RP, Daines C, Willging JP, Kaul A, Cohen AP, Wood RE, Amin RS. Advances in the diagnosis and management of chronic pulmonary aspiration in children. Eur Respir J. 2006; 28:847–61.
13. Corwin RW, Irwin RS. The lipid-laden alveolar macrophage as a marker of aspiration in parenchymal lung disease. Am Rev Respir Dis. 1985;132:576–81.
14. Krishnan U, Mitchell JD, Messina I, Day AS, Bohane TD. Assay of tracheal pepsin as a marker of reflux aspiration. J Pediatr Gastroenterol Nutr. 2002;35:303–8.
15. Farrell S, McMaster C, Gibson D, Shields MD, McCallion WA. Pepsin in bronchoalveolar lavage fluid: a specific and sensitive method of diagnosing gastro-oesophageal reflux-related pulmonary aspiration. J Pediatr Surg. 2006;41:289–93.
16. Knauer-Fischer S, Ratjen F. Lipid-laden macrophages in bronchoalveolar lavage fluid as a marker for pulmonary aspiration. Pediatr Pulmonol. 1999;27:419–22.
17. Ding Y, Simpson PM, Schellhase DE, Tryka AF, Ding L, Parham DM. Limited reliability of lipid-laden macrophage index restricts its use as a test for pulmonary aspiration: comparison with a simple semiquantitative assay. Pediatr Dev Pathol. 2002;5:551–8.
18. Vichinsky E, Williams R, Das M, Earles AN, Lewis N, Adler A, McQuitty J. Pulmonary fat embolism: a distinct cause of severe acute chest syndrome in sickle cell anemia. Blood. 1994;83:3107–12.
19. McDonald JW, Roggli VL, Bradford WD. Coexisting endogenous and exogenous lipoid pneumonia and pulmonary alveolar proteinosis in a patient with neurodevelopmental disease. Pediatr Pathol. 1994;14:505–11.
20. Midulla F, Villani A, Merolla R, Bjermer L, Sandstrom T, Ronchetti R. Bronchoalveolar lavage studies in children without parenchymal lung disease: cellular constituents and protein levels. Pediatr Pulmonol. 1995;20:112–8.

Chapter 3
Understanding Interventional Bronchoscopy

Andrew A. Colin, Joel Reiter, Giovanni A. Rossi, and Annabelle Quizon

Abstract Pediatric flexible bronchoscopy as a diagnostic modality has become a standard tool in the armamentarium of the modern pediatric pulmonologist. However the feasibility of interventions through flexible bronchoscopy is emerging slowly as it is limited not only by the size of the pediatric bronchoscope and its working channel but also by the demarcation lines between flexible and rigid bronchoscopy.

We organize this chapter on interventional bronchoscopy into the following broad topics:

1. Use of flexible bronchoscopy for acquisition of diagnostic material.
2. Bronchoscopy for removal of obstructive, noxious, or damaging materials from the airway or the lung.
3. Management of the narrowed or obstructed airway: debridement, dilation, and stenting.
4. Use of bronchoscopy for other procedures including: sealing of fistulae and pneumothorax, control of diffuse alveolar hemorrhage, and segmental bronchography.
5. New horizons: a discussion on recent reports on fetal bronchoscopy as a novel interventional approach.

A.A. Colin, M.D. (✉) • J. Reiter, M.D.
Division of Pediatric Pulmonology, Miller School of Medicine,
Batchelor Children's Research Institute, University of Miami,
1580 NW 10th Avenue, D-820, Miami, FL 33136, USA
e-mail: acolin@med.miami.edu

G.A. Rossi, M.D.
Pediatric Pulmonology and Allergy Unit, Istituto Giannina Gaslini, Largo Gaslini,
5, Genoa 16148, Italy

A. Quizon, M.D.
Section of Pediatric Pulmonology, Baystate Medical Center, 50 Wason Avenue, Springfield,
MA 01199, USA

© Springer Science+Business Media New York 2015
S.D. Davis et al. (eds.), *Diagnostic Tests in Pediatric Pulmonology*,
Respiratory Medicine, DOI 10.1007/978-1-4939-1801-0_3

Keywords Bronchoscopy • Interventional bronchoscopy • Flexible bronchoscopy • Endobronchial biopsy • Transbronchial biopsy • Airway stenting • Diffuse alveolar hemorrhage • Airway foreign body • Fetal bronchoscopy

Introduction

Over the last 3 decades, flexible bronchoscopy has replaced rigid bronchoscopy as a diagnostic tool. It is widely used for multiple diagnostic and therapeutic/interventional indications across all ages, and has become an integral component in the training and armamentarium of most pediatric pulmonologists. The routine diagnostic flexible bronchoscopy includes inspection of the airway, with the obvious advantage that its flexibility affords visualization of distal airways that cannot be reached by the rigid scope. Additionally, flexible bronchoscopy is often performed under various levels of sedation/anesthesia but mostly without the need for intubation; as such it offers an advantage over the rigid scope. Bronchoalveolar lavage (BAL) has become an integral element of routine bronchoscopy, and offers insight into inflammatory and infectious processes in the airway. This chapter does not deal with diagnostic bronchoscopy or BAL but rather with interventional procedures that constitute the demarcation line between the role of the endoscopist and the surgeon. Due to the types of pathologies and respective size of instruments, such interventional uses are much more limited in pediatrics compared to adult practice.

Our target audience is pediatric pulmonologists, who are mostly trained with flexible scopes, yet are frequently requested to weigh on decisions that are on the interface between rigid and flexible bronchoscopy. Specific circumstances that generate this discussion are the approach to retrieval of foreign bodies and placement of airway stents. These topics are broadly addressed in this chapter with the attempt to provide the most updated literature review. A recent review on the topic of Interventional Bronchoscopy in Pediatrics [1] offers a differently weighted perspective by authors whose expertise straddles both rigid and flexible bronchoscopy.

For this chapter we organize the topics into the following broader groups:

- Use of Flexible Bronchoscopy for Acquisition of Diagnostic Material.
- Bronchoscopy for Removal of Obstructive, Noxious, or Damaging Materials from the Airway or the Lung.
- Management of the Narrowed or Obstructed Airway: Debridement, Dilation, and Stenting.
- Use of Bronchoscopy for Other Procedures.
- New Horizons.

Reference is made to a book chapter on Special Procedures in a textbook of Pediatric Bronchoscopy co-authored by one of us [2], in our attempt to minimize repetition of material that has been previously addressed.

Use of Flexible Bronchoscopy for Acquisition of Diagnostic Material

Endobronchial Biopsy (EBB)

While it is unequivocal that EBB has contributed greatly to the understanding of lung diseases when used as a research tool, a careful review of the literature revealed limited documented role for EBB in clinical practice. This statement is limited to diagnostic advantage offered by EBB of tissue taken from the mucosal surface over standard BAL, and excludes biopsies taken from intraluminal lesions or lesions of the bronchial wall.

A review of the literature spanning the years since the publication of the chapter on Special Procedures in Pediatric Bronchoscopy [2], revealed no study or publication to alter the opinion expressed in the cited chapter with regard the limited utility of EBB. In a recent review on the role of rigid and flexible bronchoscopy in children, Nicolai [3] reached a similar conclusion that no clear indications have yet been identified for bronchial wall biopsies, and citing a single paper [4] commented that such role "is currently being elucidated." It is of note, however, that in the above chapter [2] as well as in a previous Editorial on Endobronchial Biopsy in Childhood [5] the authors alluded to the very same paper by Salva et al. They commented that this series of 170 children is the largest study ever published for clinical rather than research indications for EBB; the study offered no information on the clinical utility of the procedure but rather only a conclusion on safety of EBB.

Transbronchial Biopsy (TBB) and Transbronchial Needle Aspiration (TBNA)

Transbronchial biopsy (TBB) is a technique used to obtain lung tissue specimens from distal regions of the lung predominantly for histopathological examination. TBB has become the standard tool for diagnosis of acute rejection in lung transplant recipients with a high sensitivity and specificity. In a retrospective review of 61 pediatric lung transplantation patients who underwent 179 TBB; the procedure yielded clinically useful information—specific pathologic diagnosis in 54 % of cases and alteration of medical treatment in 64 %. The procedure was deemed a low-risk diagnostic procedure [6].

While intuitively attractive, the use of TBB for interstitial lung disease (ILD) is less well established; and in general, while typically including both alveolar and peribronchial tissue, sample volumes are not adequate for diagnosis [7, 8]. Interestingly, however, a questionnaire based review from 38 centers including 131 children with ILD reported utilization of TBB alone or in combination with other procedures in 19.8 % of the cases. The report does not clarify, however, to what extent TBB was a key contributor for the diagnosis [9]. In an analysis of the diagnostic methods used for children with ILD by Fan [8], TBB was used in 6 out of 30 patients, with 3 (50 %) being diagnostic for sarcoidosis and bronchiolitis obliterans. The authors did not specify the reason for choosing TBB over VATS or open lung

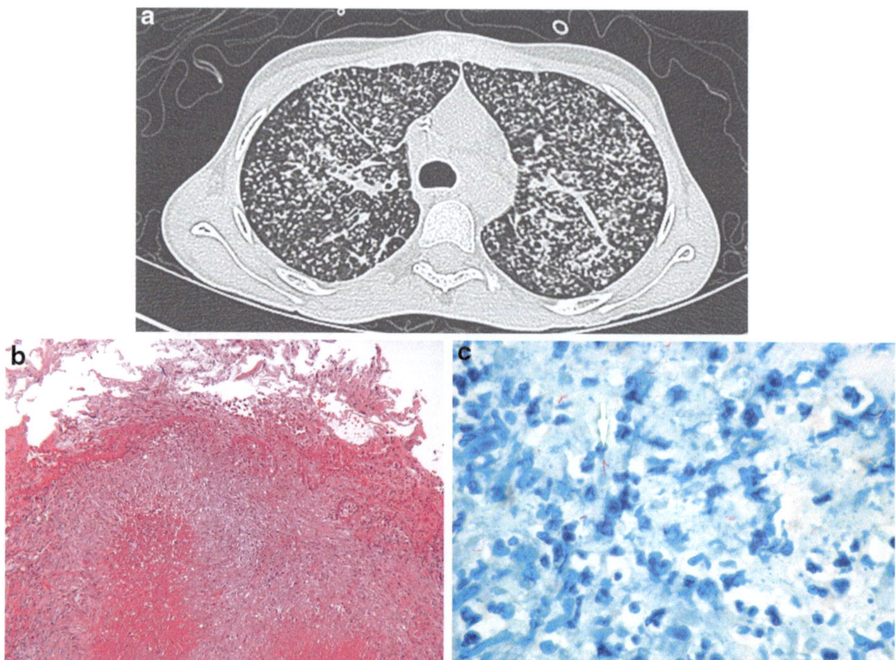

Fig. 3.1 A 21-year-old with HIV infection. (**a**) Chest CT scan with diffuse nodular disease suggestive of miliary tuberculosis. (**b**) Transbronchial biopsy specimen revealing caseating granuloma. (**c**) Ziehl–Neelsen stain revealing acid-fast bacilli

biopsy. A large prospective study of 500 consecutive patients, predominantly adults, in an ILD clinic over a 10-year period reports definitive diagnosis in 85 % of patients—60 % on the basis of invasive procedures. The diagnostic yield of TBB was limited, but 19 % of patients had their diagnosis confirmed by TBB. The yield of TBB for the few children included in this study was also disappointing [10]. Thus, the clinic's current practice is to prefer transbronchial cryo-bioptic techniques (see below) (Personal communication: Ferran Morell, MD).

The size limitation of the instrument that can be used to obtain TBB from small children imposes inherent limitations as well for tissue diagnosis in diffuse lung disease; however, Fig. 3.1 depicts an example of a transbronchial bioptic specimen obtained from an older HIV infected patient that led to conclusive diagnosis of miliary tuberculosis.

The technique, safety, and complications (e.g., pneumothorax, hemorrhage, transient pyrexia, and transient dyspnea) of TBB are beyond the scope of this chapter and are reviewed in detail by Tagliaferro et al. [11] The precautions to be kept in mind, however, are that only one lung should be sampled in order to avoid the occurrence of bilateral pneumothorax or hemorrhage [12]; it is also recommended that patients be hospitalized overnight following the procedure [11].

In a recent review article on childhood bronchoscopy [3], mention is made of new applications and techniques that are being introduced to the pediatric bronchoscopy practice such as endobronchial ultrasound and transbronchial needle biopsy of lymph nodes. The potential uses of *endobronchial ultrasound* in pediatrics was recently reviewed [13]. It is a minimally invasive technique that allows tissue sampling of peripheral lung lesions or mediastinal/hilar masses with high diagnostic accuracy and significantly lower morbidity and mortality compared to alternative approaches. Radial probe endobronchial ultrasound is used in adults for the investigation of peripheral lung lesions and could be adopted in children to achieve accurate biopsy of such lesions. Linear probe endobronchial ultrasound allows minimally invasive biopsy of mediastinal and hilar lesions.

Ultrasound-guided transbronchial needle aspiration (TBNA) of mediastinal lymph nodes is widely used in adults for cancer diagnosis [14]. This technique is not commonly utilized in pediatric patients; however, successful use of the minimally invasive technique of endobronchial ultrasound-guided transbronchial needle aspiration (EBUS-TBNA) was reported when sarcoidosis was diagnosed via material from hilar adenopathy in a 13-year-old child [15]. Given the size of the EBUS bronchoscope, application to younger children is not feasible; the largest report of pediatric TBNA for mediastinal lymphadenopathy did not use EBUS [16]. In this prospective study of 28 children (median age 41 months; range 9–168 months) guidance to the site of the biopsy was based on presence of enlarged subcarinal lymph nodes on chest CT scan reconstruction and the visual appearance of the carina. Definitive diagnosis by TBNA was found in 54 % of cases and in 36 % of the cases, cytology performed in the bronchoscopy suite led to the diagnoses. The authors concluded that TBNA is a safe procedure that adds value to flexible bronchoscopy in the diagnosis of mediastinal lymphadenopathy in children.

The limitations discussed above in regards to TBB for the diagnosis of parenchymal disease, predominantly in ILD, led to recent successful introduction of transbronchial lung biopsy by flexible cryo-probe. The technique allows acquisition of large biopsy samples of lung parenchyma that exceed the size and quality of samples obtained by forceps biopsy [17]. No pediatric reports are yet available, but in an adult study comparing historical controls to transbronchial cryo-biopsy in lung transplantation patients, no significant bleeding or pneumothorax occurred following transbronchial cryo-biopsy. The mean duration of bronchoscopy using cryo-probe was significantly shorter than the traditional forceps biopsy technique (5 vs. 8 min, respectively). The mean diameter of the specimen taken by forceps in historical controls was 2 mm compared to 10 mm obtained using the cryo-probe with no crush artifacts observed; ultimately, overall improved diagnostic value was reported [18].

Bronchoscopy for Removal of Obstructive, Noxious, or Damaging Materials from the Airway or the Lung

Bronchoscopy, both rigid and flexible, has been used for removal of various endogenous and exogenous materials in the airways that interfere with gas flow or exchange. This segment will cover in detail foreign body aspiration and also touch on less common conditions.

Bronchoscopy for Aspirated Foreign Bodies in Children

Removal of foreign bodies (FB) is by far the most common procedural challenge for the bronchoscopist. The US Centers for Disease Control (CDC) report almost 200,000 accidents per year resulting in nonfatal injury from foreign body aspiration in children less than 10 years of age [19]. These numbers may be even larger in other parts of the world, with a recent report from Algeria, where the authors state: "Foreign body aspiration is a real public health problem in Algeria" [20].

The decision about the need for intervention for suspected FB was addressed in a retrospective study of 160 children [21] aimed at exploring the best clinical and radiological predictors for finding a FB via bronchoscopy. Foreign body aspiration (FBA) was proven bronchoscopically in 122 (76 %). In multivariate analyses independent predictors of FBA were focal hyperinflation on chest radiograph, witnessed choking, and white blood cell count greater than 10,000/mL. Once there is suspicion of FBA, Martinot [22] proposed a management algorithm to assist in the decision between flexible versus rigid bronchoscopy based on the experience with 83 children. The authors propose rigid bronchoscopy to be performed first in case of asphyxia, a radiopaque FB, or association of unilaterally decreased breath sounds and obstructive emphysema. In any other case, flexible bronchoscopy is to be performed first for diagnostic purposes. They comment that if the algorithm was applied retrospectively to the 83 children in their study, it would have decreased the negative first rigid bronchoscopy rate to 4 %. They concluded that flexible bronchoscopy was a safe and cost-saving diagnostic procedure in children with suspected FB aspiration.

Rigid rather than flexible bronchoscopy has been advocated as the preferred instrument for extraction of foreign bodies since the early days of pediatric bronchoscopy [23] and continues to be the predominant practice [20]. Age appears to be a factor in decision-making. To this end, a study involving 102 infants (mean age 10.5 months, the youngest being 2 months old) with FBA, rigid bronchoscopy was used exclusively with a high success rate [24].

While the value of flexible bronchoscopy, as pointed out by Martinot et al. [22] is now widely accepted, the conventional teaching on extraction of aspirated FB points to the primacy of rigid over flexible bronchoscopy for such procedures because of its obvious advantages for visualization and instrumentation. It is conceivable, however, that this ongoing preference that emerges in literature is colored by fear of litigation if not abiding by "conventional" practice. This may create a distorted impression of limited value for flexible bronchoscopy. For the purist amongst the readers a "Cochranian" settlement of the question cannot emerge from literature that lacks any attempt for a controlled approach, neither is it likely that such evidence will emerge. The following segment attempts to provide experience on the role of flexible bronchoscopy for FBA.

Successful use of flexible bronchoscopy for extraction of FB has emerged over time, and some authors prefer flexible scopes for FBA. In a review of the Mayo Clinic Pediatric experience (1990–2001) [25] the authors preferentially used flexible bronchoscopy for extraction of FB in children. In their experience the procedure was successful and safe in children who underwent the procedure. The authors advise however that provisions be made to secure immediate rigid bronchoscope availability should the flexible bronchoscopic procedure be unsuccessful. Encouraged by previous reports of success and motivated by local circumstances or availability of relative expertise in flexible bronchoscopy, another publication [26] espoused flexible bronchoscopy for FBA. While this recommendation may be appropriate for some environments, our own experience is that we do not perform flexible bronchoscopy for suspected FB until immediate availability of rigid bronchoscopy is secured, along the lines of Swanson et al. [25].

A valid, and likely incontrovertible indication for preference of flexible over rigid bronchoscopy is FB that is lodged distally, beyond the reach of the rigid bronchoscope. Such conditions clearly justify an attempt of extraction with the more maneuverable flexible scope, yet may pose unique challenges as a result of angulation and depth of penetration into the bronchial tree with ever decreasing bronchial diameters as more distal branches are involved. Figure 3.2 depicts successful forceps extraction of a pin from a distal airway via flexible scope.

An important complicating factor can be posed by a FB that is imbedded in the surrounding tissue, often a granulation reaction, rendering the object invisible. Such circumstances may lead to surgical intervention and resection of the involved segment. Two reports however address such conditions with the use of interim procedures or techniques in an attempt to loosen the embedded foreign body, in both cases an aspirated tooth, followed by successful extraction by using urologic

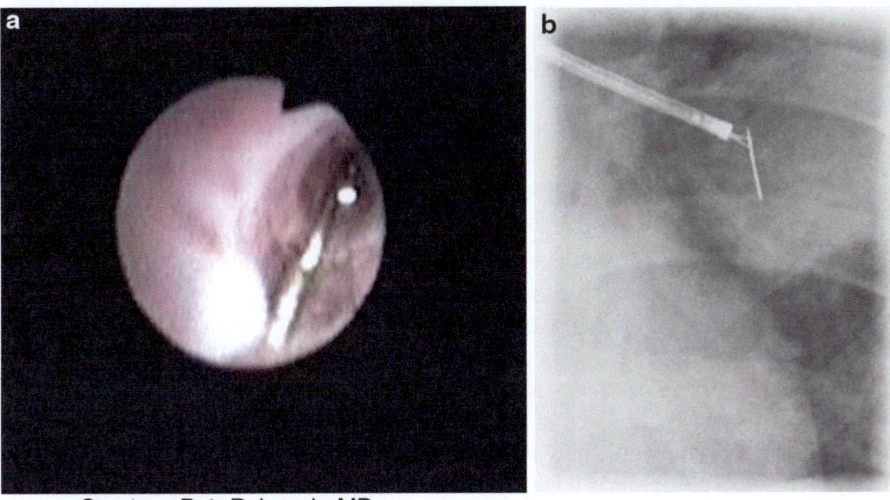

Fig. 3.2 Flexible bronchoscopic extraction of a foreign body (pin) in a 10-year-old. (**a**) Bronchoscopic image of the pin within the airway lumen. (**b**) Fluoroscopic image of bronchoscopic extraction of the pin. (Courtesy: Petr Pohunek, MD. Prague, Czech Republic)

baskets, balloon catheters or by forceps [27, 28]. These techniques included the use of topical and parenteral steroids and the use of argon plasma coagulation. The authors did not comment on late outcomes or complications of the interim procedures. The comment to make however is that these reports potentially understate the risk of dislodgement of the FB, which is often the argument cited to act with minimal delay when suspected.

With peripheral location of the FB or with bronchial lumina that are narrow in pediatric patients, visual limitation can complicate use of the flexible scope and instrumentation for extraction of a distal FB. This occurs when forceps passed through the working channel obstructs the field of vision within the narrow bronchus. Two studies describe the use of fluoroscopy [29] and image intensifier [30] to guide the grasping forceps for extraction of FB embedded in tissue past direct vision.

Sedation/Anesthesia for Foreign Body Associated Bronchoscopy

A detailed discussion on the sedation/anesthesia elements of flexible bronchoscopy is beyond the scope of this chapter. We will limit the comments on the topic to state that diagnostic procedures are mostly done through a nasal route, and recently often via laryngeal mask airway (LMA). A study of 1,947 procedures spanning the years 1988–2003 preferred use of LMA for flexible bronchoscopy in children 2 years of age and older, and complication rates were lower with the LMA (1.9 %) compared to the nasal route (3.5 %) [31].

In the context of this segment on FBA, while LMA is unlikely to be the choice approach when FBA is suspected, its use was reported in five cases in which FB was an incidental finding during a routine procedure and removed without difficulty and without the need to switch from the LMA to the conventional endotracheal tube [32].

Cast/Plastic Bronchitis

Cast or plastic bronchitis is a disorder characterized by formation of tenacious casts within the tracheobronchial tree. Spontaneously coughed up casts can draw attention to this uncommon condition. The distribution can be patchy or involving central segments of the airways when casts assume the shape of bronchial branching. Severe and sometimes life threatening obstruction can result. A comprehensive review of the topic is offered by Madsen et al. [33]. The underlying mechanisms involved in formation of casts are varied and overall not well understood; however, children with asthma who have particularly tenacious secretions may be affected and often improve with aggressive asthma therapies. At risk, albeit uncommonly, are children with various congenital heart disease, and in particular those who undergo Fontan procedures. A variety of therapies, all anecdotal, have been suggested for the cardiac-related conditions. It has been claimed that Bronchoscopy for removal of casts that obstruct large airways can be lifesaving but our experience has often found it difficult and extremely time-consuming due to the gelatinous consistency of the deposited material that renders suctioning, lavage, or removal by forceps difficult or unsuccessful.

Pulmonary Alveolar Proteinosis

Pulmonary Alveolar Proteinosis (PAP) is a rare pediatric disorder consisting of accumulation of phospholipid-proteinaceous material in the alveoli. Primary variety generally presents in infancy and early childhood and the acquired variety manifests in the older age groups. The underlying pathology is related to abnormal surfactant homeostasis and predominantly to defects in GM-CSF signaling. Shah et al. [34] and Mallory [35] comprehensively reviewed the topic. High resolution chest computerized tomographic scans (HRCT) with "crazy paving" patterns and flexible bronchoscopy with bronchoalveolar lavage are typically the key to the diagnosis when it yields milky fluid from affected segments with the extracellular substance staining with PAS [36]. The cytology is dominated by foamy macrophages [34, 35]. The most commonly considered procedure for a therapeutic intervention for PAP is a whole lung which is both challenging and time consuming. There are a number of approaches to the placement of the endotracheal tube (ETT) and isolation of the lung that is to be lavaged [37, 38]; The role of bronchoscopy is to secure the placement of the ETT and positioning of the balloon to prevent overflow of fluid into the ventilating lung. In essence a balloon catheter is placed in one main bronchus to seal off the entire lung that is to be lavaged with large amounts of saline, while ventilation is entirely dependent on the contralateral bronchus and lung. In exceptional cases where whole lung lavage is not feasible, a more arduous approach is that of direct segmental or subsegmental BAL [39, 40].

Lipoid Pneumonia

An extension of the concept of lung lavage was reported by Ciravegna et al. [41], in a case of an 8-year-old diagnosed with exogenous lipoid pneumonia due to aspiration of mineral oil that was administered for constipation. The diagnosis was supported by CT scan and BAL fluid (BALF) that was milky-appearing, yielding a high number of lipid-laden alveolar macrophages, as well as diffuse, free droplets of oil between alveolar cells on histology. Lung lavage was performed in the affected segments resulting in rapid clinical and radiologic improvement. A broader experience for the same diagnosis was reported in a study of 10 children with lipoid pneumonia secondary to mineral oil aspiration [42]. The authors took a stepwise BAL approach, which resulted in overall favorable outcomes.

Other Exogenous Foreign Material Aspiration

Sand aspiration to the lung in a 3-year-old with near-drowning was reported [43]. BAL was done when the child continued to have persistent wheezing and high ventilatory requirement and sand was detected in the BALF. Sequential lung washing followed by exogenous surfactant led to rapid improvement and subsequent recovery in PFTs. In a reported case of accidental instillation of activated charcoal into the lung by a misplaced gastric tube [44], an attempt was made to lavage the charcoal from the lung. While charcoal particles were observed in the BALF, the therapeutic effect could not be assessed since the case was complicated by severe pleural involvement.

Management of the Narrowed or Obstructed Airway: Debridement, Dilation, and Stenting

Impingement on airway lumen by tissue projecting into the lumen can result from various types of mechanical irritants and inflammatory processes both likely compounded by infection. Mechanical irritants and inflammatory processes in the airway lumen can both produce granulation tissues which with or without secondary infection can cause impingement on the airway lumen. Granulation tissue can follow irritation caused by an aspirated foreign bodies, endotracheal tubes, tracheostomy cannulas, and at surgical sites. These conditions can be approached by debridement using the forceps via flexible bronchoscope, compression by high-pressure balloon catheters and ultimately laser photoresection.

An example of granulation tissue following bronchial anastomosis in lung transplantation being treated using gentle excision by forceps via flexible bronchoscopy is presented in Fig. 3.3. Caution should be exercised since bleeding may be a complication and use of laser therapies that offer various option should be considered [1]. Soong et al. [45] described successful treatment of obstructive fibrinous tracheal pseudomembranes complicating central airways in 8 children following prolonged intubation using a combination of forceps, balloon and laser. Flexible bronchoscopic breaching, debridement, and dilation of what was assumed to be inflammation-related obstructive membranes was described in patients with CF and other post-infectious or inflammatory lesions [46, 47].

The use of *balloon dilation* for airways can be considered for a variety of conditions both congenital and acquired in which the airway wall is narrowed [48, 49]. The procedure can be done under bronchoscopic vision, but a radiologic approach has also been proposed [48]. An example of a bronchoscopic view of balloon dilation is presented in Fig. 3.4. Such pathology may recur and eventually may require stent placement. Importantly, balloon dilation can be considered for congenital narrowing of central airways such as complete tracheal rings [50]. This procedure should however be viewed as a surgical intervention since the risk of laceration and fracture of tracheal rings would require extreme caution. While evaluation of long-term outcome of balloon dilatation in adults is published, the indications and

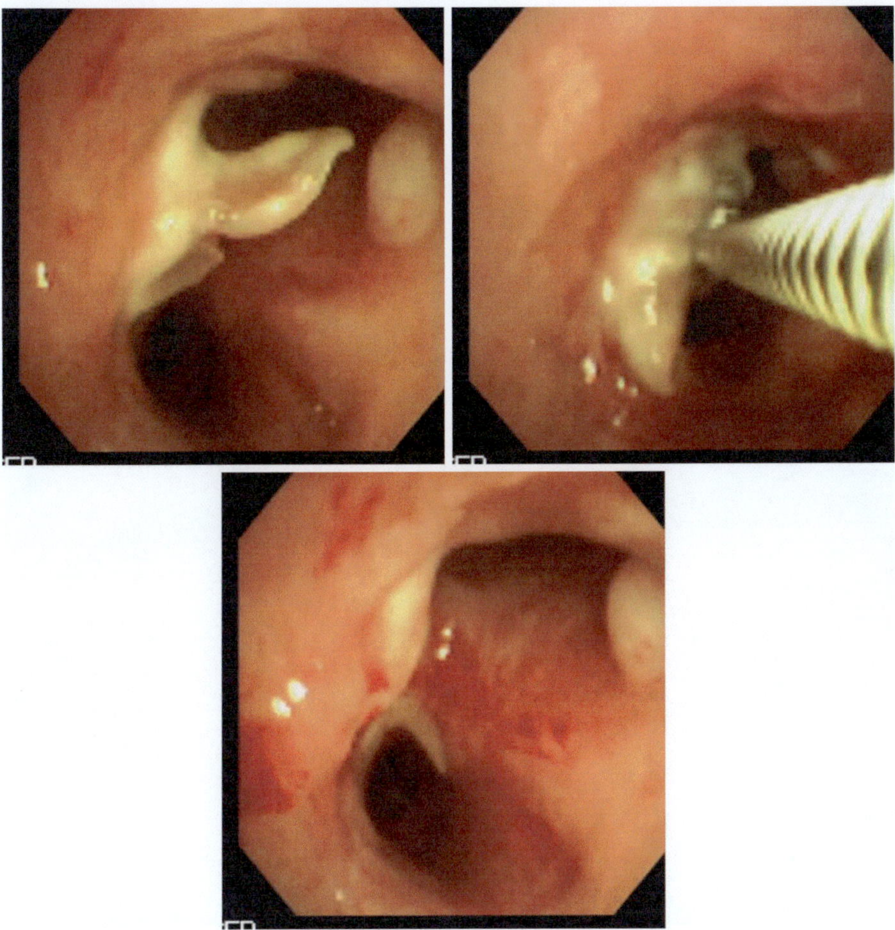

Fig. 3.3 Forceps debridement of postsurgical (anastomotic region after lung transplantation) scar tissue. The lower image shows patency of the airway lumen after the procedure

conditions of the procedure are so widely different from those in pediatric patients such that it appears unreasonable to extrapolate the results. Thus, little information about the long-term results in pediatric patients is available [51].

Placement of Stents in the Airway

Over the past two decades there has been a growing body of information on the use of tracheo-bronchial stenting in pediatrics that has slowly gained recognition as an acceptable technique for the treatment of central airway obstruction, however, there [52]. Stents though an attractive proposition continue to be a topic of discussion and debate in the pediatric pulmonary practice as their limitations generally render them unready for prime time.

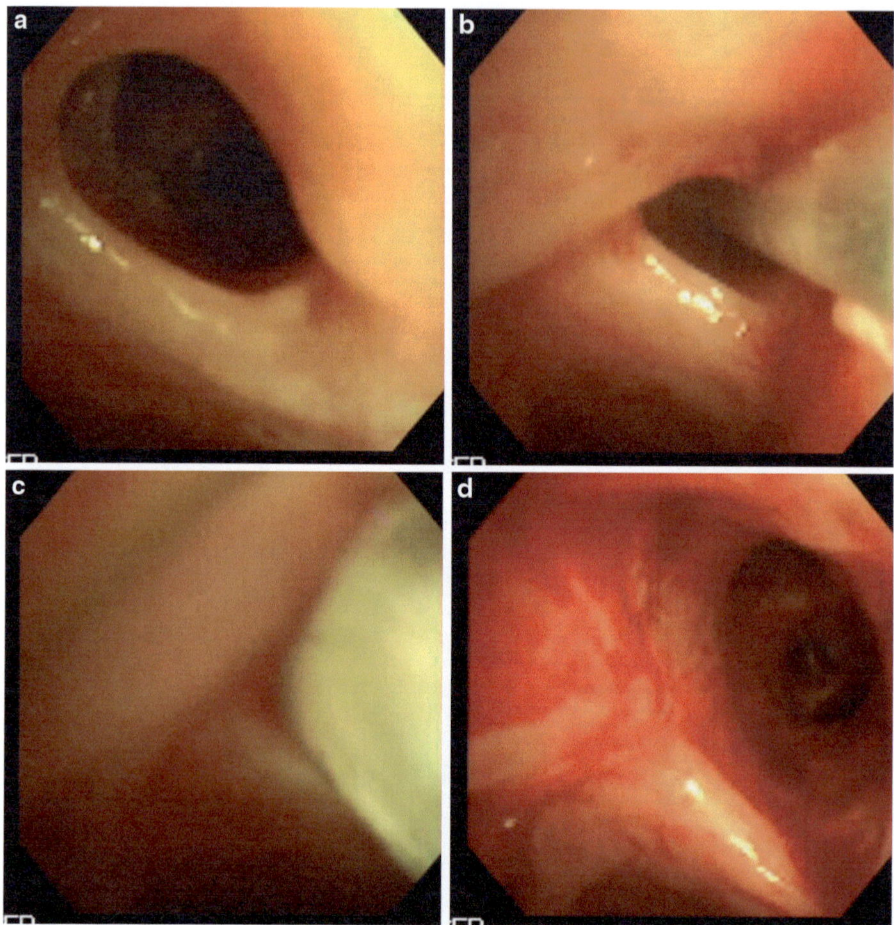

Fig. 3.4 (**a–d**) Improved patency is gained by high-pressure balloon dilation (**c** depicts balloon in place) in the narrowed bronchial anastomotic segment of a patient who underwent lung transplantation

Stenting of the airway has been used successfully in adults, and has been considered as an attractive alternative in children. Fundamental differences of pediatric compared to adult use include the benign nature of most stenoses which do not alter life expectancy, [52] the narrow and soft airways of children, that improve with airway growth and the shift of mediastinal vessels [53] and also the required long-term tolerance and adaptation to growth. These differences may significantly alter the therapeutic balance, calling into question the precise role stents play in the treatment of airway obstruction in children. However, recognition that situations exist in which no other options are available has led to increased use of this technique in pediatrics.

Obstruction of the airway is the result of abnormalities of the airway wall, intraluminal causes or extrinsic compression [48]. Prior to stent placement, the airway is typically evaluated with bronchoscopy or bronchography and the chest evaluated for causes of compression with echocardiogram, CT scan or MRI [48].

Stents may be placed by either interventional bronchoscopists or invasive radiologists with relative advantages and disadvantages to each, and often cooperation between them. Plastic/silicon stents were initially available. The first use of a metallic stent in pediatrics was reported in 1988 [54]. Currently biodegradable stents are being introduced and offer potential new horizons [55]. The advantages and disadvantages of the various stents are further discussed below.

Most reports of use of stents in pediatrics are case reports or small series. In the absence of randomized clinical trials or larger series, it is difficult to compare the efficacy and tolerance of metal versus silicone airway stents in children; furthermore mortality rates in recipients of stents are generally high given that indications for stenting are mostly options of last resort [53].

Indications

The indications for stent placement as outlined in the adult literature include: extrinsic stenosis of central airways with or without intraluminal components due to malignant or benign disorders; complex, inoperable tracheobronchial strictures, tracheobronchial malacia, palliation of recurrent intraluminal tumor growth, and central airway fistulae (esophagus, mediastinum, pleura) [56]. In pediatrics the common causes of obstruction leading to stenting are the following:

Congenital stenosis. This results from abnormal cartilage rings (small and complete), or compression by abnormal vessels, such as pulmonary artery slings. Operative repair is the standard of care, however, recurrent obstruction is often encountered, the result of malacia or restenosis. Balloon dilations and stenting is thereafter sometimes the next step [48]. It may also be the result of accumulation of metabolic products such as seen in mucopolysaccharide storage disorders [57, 58]. It is usually agreed that in cases involving vascular compression, relief of the compression is the initial step [58].

Tracheal or bronchial malacia. This usually resolves by 2 years of age; however, it may require intervention when diffuse and/or requiring treatment with long-term CPAP via tracheostomy [48]. In a series of 105 patients who underwent aortopexy for treatment of tracheo-bronchomalacia, five patients required stenting after failure of aortopexy [59]. Additionally, despite the generally favorable long term prognosis of airway malacia, severe "dying spells" [60, 61], or severe growth retardation [58] may require a temporizing procedure.

Airway obstruction at a site of previous surgery. This usually results from granulation tissue and/or fibrosis following patch repair or over suture lines [62]. This condition may occur after lung transplantation at the site of the bronchial anastomoses.

Palliative indications. Stenting is also considered for palliation. This includes patients in whom a lesion is unresectable because of anatomic constraints, metastatic disease or limitations due to overall medical condition; stent placement may be minimally invasive and may provide prolonged palliation [63]. Stenting may allow weaning of ventilatory support and subsequently allow hospital discharge, even if long term survival is not anticipated [48].

Types of Stents

There are several different types of stents with their respective advantages and disadvantages, different methods of insertion, and varying requirements for follow-up and management.

A plethora of stents have been used in the airways. They can be divided into four major groups.

1. Polymer stents (Dumon, Polyflex)
2. Mettalic stents
   Balloon expandable (Palmaz)
   Self-expanding (Wallstent)
3. Covered Mettalic stents
4. Hybrid Stents

Stents can also be grouped based on indication, insertion technique, anatomical location or whether removable or not [64]. In 2011 use of a biodegradable polydioxanone stent was first reported in children [55].

Silicone or silastic stents are long tubes that are easy to remove but have problems with luminal occlusion and to a lesser degree migration [48]. The small radii of airways of children require thin walled stents, and when made of silicon these tend to be collapsible and prone to migration [58]. The continuous, non-fenestrated tube interrupts mucociliary clearance for which humidification and inhalation, inhalation of, mucolytic agents including DNase have been suggested, but their efficacy has never been documented [58]. Insertion is with a rigid bronchoscope, a device most pediatric pulmonologist are not familiar with such that placement is done only in centers with specialists trained in this procedure. Fayon et al. reported their experience with a custom manufactured polysiloxane (Tracheobronxane) stent in 14 children with success and failure rates equal at 43 %; the latter due to migration or obstruction.

In summary, extreme caution is needed when using these stents that remain attractive mainly for short-term use in the hospital setting postoperatively. Stents with internal support structures in their walls (Polyflex) aim to resolve some of these problems; however, migration and mucous impaction remain significant and limit their use [58].

Metallic stents were initially developed for vascular lesions. They are relatively easy to deploy by bronchoscopy or bronchography, are thin walled and their mesh structure allows for continued mucociliary clearance and ventilation even when the stent covers bronchial openings [58]. Their main disadvantage is difficult removal as early as several weeks after implantation due to mucosal overgrowth [58] albeit removal has been documented up to 5 years after insertion [64]. Other problems include breaks due to material fatigue and migration into surrounding organs [58].

The most frequently used balloon expandable stent is the *Palmaz stent*. It is non-elastic and made of stainless steel. Its main advantage in pediatrics is the ability to overdilate as the child grows, while its disadvantages are fracture [48] or deformation with cough [58]. They have the advantage over the self-expanding stents (such as the Wallstent; see below) in that they do not exert constant outward pressure after placement, which is implicated in erosion and hemorrhage [58]. In a 5-year published experience with this stent; a total of 30 stents were placed via rigid bronchoscopy in 16 patients [62] with airway malacia as the most common indication. Repeat procedures were required in several patients due to obstruction, development of granulation tissue and migration.

The *Wallstent* is made of thin wire, is very flexible and compressible but re-expands after compression. Placement is not easy as it shortens by 20–40 % during placement but its flexibility renders it easily adaptable to curved airways compared with the rigid Palmaz stent [58]. It is accepted that these stents are more appropriate for compression by vascular structures where the pulsatile mass against a rigid stent, such as Palmaz, could lead to vascular erosion [48]. The disadvantage of Wallstent is that it cannot be dilated as the child grows and may therefore result in stenosis if left in the airway of an infant [48] and likewise, in the trachea of young children [58].

Nitinol stents (Ultraflex) are another form of self-expanding metal stents made of a shape-memory alloy in either covered or uncovered forms and expand at body temperature. They do not exert continuous outward pressure but dislocation is less common than with silicon stents and is proposed as the optimal material for the human airway. While fewer complications have been reported with this kind of stent, it is not clear whether this reflects veritable superiority or the relatively infrequent use [58]. They too cannot be dilated so they must be replaced as the child grows [64].

Polydioxanone biodegradable self-expanding stents were recently first reported in children [55]. Polydioxanone is a semicrystalline polymer of the polyester family. The predicted and observed degradation time was 15 weeks. These stents are inserted with a specific introducer that is too large to allow direct vision. As with the other self-expanding stents their final size is hard to predict.

Of note is that there are two stent types fraught with problems and are no longer in use: Strecker, a tantalum stent, and Gianturco a steel stent with external hooks [58].

Method of Insertion

Stents may be placed with bronchographic guidance. Bronchography has several advantages over bronchoscopy; it provides accurate measurements and can also asses the airway distal to the obstruction [48]. Bronchoscopy offers the advantage of direct visualization. The thicker silastic stents can only be inserted by rigid bronchoscopy. Imaging, usually by bronchography but also CT or MRI scans is necessary prior to the procedure for planning optimal placement and to determine the size of the stent.

The ERS/ATS published a statement with the training requirements for bronchoscopists performing stent placement. This included ample experience with rigid/flexible bronchoscopy and endotracheal intubation [56]. This implies that the procedure should only be offered in a few specialized centers [58].

Complications

Silicone stents. Occlusion and migration are the most common complications [48], the latter linked to the very nature of these stents that, in contrast to metal stents, do not become incorporated into the wall [53]. Migration was mostly encountered in the Fayon study with small caliber stents compressed by high-pressure vessels; pointing towards avoidance of the use of silicone stents in these circumstances. Granulation tissue is infrequent, moderate, and localized to the tip of the stent, and largely observed when the stent is too mobile [53].

Metallic stents. The potential for metallic stent erosion through the thin bronchial wall is a subject of discussion, but with scant documentation. Wells et al. [65] described two patients with associated heart disease and stenting of the left main stem bronchus (LMSB). Both patients presented with ruptured pseudoaneurysms adjacent to the stented bronchus; this complication was likely compounded by adjacent bronchial collateral vessels in patients with cyanotic heart disease. Stents might also erode into surrounding structures, with possible exsanguinating hemorrhage from bronchovascular fistulae [63]. Geller et al. [66] described three deaths due to massive tracheal bleeds in nine Palmaz stent placements occurring months after placement. All had concomitant tracheotomies. They concluded that tracheotomy and Palmaz stent placement in the airway might increase tracheal colonization/inflammation and hence friability and proposed that tracheotomy be viewed as contraindication to use of a Palmaz stent.

Granulation tissue formation is usually mild when the stent is placed against an intact airway wall [48]. It is best treated with intermittent ballooning, which may be insufficient. Use of lasers should be avoided due to heat transfer through metallic objects [58]. Stent fracture is a specific complication of the metallic balloon expandable—stents.

Metallic self-expandable stenting requires long-term management to correct potential stent problems that also include migration or obstruction by inspissated secretions, granulation tissue, or tumor. Peng et al. [67] in a 5-year experience emphasize the role of flexible (vs. rigid) bronchoscopy in pediatric intensive care patients with stent repair as the second most common indication for procedures.

Information regarding status of the airways after stent placement can be obtained through imaging and pulmonary function testing. The need for routine bronchoscopies to assess for complications and formation of granulation tissue is unclear, and while discouraged in adults, may be called for in pediatrics due to the smaller diameter of their airways. It remains unclear whether the finding of granulation tissue in asymptomatic patients warrants prompt treatment [58]. The risk exists that bronchoscopy through a stent may lead to its dislocation or damage [62].

Mitomycin C has been reported to inhibit fibroblast proliferation in granulation tissue formation in human cells [68] and bronchoscopic application of mitomycin C as adjuvant treatment for benign airway stenosis has been reported [69]. Curiously we have found no report of the use of this agent, for the prevention of granulation formation following stent placement, in the literature.

Since stenting is usually a last resort in patients that are a priori in critical straits, it is difficult to determine the mortality rate related directly to stent placement. A tentative estimate of 13 % mortality was stated by Nicolai [58] but remains difficult to ascertain.

Use of Bronchsocopy for Other Procedures

Sealing of Fistulae

Recurrence of tracheoesophageal fistula (TEF) after the original surgery is often difficult to demonstrate and is mostly managed by repeated surgery. Literature in recent years [1, 70, 71] points, however, to a bronchoscopic option of sealing the fistula by collagen glue, fibrin, cyanoacrylate, or sclerosing agents. To improve results preparatory mucosal priming via brush abrasion, laser or electrocautery is proposed, which is subsequently followed by the "glue." While more than one endoscopic procedure is often needed, the endoscopic repair is an attractive alternative to open surgical repair. The cited publications employ rigid bronchoscopy for the procedure. Goussard et al. [72] reported fibrin glue closure of a persistent bronchopleural fistula that complicated pneumonectomy in a 16-year-old girl with post-tuberculosis bronchiectasis. While we were unable to find reports on the use of flexible bronchoscopy for primary or secondary closure of TEF, this report may open new avenues for such repair, in particular where H-type fistulae may be involved.

Bronchoscopic Sealing of Pneumothorax

The recent emergence of necrotizing pneumonia brought about a substantial increase in complications with bronchopleural fistulae (BPF) [73], as many as 12 % of hospitalized cases with necrotizing pneumonia were reported to suffer this complication [74]. Curiously, no reports of persistent leakage or the therapeutic approach thereof has been published. Endoscopic approaches to persistent pneumothorax with various sealing materials have been reported since the 1970s [75]. To identify the bronchus leading to the air leak, a fiberoptic bronchoscope and a balloon catheter are used while diminution of the air leak with repeated inflations of the balloon is followed [76]. An interesting novel approach to identification of the leaking segment when balloon occlusion fails is the use of a capnographic catheter that is passed into the airway [77]. Once identified and with inflated balloon, the sealant can be injected through the distal port into the airway, or alternatively manipulated via forceps.

A recent review of the therapeutic transbronchial approach via use of bronchial valves [78] appears less feasible in the pediatric age group, but various sealants have been used in multiple reports of adult patients. Use of fibrin glue with rapid response was reported [76]. Wiaterek et al. [79] reported placement of several alternating layers of an absorbable hemostat (knitted fabric prepared by controlled oxidation of cellulose-Surgicel; Ethicon) within the segment of interest using bronchoscopy forceps followed by catheter injection of 3 mL of the patient's blood onto the absorbable hemostat to create an occluding blood patch. Rigid bronchoscopy is predominantly used but some of these procedures utilize flexible bronchoscopy. The youngest patient we could identify in the literature who underwent such procedure was an 11 month old who developed BPF 3 weeks after surgery for cystic adenomatoid malformation. The infant was successfully managed with porcine dermal collagen combined with fibrin glue plug [80].

Control of Diffuse Alveolar Hemorrhage

The topic of bronchoscopy for airway and pulmonary bleeding has been covered in a chapter previously alluded to [2]. At the risk of some repetition we wish, however, to highlight a novel bronchoscopic intervention for intractable lung bleeding.

Based on previous experience using systemic administration of recombinant factor VII (rFVIIa) to effectively treat patients with pulmonary bleeding, its use has been extended to direct intrapulmonary instillation of rFVIIa in recalcitrant cases of diffuse alveolar hemorrhage (DAH) [81, 82]. We recently used rFVIIa as an intervention of last resort to control unremitting diffuse pulmonary hemorrhage in two cases; a 16-year-old patient with acute myelogenous leukemia [83] and a 2-year-old patient with relapsed acute lymphoblastic leukemia [84]. We used the protocol proposed by Heslet [81] that entailed administration of rFVIIa into both main stem bronchi at a dose of 50 mcg/kg diluted in 50 mL of normal saline; for the smaller or younger patient, we opted to dilute in 25 mL of normal saline. The dose was divided in two equal aliquots and separately instilled to the main bronchi. To cite directly from our report: "Hemorrhage was visualized bronchoscopically, and its resolution following the treatment was immediate, unequivocal, and definitive" [83]. In a recent review of the topic, emphasis is made that multiple reported cases have been shown to respond promptly with the added safety of absence of thromboembolic complications when rFVIIa is administered bronchoscopically as opposed to systemically [85].

Segmental Bronchography

Bronchography is rarely used in the era of CT scan, and in particular since the advent of 3-D reconstruction. However, Bramson et al. [86] reported the use of flexible bronchoscopy and instillation of contrast material via the bronchoscope channel. They pointed out that bronchogram elucidated findings that were unclear from other imaging procedures. A more recent study [48] of bronchography via flexible bronchoscopy emphasized the advantage of the procedure particularly when a laryngeal mask airway is used. In our previous publication [2], we stated the utility of segmental bronchography for cases in which CT scan failed to elucidate details of the finer internal structure of bronchi or their connections. The flexible bronchoscope was advanced peripherally and wedged into the bronchus feeding the area of interest, and the dye was injected through the working channel under fluoroscopy with images taken in rapid sequence.

In the study by Bramson et al. [86], Dionsil—a lipid based contrast material was used. This agent is not readily available at present; instead contrast materials used in arteriography such as Ioversol (Optiray, Mallinckrodt, Inc.) is used. McLaren et al. [48] report use of very small volumes of contrast, as little as 1 mL or less, for diagnostic bronchography in small children, except for interventional procedures where larger volumes of contrast (5 mL or more) may be required. They recommend isotonic contrast such as iotrolan (Isovist, Schering, Burgess Hill, UK), but point to safety of widely available, moderately hypertonic agents (such as Omnipaque, Nycomed, Nycoveien, Norway). In our experience the resolution of images with the non-lipid contrast materials is inferior to that achieved with the older materials;

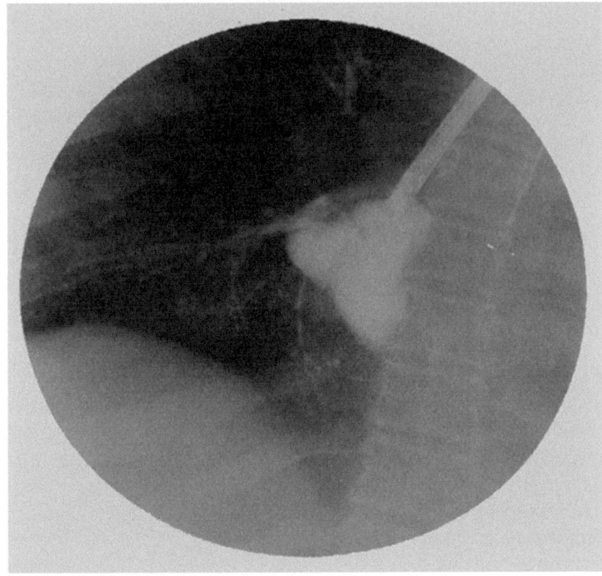

Fig. 3.5 Segmental bronchography. Contrast material is injected via a wedged bronchoscope to establish airway connection, in this case revealing a cardiac bronchus

moreover, they fade rapidly, but with rapid sequence image acquisition, the information sought can usually be obtained. Figure 3.5 exemplifies segmental bronchography that established the diagnosis of unsuspected cardiac bronchus.

New Horizons

Fetal Bronchoscopy

A distinctly novel horizon in pediatric bronchoscopy is a recent report by Quintero et al. [87] of a first fetal bronchoscopy. This in utero bronchoscopy was undertaken with the hope of salvaging the lungs of a 32-week gestation fetus diagnosed with congenital lung abnormalities that were deemed incompatible with extrauterine survival. The left lung was taken up by a mass that caused mediastinal shift and as a result, extremely small right lung (Fig. 3.6). Ultrasound and fetal MRI suggested the possible presence of bronchial atresia or congenital cystic adenomatoid malformation (CCAM). Bronchoscopy resulted in intraoperative expansion of normal lung parenchyma in both the right and left lungs, with dramatically improved and normalized lung growth until birth. Postnatal CT and MRI were suggestive of extralobar pulmonary sequestration with cystic areas, with a feeding vessel stemming from the descending aorta. The lesions were eventually resected at 10 months of age confirming the presumptive diagnoses. The authors submit that the bronchoscopy established airway patency in obstructed airways and restored amniotic fluid flow to the lung periphery—a key element in lung development. This notion is

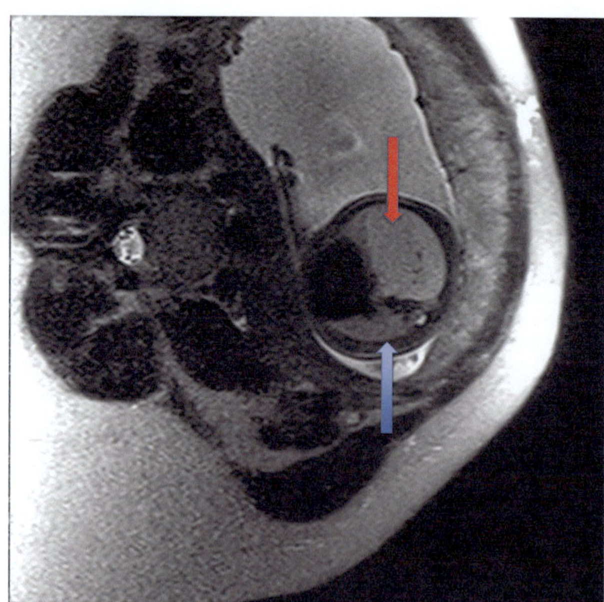

Fig. 3.6 MRI of maternal abdomen with transverse section of fetal lungs in the uterus. *Upper arrow* points to a large left lung mass. *Lower arrow* points to a markedly diminished, normally structured right lung

based on increasing recognition that bronchial obstruction may be the common pathway to the frequently overlapping congenital anomalies of the lung, including CCAM, intralobar sequestration (ILS), extralobar sequestration (ELS), and lobar emphysema (LE). Several studies support bronchial atresia as the unifying mechanism responsible for these malformations, termed "bronchial atresia sequence" [88, 89]. This was corroborated by a report [90] stating that lesions already diagnosed with peripheral bronchial atresia (radiologically and/or pathologically) were found to have frequent microcystic changes consistent with small cyst type CCAM.

The same authors [91] reported a second fetal bronchoscopy at 30 weeks gestation with similar presentation based on US and MRI findings. In this case the therapeutic effect of the intervention was not as obvious, and only minor improvement occurred until delivery at 40 weeks. Perinatal CT-angiography demonstrated LUL congenital lobar emphysema (CLE), which was subsequently confirmed by pathology after postnatal resection.

In another study fetal intervention using the fetoscope (vs. bronchoscope) was undertaken to surgically breach an atretic bronchus in utero [92]. While the results are reported to have been favorable, little detail is provided regarding the technical elements of the intervention.

It is not possible to draw conclusion regarding the role of fetal bronchoscopy from this limited reported experience. It appears to be technically feasible with current instrumentation, and since fetal oxygenation is not dependent on the fetal lung, desaturation during the procedure is not a limiting factor. Cognizant that the intrauterine course of congenital pulmonary lesions is not easy to predict, we think that fetal bronchoscopy should be reserved for cases in which the size or complexity of the lesion makes extrauterine viability unlikely. It is hoped that further experience will better define the potential role of improving or reversing progression of intrauterine congenital anomalies with use of this novel intervention.

References

1. Donato LL, Mai Hong Tran T, Ammouche C, Musani AI. Pediatric interventional bronchoscopy. Clin Chest Med. 2013;34:569–82.
2. Colin AA, Walz DA. Techniques and technical issues: special procedures. In: Priftis KN, Anthracopoulos MB, Eber E, Koumbourlis A, Wood RE, editors. Paediatric bronchoscopy. Basel: Karger AG; 2010. p. 42–53.
3. Nicolai T. The role of rigid and flexible bronchoscopy in children. Paediatr Respir Rev. 2011;12:190–5.
4. Salva PS, Theroux C, Schwartz D. Safety of endobronchial biopsy in 170 children with chronic respiratory symptoms. Thorax. 2003;58:1058–60.
5. Colin AA, Ali-Dinar T. Endobronchial biopsy in childhood. Chest. 2007;131:1626–7.
6. Greene CL, Reemtsen B, Polimenakos A, Horn M, Wells W. Role of clinically indicated transbronchial lung biopsies in the management of pediatric post-lung transplant patients. Ann Thorac Surg. 2008;86:198–203.
7. Whitehead B, Scott JP, Helms P, et al. Technique and use of transbronchial biopsy in children and adolescents. Pediatr Pulmonol. 1992;12:240–6.

8. Fan LL, Kozinetz CA, Wojtczak HA, Chatfield BA, Cohen AH, Rothenberg SS. Diagnostic value of transbronchial, thoracoscopic, and open lung biopsy in immunocompetent children with chronic interstitial lung disease. J Pediatr. 1997;131:565–9.

9. Barbato A, Panizzolo C, Cracco A, de Blic J, Dinwiddie R, Zach M. Interstitial lung disease in children: a multicentre survey on diagnostic approach. Eur Respir J. 2000;16:509–13.

10. Morell F, Reyes L, Domenech G, De Gracia J, Majo J, Ferrer J. Diagnoses and diagnostic procedures in 500 consecutive patients with clinical suspicion of interstitial lung disease. Arch Bronconeumol. 2008;44:185–91.

11. Tagliaferro T, Michelin E, Snijders D, Barbato A. Endobronchial and transbronchial biopsies in children. Expert Rev Respir Med. 2008;2:245–51.

12. Barbato A, Panizzolo C. Chronic interstitial lung disease in children. Paediatr Respir Rev. 2000;1:172–8.

13. Steinfort DP, Wurzel D, Irving LB, Ranganathan SC. Endobronchial ultrasound in pediatric pulmonology. Pediatr Pulmonol. 2009;44:303–8.

14. Dango S, Cucuruz B, Mayer O, et al. Detection of disseminated tumour cells in mediastinoscopic lymph node biopsies and endobronchial ultrasonography-guided transbronchial needle aspiration in patients with suspected lung cancer. Lung Cancer. 2010;68:383–8.

15. Wurzel DF, Steinfort DP, Massie J, Ryan MM, Irving LB, Ranganathan SC. Paralysis and a perihilar protuberance: an unusual presentation of sarcoidosis in a child. Pediatr Pulmonol. 2009;44:410–4.

16. Goussard P, Gie RP, Kling S, et al. The diagnostic value and safety of transbronchial needle aspiration biopsy in children with mediastinal lymphadenopathy. Pediatr Pulmonol. 2010;45:1173–9.

17. Babiak A, Hetzel J, Krishna G, et al. Transbronchial cryobiopsy: a new tool for lung biopsies. Respiration. 2009;78:203–8.

18. Fruchter O, Fridel L, Rosengarten D, Raviv Y, Rosanov V, Kramer MR. Transbronchial cryobiopsy in lung transplantation patients: first report. Respirology. 2013;18:669–73.

19. Leading causes of death reports. 10 leading causes of nonfatal unintentional injury, United States 2007, all races, both sexes, ages <1. Web-based injury statistics query and reporting system (WISQARS) 2007. Center for Disease Control, 2007. http://www.cdc.gov/ncipc/wisqars

20. Boufersaoui A, Smati L, Benhalla KN, et al. Foreign body aspiration in children: experience from 2624 patients. Int J Pediatr Otorhinolaryngol. 2013;77:1683–8.

21. Heyer CM, Bollmeier ME, Rossler L, et al. Evaluation of clinical, radiologic, and laboratory prebronchoscopy findings in children with suspected foreign body aspiration. J Pediatr Surg. 2006;41:1882–8.

22. Martinot A, Closset M, Marquette CH, et al. Indications for flexible versus rigid bronchoscopy in children with suspected foreign-body aspiration. Am J Respir Crit Care Med. 1997;155:1676–9.

23. Wood RE. Flexible bronchoscopy to remove foreign bodies in children – yes, maybe – but… J Bronchol. 1994;1:87.

24. Shubha AM, Das K. Tracheobronchial foreign bodies in infants. Int J Pediatr Otorhinolaryngol. 2009;73:1385–9.

25. Swanson KL, Prakash UB, Midthun DE, et al. Flexible bronchoscopic management of airway foreign bodies in children. Chest. 2002;121:1695–700.

26. Mehta D, Mehta C, Bansal S, Singla S, Tangri N. Flexible bronchoscopic removal of a three piece foreign body from a child's bronchus. Australas Med J. 2012;5:227–30.

27. Lando T, Cahill AM, Elden L. Distal airway foreign bodies: importance of a stepwise approach, knowledge of equipment and utilization of other services' expertise. Int J Pediatr Otorhinolaryngol. 2011;75:968–72.

28. Jabbardarjani H, Kiani A, Arab A, Masjedi M. Foreign body removal using bronchoscopy and argon plasma coagulation. Arch Iran Med. 2010;13:150–2.

29. Hockstein NG, Jacobs IN. Flexible bronchoscopic removal of a distal bronchial foreign body with cinefluoroscopic guidance. Ann Otol Rhinol Laryngol. 2004;113:863–5.

30. Nwaejike N, Khan Z, Villaquiran J, Awan YM, Rahamim J. Use of an image intensifier to remove a challenging foreign body in a segmental bronchiole. Ann R Coll Surg Engl. 2010;92:W38–40.
31. Naguib ML, Streetman DS, Clifton S, Nasr SZ. Use of laryngeal mask airway in flexible bronchoscopy in infants and children. Pediatr Pulmonol. 2005;39:56–63.
32. Avital A, Gozal D, Uwyyed K, Springer C. Retrieval of spirated foreign bodies in children using a flexible bronchoscope and a laryngeal mask airway. J Bronchol. 2002;9:6–9.
33. Madsen P, Shah SA, Rubin BK. Plastic bronchitis: new insights and a classification scheme. Paediatr Respir Rev. 2005;6:292–300.
34. Shah PL, Hansell D, Lawson PR, Reid KB, Morgan C. Pulmonary alveolar proteinosis: clinical aspects and current concepts on pathogenesis. Thorax. 2000;55:67–77.
35. Mallory Jr GB. Surfactant proteins: role in lung physiology and disease in early life. Paediatr Respir Rev. 2001;2:151–8.
36. Rossi GA. Bronchoalveolar lavage in the investigation of disorders of the lower respiratory tract. Eur J Respir Dis. 1986;69:293–315.
37. Wood RE. Whole Lung Lavage. In: Priftis KN, Anthracopoulos MB, Eber E, Koumbourlis A, Wood RE, editors. Paediatric bronchoscopy. Basel: Karger; 2010. p. 75–82.
38. Reiter K, Schoen C, Griese M, Nicolai T. Whole-lung lavage in infants and children with pulmonary alveolar proteinosis. Paediatr Anaesth. 2010;20:1118–23.
39. Mahut B, Delacourt C, Scheinmann P, et al. Pulmonary alveolar proteinosis: experience with eight pediatric cases and a review. Pediatrics. 1996;97:117–22.
40. Dogru D, Yalcin E, Aslan AT, et al. Successful unilateral partial lung lavage in a child with pulmonary alveolar proteinosis. J Clin Anesth. 2009;21:127–30.
41. Ciravegna B, Sacco O, Moroni C, et al. Mineral oil lipoid pneumonia in a child with anoxic encephalopathy: treatment by whole lung lavage. Pediatr Pulmonol. 1997;23:233–7.
42. Sias SM, Daltro PA, Marchiori E, et al. Clinic and radiological improvement of lipoid pneumonia with multiple bronchoalveolar lavages. Pediatr Pulmonol. 2009;44:309–15.
43. Kapur N, Slater A, McEniery J, Greer ML, Masters IB, Chang AB. Therapeutic bronchoscopy in a child with sand aspiration and respiratory failure from near drowning-case report and literature review. Pediatr Pulmonol. 2009;44:1043–7.
44. Godambe SA, Mack JW, Chung DS, Lindeman R, Lillehei CW, Colin AA. Iatrogenic pleuropulmonary charcoal instillation in a teenager. Pediatr Pulmonol. 2003;35:490–3.
45. Soong WJ, Jeng MJ, Lee YS, Tsao PC, Yang CF, Soong YH. Pediatric obstructive fibrinous tracheal pseudomembrane-characteristics and management with flexible bronchoscopy. Int J Pediatr Otorhinolaryngol. 2011;75:1005–9.
46. Colin AA, Tsiligiannis T, Nose V, Waltz DA. Membranous obliterative bronchitis: a proposed unifying model. Pediatr Pulmonol. 2006;41:126–32.
47. Quizon A, Minic P, Pohunek P, Tal A, Colin AA. Obliterative lower airway lesions in childhood: Bronchoscopic diagnosis and clinical spectrum. Pediatr Pulmonol. 2014;49(3):E27–34 doi:10.1002/ppul.22775.
48. McLaren CA, Elliott MJ, Roebuck DJ. Tracheobronchial intervention in children. Eur J Radiol. 2005;53:22–34.
49. Meng C, Yu HF, Ni CY, et al. Balloon dilatation bronchoplasty in management of bronchial stenosis in children with mycoplasma pneumonia. Zhonghua Er Ke Za Zhi. 2010;48:301–4.
50. Hebra A, Powell DD, Smith CD, Othersen Jr HB. Balloon tracheoplasty in children: results of a 15-year experience. J Pediatr Surg. 1991;26:957–61.
51. Shitrit D, Kuchuk M, Zismanov V, Rahman NA, Amital A, Kramer MR. Bronchoscopic balloon dilatation of tracheobronchial stenosis: long-term follow-up. Eur J Cardiothorac Surg. 2010;38:198–202.
52. Lund ME, Force S. Airway stenting for patients with benign airway disease and the food and drug administration advisory: a call for restraint. Chest. 2007;132:1107–8.
53. Fayon M, Donato L, de Blic J, et al. French experience of silicone tracheobronchial stenting in children. Pediatr Pulmonol. 2005;39:21–7.

54. Loeff DS, Filler RM, Gorenstein A, et al. A new intratracheal stent for tracheobronchial reconstruction: experimental and clinical studies. J Pediatr Surg. 1988;23:1173–7.
55. Vondrys D, Elliott MJ, McLaren CA, Noctor C, Roebuck DJ. First experience with biodegradable airway stents in children. Ann Thorac Surg. 2011;92:1870–4.
56. Bolliger CT, Mathur PN, Beamis JF, et al. ERS/ATS statement on interventional pulmonology. European Respiratory Society/American Thoracic Society. Eur Respir J. 2002;19:356–73.
57. Shinhar SY, Zablocki H, Madgy DN. Airway management in mucopolysaccharide storage disorders. Arch Otolaryngol Head Neck Surg. 2004;130:233–7.
58. Nicolai T. Airway stents in children. Pediatr Pulmonol. 2008;43:330–44.
59. Calkoen EE, Gabra HO, Roebuck DJ, Kiely E, Elliott MJ. Aortopexy as treatment for tracheobronchomalacia in children: an 18-year single-center experience. Pediatr Crit Care Med. 2011;12:545–51.
60. Kothari SS, Roy A, Sharma S, Bhan A. An infant with "dying spells". Indian Heart J. 2003;55:78–80.
61. Friedman E, Kennedy A, Neitzschman HR. Innominate artery compression of the trachea: an unusual cause of apnea in a 12-year-old boy. South Med J. 2003;96:1161–4.
62. Filler RM, Forte V, Chait P. Tracheobronchial stenting for the treatment of airway obstruction. J Pediatr Surg. 1998;33:304–11.
63. Stephens Jr KE, Wood DE. Bronchoscopic management of central airway obstruction. J Thorac Cardiovasc Surg. 2000;119:289–96.
64. Anton-Pacheco JL, Cabezali D, Tejedor R, et al. The role of airway stenting in pediatric tracheobronchial obstruction. Eur J Cardiothorac Surg. 2008;33:1069–75.
65. Wells WJ, Hussain NS, Wood JC. Stenting of the mainstem bronchus in children: a word of caution. Ann Thorac Surg. 2004;77:1420–2.
66. Geller KA, Wells WJ, Koempel JA, St John MA. Use of the Palmaz stent in the treatment of severe tracheomalacia. Ann Otol Rhinol Laryngol. 2004;113:641–7.
67. Peng YY, Soong WJ, Lee YS, Tsao PC, Yang CF, Jeng MJ. Flexible bronchoscopy as a valuable diagnostic and therapeutic tool in pediatric intensive care patients: a report on 5 years of experience. Pediatr Pulmonol. 2011;46:1031–7.
68. Chen N, Zhang J, Xu M, Wang YL, Pei YH. Inhibitory effect of mitomycin C on proliferation of primary cultured fibroblasts from human airway granulation tissues. Respiration. 2013;85:500–4.
69. Rojas-Solano J, Becker HD. Bronchoscopic application of mitomycin-C as adjuvant treatment for benign airway stenosis. J Bronchol Interv Pulmonol. 2011;18:53–5.
70. Meier JD, Sulman CG, Almond PS, Holinger LD. Endoscopic management of recurrent congenital tracheoesophageal fistula: a review of techniques and results. Int J Pediatr Otorhinolaryngol. 2007;71:691–7.
71. Richter GT, Ryckman F, Brown RL, Rutter MJ. Endoscopic management of recurrent tracheoesophageal fistula. J Pediatr Surg. 2008;43:238–45.
72. Goussard P, Gie RP, Kling S, et al. Fibrin glue closure of persistent bronchopleural fistula following pneumonectomy for post-tuberculosis bronchiectasis. Pediatr Pulmonol. 2008;43:721–5.
73. Hoffer FA, Bloom DA, Colin AA, Fishman SJ. Lung abscess versus necrotizing pneumonia: implications for interventional therapy. Pediatr Radiol. 1999;29:87–91.
74. Sawicki GS, Lu FL, Valim C, Cleveland RH, Colin AA. Necrotising pneumonia is an increasingly detected complication of pneumonia in children. Eur Respir J. 2008;31:1285–91.
75. Ratliff JL, Hill JD, Tucker H, Fallat R. Endobronchial control of bronchopleural fistulae. Chest. 1977;71:98–9.
76. Finch CK, Pittman AL. Use of fibrin glue to treat a persistent pneumothorax with bronchopleural fistula. Am J Health Syst Pharm. 2008;65:322–4.
77. Moody GN, Zeno BR. Localization and treatment of bronchopleural fistula through capnography. J Bronchol Interv Pulmonol. 2010;17:261–3.
78. Wood DE, Cerfolio RJ, Gonzalez X, Springmeyer SC. Bronchoscopic management of prolonged air leak. Clin Chest Med. 2010;31:127–33. Table of Contents.

79. Wiaterek G, Lee H, Malhotra R, Shepherd W. Bronchoscopic blood patch for treatment of persistent alveolar-pleural fistula. J Bronchol Interv Pulmonol. 2013;20:171–4.
80. Ruttenstock E, Saxena AK, Hollwarth ME. Closure of bronchopleural fistula with porcine dermal collagen and fibrin glue in an infant. Ann Thorac Surg. 2012;94:659–60.
81. Heslet L, Nielsen JD, Levi M, Sengelov H, Johansson PI. Successful pulmonary administration of activated recombinant factor VII in diffuse alveolar hemorrhage. Crit Care. 2006; 10:R177.
82. Estella A, Jareno A, Perez-Bello Fontaina L. Intrapulmonary administration of recombinant activated factor VII in diffuse alveolar haemorrhage: a report of two case stories. Cases J. 2008;1:150.
83. Colin AA, Shafieian M, Andreansky M. Bronchoscopic instillation of activated recombinant factor VII to treat diffuse alveolar hemorrhage in a child. Pediatr Pulmonol. 2010;45(4):411.
84. Ali-Dinar T, Colin AA, Andreansky M, Reiter L. Direct pulmonary instillation of recombinant factor VII (rFVIIa) for treatment of diffuse alveolar hemorrhage (DAH) in a 2 year old: the youngest pediatric case reported. Paediatr Respir Rev. 2013;14 Suppl 2:S77.
85. Heslet L, Nielsen JD, Nepper-Christensen S. Local pulmonary administration of factor VIIa (rFVIIa) in diffuse alveolar hemorrhage (DAH) – a review of a new treatment paradigm. Biologics. 2012;6:37–46.
86. Bramson RT, Sherman JM, Blickman JG. Pediatric bronchography performed through the flexible bronchoscope. Eur J Radiol. 1993;16:158–61.
87. Quintero RA, Kontopoulos E, Reiter J, Pedreira WL, Colin AA. Fetal bronchoscopy: its successful use in a case of extralobar pulmonary sequestration. J Matern Fetal Neonatal Med. 2012;25:2354–8.
88. Langston C. New concepts in the pathology of congenital lung malformations. Semin Pediatr Surg. 2003;12:17–37.
89. Riedlinger WF, Vargas SO, Jennings RW, et al. Bronchial atresia is common to extralobar sequestration, intralobar sequestration, congenital cystic adenomatoid malformation, and lobar emphysema. Pediatr Dev Pathol. 2006;9:361–73.
90. Peranteau WH, Merchant AM, Hedrick HL, et al. Prenatal course and postnatal management of peripheral bronchial atresia: association with congenital cystic adenomatoid malformation of the lung. Fetal Diagn Ther. 2008;24:190–6.
91. Reiter J, Colin AA, Kontopoulos EV, Shahzeidi S, Quintero RA. Fetal bronchoscopy for treatment of congenital pulmonary anomalies. Eur Respir J. 2013;42 Suppl 57:1062s.
92. Rada AG. Girl who had surgery to correct bronchial atresia in utero is healthy. BMJ. 2012;344:e2193.

Chapter 4
Nasal Nitric Oxide and Ciliary Videomicroscopy: Tests Used for Diagnosing Primary Ciliary Dyskinesia

Adam J. Shapiro, Mark A. Chilvers, Stephanie D. Davis, and Margaret W. Leigh

Abstract Primary ciliary dyskinesia (PCD) is a rare disease affecting approximately 1/15,000 to 1/30,000 persons. In this disease, respiratory cilia are dysmotile and mucociliary clearance is decreased; thereby, leading to chronic respiratory tract infections. Primary ciliary dyskinesia is difficult to diagnose, and there is no gold standard test that will detect all cases of PCD. Screening with nasal nitric oxide measurement is a rapid, sensitive, and noninvasive method that allows physicians to make proper referrals for further PCD investigations. High speed digital videomicroscopy is a powerful tool which allows for detailed assessment of ciliary beat pattern and can detect novel forms of PCD which may be missed on electron microscopy. With the rapidly expanding knowledge of genetic mutations causing PCD, both nasal nitric oxide and ciliary videomicroscopy testing will require future correlation and validation with genetic mutations in PCD patients.

Keywords Primary ciliary dyskinesia • Nitric oxide • Videomicroscopy • Cilia beat

A.J. Shapiro, M.D. (✉)
Pediatric Respiratory Medicine, Montréal Children's Hospital, McGill University,
2300 Rue Tupper, D-380, Montréal, QC, Canada H3H 1P3
e-mail: adam.shapiro@muhc.mcgill.ca

M.A. Chilvers, M.D.
Division of Pediatric Respiratory Medicine, British Columbia's Children's Hospital,
University of British Columbia, 4480 Oak Street, Vancouver, BC, Canada V6L 1T2
e-mail: MChilvers@cw.bc.ca

S.D. Davis, M.D.
Section of Pediatric Pulmonology, Allergy and Sleep Medicine, Riley Hospital for Children,
Indiana University School of Medicine, 705 Riley Hospital Drive, ROC 4270,
Indianapolis, IN 46202, USA
e-mail: sddavis3@iu.edu

M.W. Leigh, M.D.
Pediatric Pulmonology Division, Department of Pediatrics, UNC Hospitals,
University of North Carolina, 450 MacNider, CB#7217, Chapel Hill, NC 27599-7217, USA
e-mail: Margaret_leigh@med.unc.edu

© Springer Science+Business Media New York 2015

S.D. Davis et al. (eds.), *Diagnostic Tests in Pediatric Pulmonology*,
Respiratory Medicine, DOI 10.1007/978-1-4939-1801-0_4

Introduction

Primary ciliary dyskinesia (PCD) is a rare, autosomal recessive disease affecting approximately 1/15,000 to 1/30,000 persons [1]. In this disease, respiratory cilia are dysmotile and mucociliary clearance is decreased; thereby, leading to chronic respiratory tract infections. Classic PCD symptoms include chronic nasal congestion and sinusitis; recurrent otitis media; daily wet cough; recurrent pneumonia or bronchitis; and neonatal respiratory distress, with each occurring in greater than 75 % of the diseased population [2]. Fifty percent have laterality defects (typically situs inversus totalis, but in some cases, situs ambiguous or heterotaxy have been reported) [3]. Bronchiectasis develops with advancing lung disease and has been reported in some children <5 years of age [4]. The gold standard test for diagnosing PCD has been transmission electron microscopy (EM) of ciliated epithelial cells. This diagnostic tool evaluates pathologic ultrastructural changes in the ciliary outer dynein arms, inner dynein arms, radial spokes, or central apparatus (Fig. 4.1).

Accurately processing and interpreting ciliary samples with EM requires training and expertise [5]. A standardized approach for processing these samples is limited to only a few tertiary care centers. Recent studies have demonstrated that ciliary ultrastructure may be normal in some cases of PCD confirmed by genetic testing [6]. Therefore, more emphasis has been placed on other tests, such as nasal nitric oxide measurement and functional ciliary analysis with videomicroscopy, that were originally used as "screening tests" for PCD and now are gaining momentum as "adjunctive diagnostic tests" for PCD at specialized PCD Research and Clinical Centers. With further standardization, nasal nitric oxide testing and/or functional ciliary analysis could be extended to other clinical centers.

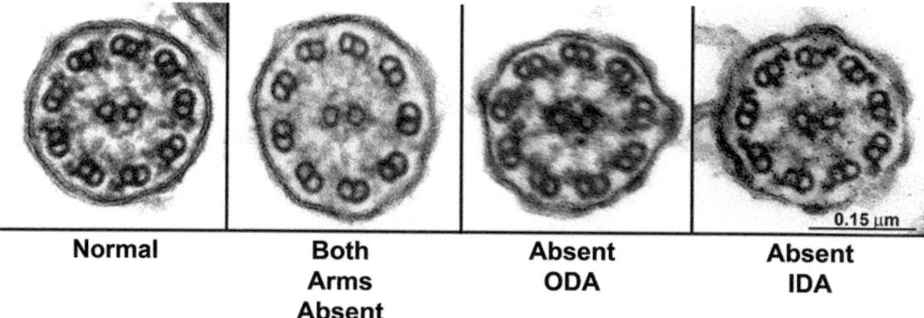

Fig. 4.1 Ciliary electron microscopy showing a normal cross section and various ultrastructural defects causing PCD. *ODA* outer dynein arm, *IDA* inner dynein arm. Reprinted from Leigh MW, Pittman JE, Carson JL, Ferkol TW, Dell SD, Davis SD, et al. Clinical and genetic aspects of primary ciliary dyskinesia/Kartagener syndrome. Genet Med. 2009 Jul;11(7):473–87, with permission of Nature Publishing Group

Nasal Nitric Oxide

Nitric oxide, a colorless, odorless gas, is produced in numerous cells throughout the body, including upper and lower airway epithelial cells, vascular endothelial cells, neuronal cells, smooth muscle cells, fibroblasts, and macrophages. Nitric oxide gas is formed when L-arginine is oxidized to L-citrulline through the enzymatic action of nitric oxide synthase and a cofactor of nicotinamide adenine dinucleotide phosphate (NADPH). Concentrations of nitric oxide within the nasal cavity and paranasal sinuses are typically 10- to 100-fold greater than exhaled nitric oxide concentrations from the lower airways [7]. In PCD, exhaled and nasal nitric oxide levels are frequently quite low in comparison to healthy controls. A variety of other disorders may be associated with increased or decreased nitric oxide levels. Respiratory tract inflammation due to asthma can cause elevations in both exhaled and nasal nitric oxide levels, while inflammation due to idiopathic bronchiectasis can be associated with increased exhaled nitric oxide levels but nasal nitric oxide may be either increased or decreased [8]. In cystic fibrosis, some patients may have low nasal and exhaled nitric oxide values compared to healthy controls [9]. Sinusitis can increase or decrease nasal nitric oxide levels depending on underlying mechanisms [10, 11].

Evidence for Utility as a Test for PCD

In clinical medicine, nasal nitric oxide measurement is largely limited to evaluation of primary ciliary dyskinesia, as patients afflicted with this disease have consistently low levels. In older children (>5 years of age who can cooperate with testing) and adults with classic PCD, nasal nitric oxide levels are typically well below 77 nL/min [12], while healthy controls typically have levels above 250 nL/min [13, 14] (Fig. 4.2).

Despite intensive research evaluating the etiology for low nasal nitric oxide levels in PCD, the exact mechanism leading to this phenomenon remains unknown [15]. Possible explanations include sinus cavity hypoplasia, increased breakdown of nitric oxide by specific bacteria, decreased production of nitric oxide, or entrapment of nitric oxide in obstructed sinus passages. Others have speculated that decreased expression of inducible nitric oxide synthase, the isoenzyme most responsible for nitric oxide production in airway epithelial cells, may be responsible for the low levels in PCD; however, the etiology for diminished nasal nitric oxide remains inconclusive [16, 17]. Nasal nitric oxide may serve as a fuel for ciliary movement, but no definitive evidence exists to fully support this theory [18]. After administering the nitric oxide precursor L-arginine to cystic fibrosis and PCD patients [19, 20], ciliary activity increased; however, nitric oxide did not increase to normal levels, and pulmonary function did not improve [21]. Future treatment strategies for PCD may include techniques to increase airway nitric oxide levels if a beneficial effect can be demonstrated.

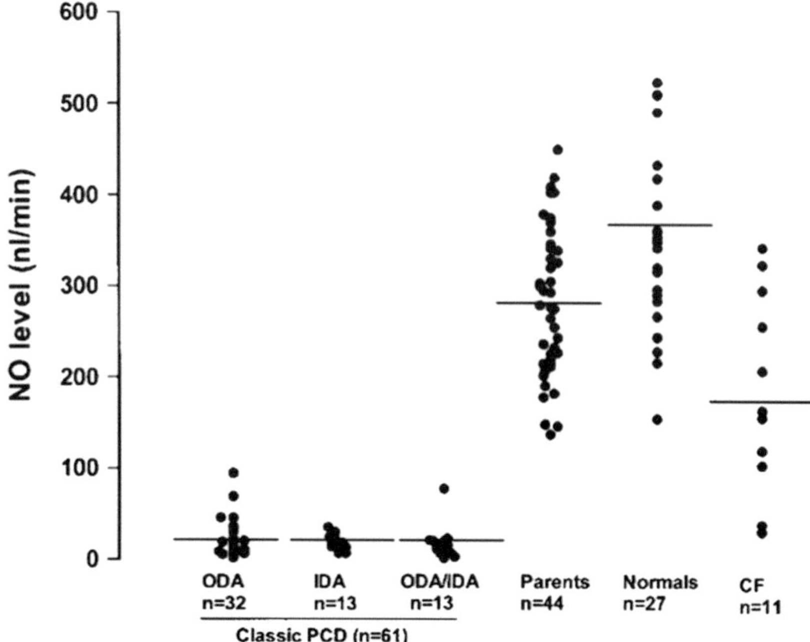

Fig. 4.2 Nasal nitric oxide levels in classic PCD with defects in outer dynein arms (ODA), inner dynein arms (IDA) or both (ODA/IDA) on electron microscopy, Parents of PCD patients, normal healthy controls, and cystic fibrosis (CF). All confirmed PCD cases, but none of healthy controls, fall below 100 nL/min; a few CF patients have values that overlap with PCD. Reprinted with permission of the American Thoracic Society. Copyright © 2013 American Thoracic Society. Noone PG, Leigh MW, Sannuti A, Minnix SL, Carson JL, Hazucha M, et al. Primary ciliary dyskinesia: diagnostic and phenotypic features. Am J Respir Crit Care Med. 2004 Feb 15;169(4):459–67. Official Journal of the American Thoracic Society

Numerous prospective studies have shown extremely low nasal nitric oxide levels in PCD patients; therefore, this test is now an accepted clinical screening method for PCD in Europe [22–24]. A consensus statement by the European Respiratory Society now includes measurement of nasal nitric oxide in children over 5 years old as a recommended screening test for PCD [25]. Nasal nitric oxide testing is approved for clinical use in Canada, Great Britain, and throughout continental Europe (CE MDD mark). Unfortunately, nasal nitric oxide measurement devices are not yet FDA approved for clinical use in the USA, but this tool is actively used in PCD research centers.

Since its clinical debut, measurement of nasal nitric oxide is becoming a more widespread screening test for PCD. Nasal nitric oxide levels below 62.5–126 nL/min have been reported to have high sensitivity for a PCD diagnosis proven with EM [9, 12, 26, 27]. While nasal nitric oxide is a highly sensitive screening test for PCD, the specificity varies depending on the chosen cutoff value. Current diagnostic strategies set a cutoff value for a positive screening test below 60–100 nL/min in children >5 years old who can comply with blowing into a resistor [12, 27, 28]. Studies have examined various other techniques for nasal nitric oxide sampling, including humming, breath holding, and tidal breathing with the mouth open or closed. All of these techniques can discriminate PCD from non-PCD patients, but each technique requires a different cutoff value for a positive PCD screen [29]. Cutoff values for children <5 years old using the tidal breathing technique are age-dependent and are currently being investigated [29–31].

A low nasal nitric oxide level coupled with the classic phenotype of PCD provides strong support for the diagnosis of PCD that may be confirmed by further diagnostic testing (EM of the cilia and/or genetic testing). This approach can be especially helpful in cases where patients have a PCD causing gene defect with normal EM results, such as in DNAH11 mutations [6]. However, physicians must be aware that other diseases can have similarly low nasal nitric oxide levels. In cystic fibrosis, nasal nitric oxide values can consistently fall below PCD cutoff ranges [8, 9, 19]. Therefore, negative sweat chloride testing or genetic testing for cystic fibrosis is essential when using nasal nitric oxide to guide clinical decision making. Nasal nitric oxide levels can also transiently fall below PCD cutoff ranges in acute respiratory illness, acute sinusitis, diffuse panbronchiolitis, HIV, and nasal polyposis [8–11, 32, 33]. Thus, repeat testing during a healthy time period is also critical to assure that the nasal nitric oxide values are consistent. Perhaps of equal importance, a nasal nitric oxide value that is well in the normal range significantly decreases the likelihood of PCD and should guide the clinician to investigate other diagnoses in the differential.

Equipment

The initial purchase cost for a stationary nasal nitric oxide machine using chemiluminescence technology may exceed $50,000 USD; however, after this initial purchase, nasal nitric oxide testing is relatively inexpensive from a disposable material per test standpoint. Only chemiluminescence technology has been prospectively used and proven effective in PCD screening with nasal nitric oxide. Less expensive electrochemical nitric oxide analyzers have been used to measure exhaled nitric oxide, but their agreement with stationary chemiluminescence analyzers in healthy controls has been inconsistent [34–36]. Efforts are underway to adapt these electrochemical analyzers to measure nasal nitric oxide; however, potential utility as a test for PCD has not yet been fully defined [37]. Use of these electrochemical analyzers requires more patient cooperation to perform controlled expiratory breathing maneuvers; therefore, these electrochemical nitric oxide analyzers have limited utility in children.

Technique

On-line nasal nitric oxide measurement is a rapid and noninvasive screening test for PCD. The entire procedure takes approximately 10 min and results are immediately available. To perform this test, a plastic catheter with a surrounding soft nasal sponge or olive is placed just deep enough into one nare to ensure an air-tight seal. Children who are able to comply with directions (typically over 5 years old)

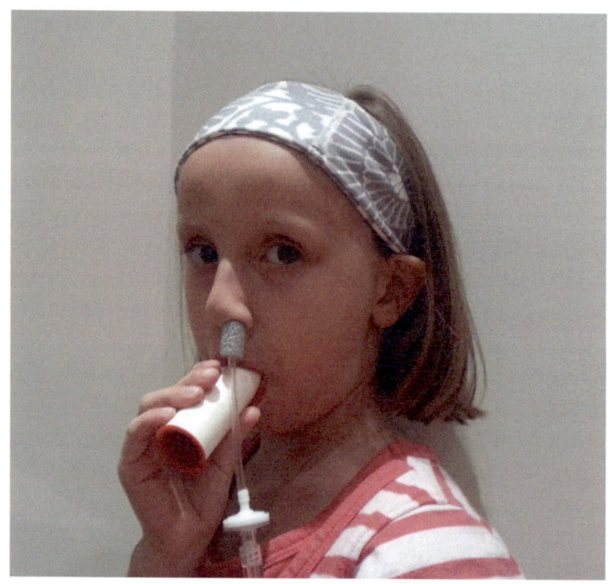

Fig. 4.3 Subject performing a nasal nitric oxide measurement by blowing into a resistor while the probe is securely in the naris. Provided by A. Shapiro, Montreal Children's Hospital

perform maneuvers to close their velum, which prevents dilution of nasal gas (containing much higher nitric oxide) with gas from the lower airways. These maneuvers include blowing into a resistor or a child's party favor which is partially sealed at the end for at least 10 s. Alternative approaches to decrease dilution of nasal gases that can be used in cooperative children and adults include a 30 s breath hold, pursed lip exhalation via the mouth, or voluntarily closing the velum by making a repeated "ka" sound [24] (Fig. 4.3). This technique produces an initial washout phase followed by a nitric oxide concentration plateau phase, which signifies steady state nitric oxide sampling from the nasal cavity (Fig. 4.4).

The same procedure is repeated in the contralateral naris; values are expressed in nanoliters per minute, which are a product of the concentration (in parts per billion) and the flow rate of transnasal airflow in the sampling catheter (in liters/minute) yielding nasal nitric oxide production values (in nL/min). The mean of three separate plateau measurements is calculated for each naris, followed by calculation of the mean for both nares together to yield a final test result. Reporting nasal nitric oxide values as a volume per unit time rather than a simple concentration is preferred [24]. Current chemiluminescence devices have various flow sampling rates that establish a steady state phase of nitric oxide in the sampling tube; nasal nitric oxide concentration is inversely proportional to transnasal flow rates [38]. Very high airflow rates can cause airflow turbulence, which can significantly alter the nitric oxide sampling results [39]. Thus, a standard transnasal airflow sampling rate (0.25–0.5 L/min in children) is currently recommended [24].

Several other testing parameters must be monitored in order to ensure adequate results. An air-tight seal of the nasal olive is essential to prevent dilution with ambient air which would result in a falsely low nitric oxide value. Rhythmic movement

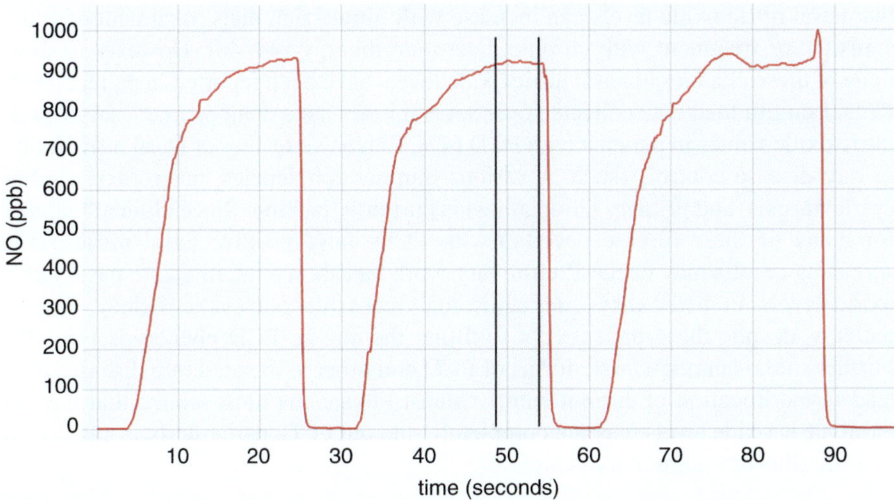

Fig. 4.4 Nitric oxide concentration (parts per billion) versus time (seconds) graph of a nasal nitric oxide measurement obtained while blowing into a resistor. Note the concentration reaches a plateau of at least 3 s, where the measurement is obtained (delineated by the *vertical lines*). Provided by A. Shapiro, Montreal Children's Hospital

of the olive in and out of the naris with each breath may signify air leak. Operators may need to hold the olive steady to avoid this movement. Occlusion of the nasal catheter by secretions may cause an abrupt drop in nitric oxide concentration; therefore, operators should monitor for this problem. In children with nasal congestion (a common feature in PCD), secretions may be aspirated into the catheter necessitating several catheter changes during the course of a test. Given this issue, nasal nitric oxide measurements should ideally be performed when the patient is at his or her respiratory baseline. In addition, ambient nitric oxide values should be monitored to ensure that there is no artificial elevation of nitric oxide that could lead to false negative results. Ambient concentrations of nitric oxide should be recorded prior to each test. This screening test should only be performed when subjects are free of viral illness, as viral respiratory infection may affect nasal nitric oxide levels as noted above [40]. Lastly, there may be a normal circadian change in nasal nitric oxide levels, with significantly lower values in the morning and evening [41]. Nasal steroids, nasal decongestants, topical nasal lidocaine, systemic antibiotics, and cigarette smoke may also variably influence nasal nitric oxide levels [42].

Limitations

Recent reports identifying PCD cases with definite ultrastructural defects, but nasal nitric oxide values higher than the usual cutoff levels, have led investigators to consider the possibility of variant forms of PCD [43]. In addition, research has shown that nasal nitric oxide levels can increase with nitrate rich diets, treatment of acute sinusitis, or treatment with chronic macrolide therapy [44–46]. However to date, none of these changes in nasal nitric oxide levels have been reported in patients with PCD. Longitudinal data collected over several years have demonstrated stable nasal nitric oxide values in patients with PCD [47]. Extensive testing of nasal nitric oxide in rare disease controls (such as various immunodeficiencies, heterotaxy, variant cystic fibrosis, and primary ciliopathies) is currently lacking. Since clinical features for many of these diseases overlap with PCD, false positive nasal nitric oxide screening results may occur. Preliminary work has shown intermediate nasal nitric oxide levels in heterotaxy and autosomal recessive polycystic kidney disease patients, despite these patients not fulfilling the classic PCD phenotype [48, 49]. Further studies in non-classic forms of PCD and other associated rare diseases may lead to modification of current cutoff values. Physicians must realize that normal nasal nitric oxide levels may not completely rule out PCD, particularly in cases with chronic sino-oto-pulmonary symptoms.

Next Steps

Employing nasal nitric oxide as a screening test in children under 5 years of age, who cannot cooperate with expiratory resistance maneuvers, will allow for earlier diagnosis and treatment of PCD at a younger age. Earlier treatment may improve long term respiratory outcomes [50]. Tidal breathing measurement techniques are feasible and sensitive for PCD screening in children under 5 years old, but normal nasal nitric oxide values spanning the entire age range of this group are still being determined [29, 51, 52]. Tidal breathing procedural guidelines are also needed to successfully expand nasal nitric oxide testing to this younger population (Fig. 4.5). Children less than 5 years of age have varying normal levels of nasal nitric oxide, with age-dependant production possibly following the degree of paranasal sinus development [53, 54]. Healthy infants have a much lower nasal nitric oxide level than healthy toddlers and preschoolers, but nasal nitric oxide values become age-independent after approximately 5 years of age. Normal values for nasal nitric oxide in healthy infants under 1 year of age often fall within PCD cutoff ranges, which may preclude nasal nitric oxide as an effective screening test in this age group [53].

For children older than 5 years of age, standardized procedures for analyzer calibration and quality control are critical. Standardization of acceptable test maneuvers and maximal allowable ambient nitric oxide concentration are also needed for broad implementation of nasal nitric oxide screening in children. Well-defined exclusion criteria for clinical testing, such as recent epistaxis or acute viral infection, should also be established. Lastly, Food and Drug Administration approval of chemiluminescence nasal nitric oxide analyzers for clinical use in the USA is a major obstacle preventing widespread use of this test in PCD.

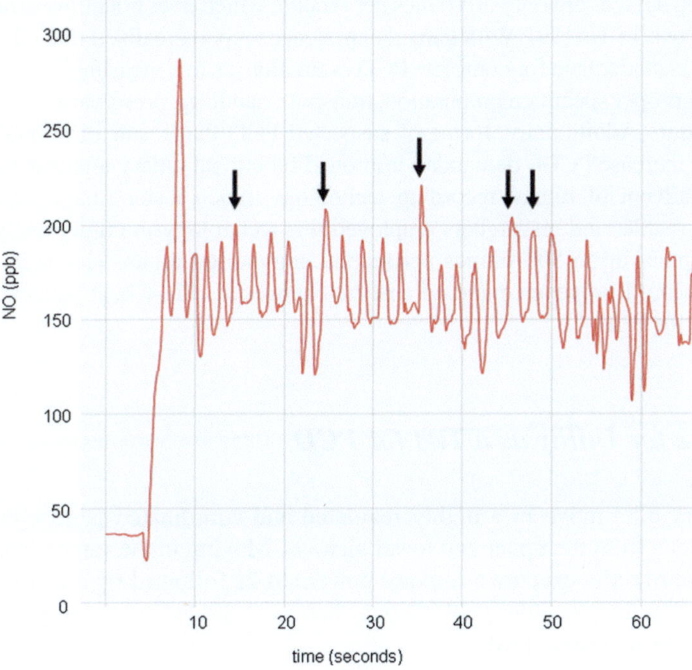

Fig. 4.5 Nitric oxide concentration (parts per billion) versus time (seconds) graph of a nasal nitric oxide measurement obtained during tidal breathing in a child <5 years old. Note the repetitive peaks (*arrows*), all approximately of the same value, of which 5 will be used to calculate the mean value for one naris. Provided by A. Shapiro, Montreal Children's Hospital

Ciliary Videomicroscopy

Functional analysis of ciliary movement with videomicroscopy has become an integral part of PCD diagnosis in several specialized centers. Although functional analysis has been in practice for many years, older diagnostic techniques relied mainly upon calculation of ciliary beat frequency (CBF) [55]. Many clinical centers continue to use subjective light microscopy examination and/or CBF calculation as a screening test for PCD [56]. This methodology can be an arduous process when done manually, thus digital image capture software with automated whole-field analysis is often purchased to calculate CBF [57]. Photomultiplier and photodiode devices, which analyze changes in light intensity passing through beating cilia, also help to automate this meticulous process, but may underestimate CBF [58]. In addition, these automated programs only provide a CBF value and do not analyze ciliary beat pattern.

Clinicians performed initial videomicroscopy beat pattern studies with analog video recorders, which provided vast amounts of recording data and often required days or even weeks of painstaking visual interpretation per study. Maximum recording rates with analog devices are only 30 frames per second, which does not allow measurement of CBF above 15 Hz [59]. With gained experience, experts realized that CBF calculation alone is inadequate for complete PCD evaluation, as this measure is subject to bias through improper specimen preparation, transport, handling, preservation and intercurrent infection. Additionally, forms of suspected PCD that result in normal EM and normal or increased CBF demanded improved functional ciliary analysis techniques. With the advent of digital recording technology, much faster image capture rates became possible, and researchers employed this technology in ciliary analysis. Now able to capture up to 500 frames per second, high speed digital videomicroscopy is used in several European centers to analyze changes in ciliary beat pattern as a diagnostic test for PCD.

Evidence for Utility as a Test for PCD

Respiratory cilia move in a highly regulated and coordinated pattern in order to sweep mucus from the upper and lower airways. Moving in the same plane forward and backward, cilia execute a forward power stroke followed by a recovery stroke (Fig. 4.6). Contrary to older publications, there is no sideways recovery stroke causing a metachronal wave [58].

Experts now appreciate that some ciliary movement is present in most forms of PCD, but that movement is dyskinetic (Fig. 4.7). Cilia from patients with "classic" defects in outer dynein arms (+/− accompanying inner dynein arm defects) are largely immotile, and if movement is present, it is restricted to a slow, short, stiff flickering motion with a CBF <1 Hz. Inner dynein arm defects (+/− radial spoke defects) have a very abnormal stiff forward power stroke with a markedly reduced amplitude, where cilia fail to bend along the length of the axoneme. Approximately 10–30 % of cilia are fully immotile with inner dynein arm or radial spoke defects, and the remainder can actually have a CBF at the lower end of normal. Central apparatus defects (transposition defect) cause circular ciliary motion when viewed from above, but can appear normal when viewed from the side and move with a normal CBF [60]. Lastly, PCD causing genetic defects in DNAH11 result in reduced bending capacity of cilia, with reduced amplitudes and recovery strokes, despite a greater than normal ciliary beat frequency and normal ciliary ultrastructure on electron microscopy [61].

High speed videomicroscopy is clearly superior for PCD diagnosis over CBF calculation alone or subjective light microscopy analysis. When making a PCD diagnosis, direct comparison of CBF alone against digital high speed videomicroscopy with beat pattern analysis confirms that using CBF alone will give a false negative result in approximately 15 % of samples [62]. The benefits of high speed videomicroscopy with beat pattern analysis include the ability to capture extremely fast frame rates, which can then be slowed down at a later time for detailed review of ciliary waveforms. Clinicians can actually examine frame-by-frame ciliary motion to detect subtle alterations in ciliary beat pattern. For instance, cilia with inner

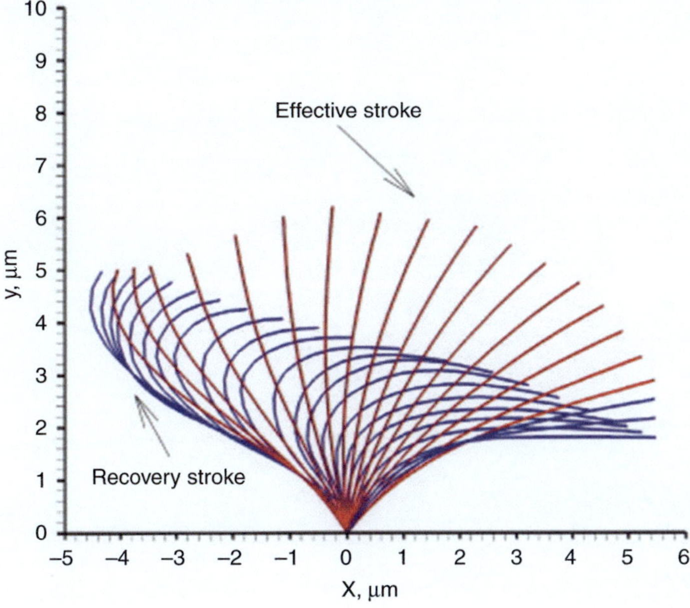

Fig. 4.6 Normal ciliary waveform pattern seen in side profile, demonstrating forward power stroke and recovery stroke. Reprinted from Jayathilake PG, Zhijun T, Le DV, Lee HP, Khoo BC, Three-dimensional numerical simulations of human pulmonary cilia in the periciliary liquid layer by the immersed boundary method, Computers & Fluids, Volume 67, 30 August 2012, Pages 130–137, with permission of Elsevier

dynein arm defects, which can be difficult to diagnose even on EM ciliary studies, have abnormal and stiff forward power strokes with reduced beat amplitudes on videomicroscopy [60]. Furthermore, digital videomicroscopy can detect very subtle changes in ciliary waveforms even when EM is completely normal. This technology was essential in discovering the abnormal ciliary beat patterns associated with DNAH11 gene mutations mentioned above [61]. As newer candidate PCD genes are validated, there will likely be more PCD cases with normal EM and normal CBF; thereby, requiring digital videomicroscopy for complete phenotyping.

Equipment

The initial equipment required to perform ciliary videomicroscopy analysis includes a standard light microscope with 100× magnification capability, a heat source to maintain ciliated epithelial cells at body temperature, an anti-vibration stand, and a high speed digital video camera. Additionally, video playback and digital storage devices are necessary. Total start-up costs vary from $30,000 to $50,000 USD for the above listed hardware (Fig. 4.8).

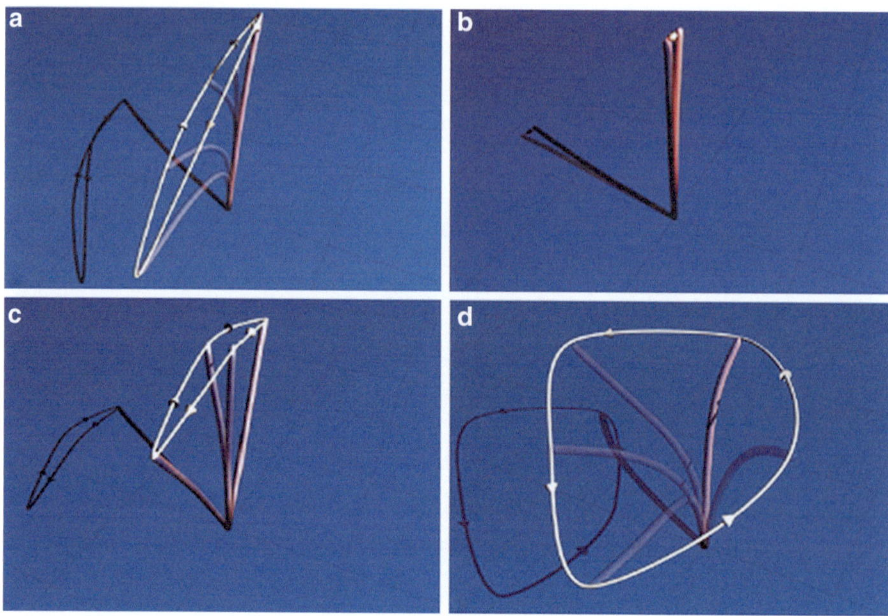

Fig. 4.7 Various ciliary beat patterns as seen on high speed videomicroscopy. (**a**) Normal ciliary beat pattern; (**b**) ciliary beat pattern with outer dynein arm defect or outer plus inner dynein arm defects; (**c**) ciliary beat pattern with inner dynein arm or radial spoke defect; (**d**) ciliary beat pattern with transposition defect affecting the central apparatus. Reprinted from Chilvers MA, Rutman A, O'Callaghan C. Ciliary beat pattern is associated with specific ultrastructural defects in primary ciliary dyskinesia. J Allergy Clin Immunol. 2003 Sep;112(3):518–24, with permission of Elsevier

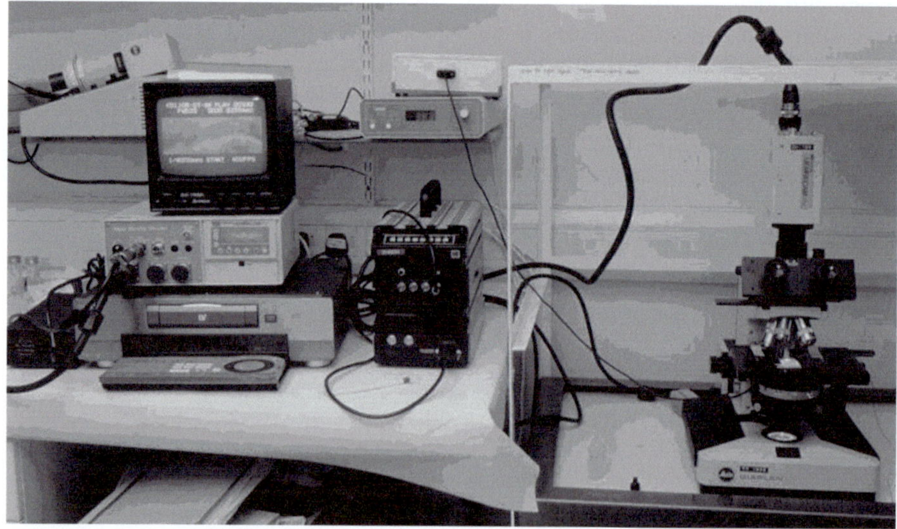

Fig. 4.8 High speed ciliary videomicroscopy equipment setup. Courtesy of M. Chilvers, University of British Columbia

Technique

To perform a high speed digital videomicroscopic analysis, an appropriate ciliary sample is procured with a biopsy brush from the posterior two-thirds of the inferior nasal turbinate or from the lower airways during bronchoscopy. The sample is immediately placed in a transport fluid (such as Medium 199, containing various antibiotics, salts, and amino acids). Strips of ciliated epithelium are suspended in a chamber created by the separation of a cover slip and glass slide by two adjacent cover slips. Specimens are heated to body temperature (37 °C), and examined with a standard light microscope at 100× magnification. Beating cilia are then viewed in three planes: from the side profile, beating toward the observer, and from above. For interpretation, only samples of epithelium longer than 50 µm are considered. Beating ciliary edges are recorded at a rate of 400 frames per second with a digital high speed video camera attached to the microscope. CBF can be determined with digital videomicroscopy by counting the number of frames required to complete ten beat cycles, and dividing the frame rate by this number multiplied by a factor of 10 [58].

If the ciliary brush sample is obtained in an improper manner, mishandled during transport, or poorly preserved before filming, ciliary edges may be damaged (with protrusion of epithelial cells). Due to this damage, it is impossible to know if the resulting dyskinetic movement and slow CBF is to due to underlying PCD or due to the disrupted ciliary edges. Therefore, another biopsy sample should be obtained, as beat pattern analysis and CBF are not reliable [63]. Similarly, in the presence of a viral respiratory infection, which can occur without overt clinical symptoms, ciliary surfaces can be disrupted, resulting in secondary ciliary dyskinesia upon beat pattern analysis [64]. Therefore, another biopsy should be obtained after full recovery from the viral infection. The temperature at which beat pattern analysis is performed can also affect videomicroscopy findings and interpretations. Colder temperatures can completely halt ciliary activity, but beating should resume once warmed to at least 10 °C. When performing videomicroscopy and interpretation at body temperature (37 °C), the rapid ciliary beat frequency can make interpretation of the video difficult, even with frame-by-frame slow motion review. However, by cooling cilia to 2 °C, CBF is greatly decreased, but ciliary beat pattern is unaffected. This may allow interpretation of cilia beat pattern under a light microscope without the need for digital high speed videomicroscopy [65]. Yet, this method has only been used in healthy controls, has never been used prospectively for PCD diagnosis, and other publications have indeed demonstrated abnormal ciliary beat pattern as cilia are cooled [66].

After preparing an adequate sample and obtaining video recordings, proper interpretation of ciliary waveforms is essential to avoid an incorrect diagnosis. Qualitative analysis is often a first line technique, where grossly abnormal ciliary beat patterns (immotile or highly dyskinetic) are easily identified. However, the subjective nature of this analysis makes definitive diagnosis difficult when only subtle changes are noted in the beat pattern [67]. Thus, several scoring systems have been developed to allow for quantitative analysis of videomicroscopy images: (1) A cilia immotility index is calculated by dividing the number of immotile cilia edge readings by the total number of readings per sample; (2) A ciliary dyskinesia score is calculated by subjectively grading the amount of dyskinetic cilia per cell edge on a scale from 0 to 3, with 0 for normal movement, and 3 for dyskinesia of all cilia. (3) The absolute percentage of edges demonstrating dyskinetic cilia. A ciliary dyskinesia score above 2 or having at least 90 % dyskinetic edges have sensitivities of 93 % and 97 % respectively for a diagnosis of PCD confirmed on EM [62]. Recently, a more detailed 12-point quantitative scoring system for high speed videomicroscopy was proposed, examining CBF, beat cycle duration, pauses between beat cycles, angle of ciliary beat, cilia length, distance traveled by cilia tip per second, and area of sweep per second. Of all these measured parameters, the weighted distance traveled by cilia tip per second showed the best sensitivity and specificity (96 and 95 %) when compared against the combined gold standard of EM with nasal nitric oxide measurement [67]. This combination of 12 parameters can be assessed in a clinical setting in approximately 1 h, but calculations require a great deal of expertise in functional ciliary analysis.

Limitations

Limitations in using digital high speed videomicroscopy for PCD analysis include expensive start-up costs for equipment and complicated procedural and interpretation techniques. These techniques require extensive training and experience. Currently, there is no commercially available computer software to assist in ciliary beat pattern analysis. The lack of an automated program for beat pattern analysis limits widespread use of this test to only a few clinical centers with a great deal of expertise in beat pattern analysis.

Future Direction

Computer programs capable of performing automated ciliary beat pattern analysis will greatly expand the clinical role of high speed ciliary videomicroscopy in the future. Designing these programs will require intensive software engineering, but would make widespread clinical use of this test much more feasible. Standard operating procedures and sample preparation protocols are also needed to expand this test for everyday clinical use. Lastly, acceptability standards for ciliary samples need to be established to ensure videomicroscopy results are accurate.

Aside from primary ciliary defects, ciliary beat pattern can be abnormal due to secondary cilia dyskinesia, which occurs with infection, inflammation, or toxic exposure [68]. All of these insults can also alter ciliary ultrastructure on EM. Growth of ciliated cells in culture with repeat analysis has shown that both ultrastructural and beat pattern abnormalities from secondary ciliary dyskinesia may resolve [69–71]; however, the potential for culture artifact cannot be excluded. Thus, the diagnosis of PCD by EM or beat pattern analysis after ciliogenesis in culture may improve specificity and sensitivity; however, the time, expense, and laboratory expertise required for this process have precluded its widespread use in clinical medicine to date [72].

Conclusion

Primary ciliary dyskinesia is difficult to diagnose, and there is no gold standard test that will detect all cases of PCD. Outside of centers with extensive experience in PCD diagnosis, screening with nasal nitric oxide measurement is a rapid, sensitive, and noninvasive method that allows physicians to make proper referrals for further PCD investigations. High speed digital videomicroscopy is a powerful tool which allows for a detailed assessment of ciliary beat pattern and can detect novel forms of PCD which may be missed on electron microscopy. Inexperience with laboratory techniques and video interpretation make this a difficult test to employ outside of highly specialized centers. Lastly, with the rapidly expanding knowledge of genetic mutations causing PCD, both nasal nitric oxide and ciliary videomicroscopy testing will require future correlation and validation with genetic mutations in PCD patients.

References

1. Katsuhara K, Kawamoto S, Wakabayashi T, et al. Situs inversus totalis and Kartagener's syndrome in a Japanese population. Chest. 1972;61:56–61.
2. Knowles MR, Daniels LA, Davis SD, Zariwala MA, Leigh MW. Primary ciliary dyskinesia. Recent advances in diagnostics, genetics, and characterization of clinical disease. Am J Respir Crit Care Med. 2013;188(8):913–22. doi:10.1164/rccm.201301-0059CI.
3. Shapiro AJ, Davis SD, Ferkol T, Dell SD, Rosenfeld M, Olivier KN, et al. Laterality defects other than situs inversus totalis in primary ciliary dyskinesia: insights into situs ambiguus and heterotaxy. Chest. 2014. doi: 10.1378/chest.13-1704. [Epub ahead of print].
4. Brown DE, Pittman JE, Leigh MW, Fordham L, Davis SD. Early lung disease in young children with primary ciliary dyskinesia. Pediatr Pulmonol. 2008;43(5):514–6.
5. Olin JT, Burns K, Carson JL, Metjian H, Atkinson JJ, Davis SD, et al. Diagnostic yield of nasal scrape biopsies in primary ciliary dyskinesia: a multicenter experience. Pediatr Pulmonol. 2011;46:483–8.
6. Knowles MR, Leigh MW, Carson JL, Davis SD, Dell SD, Ferkol TW, et al. Mutations of DNAH11 in patients with primary ciliary dyskinesia with normal ciliary ultrastructure. Thorax. 2012;67(5):433–41.
7. Lundberg JO. Nitric oxide and the paranasal sinuses. Anat Rec. 2008;291:1479–84.
8. Narang I, Ersu R, Wilson NM, Bush A. Nitric oxide in chronic airway inflammation in children: diagnostic use and pathophysiological significance. Thorax. 2002;57(7):586–9.
9. Balfour-Lynn IM, Laverty A, Dinwiddie R. Reduced upper airway nitric oxide in cystic fibrosis. Arch Dis Child. 1996;75(4):319–22.
10. Arnal JF, Flores P, Rami J, et al. Nasal nitric oxide concentration in paranasal sinus inflammatory diseases. Eur Respir J. 1999;13(2):307–12.
11. Bommarito L, Guida G, Heffler E, et al. Nasal nitric oxide concentration in suspected chronic rhinosinusitis. Ann Allergy Asthma Immunol. 2008;101(4):358–62.

12. Leigh MW, Hazucha MJ, Chawla KK, Baker BR, Shapiro AJ, Brown DE, et al. Standardizing nasal nitric oxide measurement as a test for primary ciliary dyskinesia. Ann Am Thorac Soc. 2013;10(6):574–81. doi:10.1513/AnnalsATS.201305-110OC.
13. Lundberg JON, Weitzberg E, Nordvall SL, et al. Primary nasal origin of exhaled nitric oxide and absence in Kartegener's syndrome. Eur Respir J. 1994;7:1501–4.
14. Karadag B, James AJ, Gültekin E, et al. Nasal and lower airway level of nitric oxide in children with primary ciliary dyskinesia. Eur Respir J. 1999;13(6):1402–5.
15. Walker WT, Jackson CL, Lackie PM, et al. Nitric oxide in primary ciliary dyskinesia. Eur Respir J. 2012;40:1024–32.
16. Degano B, Valmary S, Serrano E, et al. Expression of nitric oxide synthases in primary ciliary dyskinesia. Hum Pathol. 2011;42:1855–61.
17. Pifferi M, Bush A, Maggi F, et al. Nasal nitric oxide and nitric oxide synthase expression in primary ciliary dyskinesia. Eur Respir J. 2011;37:572–7.
18. Jain B, Rubinstein I, Robbins RA, Leise KL, Sisson JH. Modulation of airway epithelial cell ciliary beat frequency by nitric oxide. Biochem Biophys Res Commun. 1993;191:83–8.
19. Grasemann H, Kurtz F, Ratjen F. Inhaled L-arginine improves exhaled nitric oxide and pulmonary function in patients with cystic fibrosis. Am J Respir Crit Care Med. 2006;174(2):208–12.
20. Loukides S, Kharitonov S, Wodehouse T, Cole PJ, Barnes PJ. Effect of arginine on mucociliary function in primary ciliary dyskinesia. Lancet. 1998;352(9125):371–2.
21. Grasemann H, Gärtig SS, Wiesemann HG, Teschler H, Konietzko N, Ratjen F. Effect of L-arginine infusion on airway NO in cystic fibrosis and primary ciliary dyskinesia syndrome. Eur Respir J. 1999;13(1):114–8.
22. Wodehouse T, Kharitonov SA, Mackay IS, et al. Nasal nitric oxide measurements for the screening of primary ciliary dyskinesia. Eur Respir J. 2003;21(1):43–7.
23. Piacentini GL, Bodini A, Peroni D, et al. Nasal nitric oxide for early diagnosis of primary ciliary dyskinesia: practical issues in children. Respir Med. 2008;102(4):541–7.
24. American Thoracic Society; European Respiratory Society. ATS/ERS recommendations for standardized procedures for the online and offline measurement of exhaled lower respiratory nitric oxide and nasal nitric oxide, 2005. Am J Respir Crit Care Med. 2005;171(8):912–30.
25. Barbato A, Frischer T, Kuehni CE, et al. Primary ciliary dyskinesia: a consensus statement on diagnostic and treatment approaches in children. Eur Respir J. 2009;34:1264–76.
26. Corbelli R, Bringolf-Isler B, Amacher A, et al. Nasal nitric oxide measurements to screen children for primary ciliary dyskinesia. Chest. 2004;126(4):1054–9.
27. Noone PG, Leigh MW, Sannuti A, Minnix SL, Carson JL, Hazucha M, et al. Primary ciliary dyskinesia: diagnostic and phenotypic features. Am J Respir Crit Care Med. 2004;169(4):459–67.
28. Marthin JK, Petersen N, Skovgaard LT, Nielsen KG. Lung function in patients with primary ciliary dyskinesia: a cross-sectional and 3-decade longitudinal study. Am J Respir Crit Care Med. 2010;181(11):1262–8.
29. Mateos-Corral D, Coombs R, Grasemann H, Ratjen F, Dell SD. Diagnostic value of nasal nitric oxide measured with non-velum closure techniques for children with primary ciliary dyskinesia. J Pediatr. 2011;159(3):420–4.
30. Leigh MW, Chawla KK, Baker BR, Hazucha MJ, Brown DE, LaVange LM, et al. Standardization of nasal nitric oxide as screening test for primary ciliary dyskinesia. Am J Respir Crit Care Med. 2012;185:A3898.
31. Pittman JE, Rosenfeld M, LaFave C, Ferkol T, Milla C, Sagel S, et al. Characteristics of primary ciliary dyskinesia in children under 5 years of age. Am J Respir Crit Care Med. 2011;183:A1213.
32. Palm J, Lidman C, Graf P, Alving K, Lundberg J. Nasal nitric oxide is reduced in patients with HIV. Acta Otolaryngol. 2000;120(3):420–3.
33. Nakano H, Ide H, Imada M, Osanai S, Takahashi T, Kikuchi K, et al. Reduced nasal nitric oxide in diffuse panbronchiolitis. Am J Respir Crit Care Med. 2000;162(6):2218–20.
34. Kim SH, Moon JY, Kwak HJ, et al. Comparison of two exhaled nitric oxide analyzers: the NIOX MINO hand-held electrochemical analyzer and the NOA280i stationary chemiluminescence analyzer. Respirology. 2012;17:830–4.

35. Boot JD, de Ridder L, de Kam ML, et al. Comparison of exhaled nitric oxide measurements between NIOX MINO electrochemical and Ecomedics chemiluminescence analyzer. Respir Med. 2008;102(11):1667–71.
36. Korn S, Telke I, Kornmann O, et al. Measurement of exhaled nitric oxide: comparison of different analysers. Respirology. 2010;15:1203–8.
37. Montella S, Alving K, Maniscalco M, Sofia M, De Stefano S, Raia V, et al. Measurement of nasal nitric oxide by hand-held and stationary devices. Eur J Clin Invest. 2011;41(10):1063–70. doi:10.1111/j.1365-2362.2011.02501.x. Epub 2011 Mar 17.
38. Imada M, Iwamoto J, Nonaka S, Kobayashi Y, Unno T. Measurement of nitric oxide in human nasal airway. Eur Respir J. 1996;9(3):556–9.
39. Djupesland PG, Chatkin JM, Qian W, Cole P, Zamel N, McClean P, et al. Aerodynamic influences on nasal nitric oxide output measurements. Acta Otolaryngol. 1999;119(4):479–85.
40. Maniscalco M, Lundberg JO. Nasal nitric oxide in European Respiratory Monograph 49: exhaled biomarkers by I Horvath and JC de Jongst. Switzerland: European Respiratory Society; 2010. p. 67–78.
41. Dressel H, Bihler A, Jund F, de la Motte D, Nowak D, Jörres RA, et al. Diurnal variation of nasal nitric oxide levels in healthy subjects. J Investig Allergol Clin Immunol. 2008;18(4):316–7.
42. Jorissen M, Lefevere L, Willems T. Nasal nitric oxide. Allergy. 2001;56:1026–33.
43. Marthin JK, Nielsen KG. Choice of nasal nitric oxide technique as first-line test for primary ciliary dyskinesia. Eur Respir J. 2011;37(3):559–65.
44. Olin AC, Aldenbratt A, Ekman A, Ljungkvist G, Jungersten L, Alving K, et al. Increased nitric oxide in exhaled air after intake of a nitrate-rich meal. Respir Med. 2001;95(2):153–8.
45. Baraldi E, Azzolin NM, Biban P, Zacchello F. Effect of antibiotic therapy on nasal nitric oxide concentration in children with acute sinusitis. Am J Respir Crit Care Med. 1997;155(5):1680–3.
46. Cervin A, Kalm O, Sandkull P, Lindberg S. One-year low-dose erythromycin treatment of persistent chronic sinusitis after sinus surgery: clinical outcome and effects on mucociliary parameters and nasal nitric oxide. Otolaryngol Head Neck Surg. 2002;126(5):481–9.
47. Chawla K, Hazucha M, Dell S, Ferkol T, Sagel S, Rosenfeld M, et al. A multi-center longitudinal study of nasal nitric oxide in children with primary ciliary dyskinesia. Am J Respir Crit Care Med. 2010;181:A6726.
48. Shapiro A, Chawla K, Baker B, Minnix S, Davis S, Knowles M, et al. Nasal nitric oxide and clinical characteristics of patients with heterotaxy: comparison to primary ciliary dyskinesia. Am J Respir Crit Care Med. 2011;183:A1209.
49. Root HB, Gunay-Aygun M, Olivier KN. Screening for respiratory ciliary dysfunction in autosomal recessive polycystic kidney disease. Am J Respir Crit Care Med. 2011;183:A6346.
50. Ellerman A, Bisgaard H. Longitudinal study of lung function in a cohort of primary ciliary dyskinesia. Eur Respir J. 1997;10(10):2376–9.
51. Piacentini GL, Bodini A, Peroni DG, Sandri M, Brunelli M, Pigozzi R, et al. Nasal nitric oxide levels in healthy pre-school children. Pediatr Allergy Immunol. 2010;21(8):1139–45.
52. Gupta R, Gupta N, Turner SW. A methodology for measurements of nasal nitric oxide in children under 5 yr. Pediatr Allergy Immunol. 2008;19(3):233–8.
53. Chawla KK, Shapiro A, Hazucha MJ, Brown DE, Pittman JE, Minnix SL, et al. Nasal nitric oxide during tidal breathing in children under 6 years of age. Am J Respir Crit Care Med. 2009;179:A3673.
54. Pifferi M, Bush A, Caramella D, Di Cicco M, Zangani M, Chinellato I, et al. Agenesis of paranasal sinuses and nasal nitric oxide in primary ciliary dyskinesia. Eur Respir J. 2011;37(3):566–71.
55. Bush A, Cole P, Hariri M, Mackay I, Phillips G, O'Callaghan C, et al. Primary ciliary dyskinesia: diagnosis and standards of care. Eur Respir J. 1998;12(4):982–8.
56. Josephson GD, Patel S, Duckworth L, Goldstein J. High yield technique to diagnose immotile cilia syndrome: a suggested algorithm. Laryngoscope. 2010;120 Suppl 4:S240.
57. Sisson JH, Stoner JA, Ammons BA, Wyatt TA. All-digital image capture and whole-field analysis of ciliary beat frequency. J Microsc. 2003;211(Pt 2):103–11.

58. Chilvers MA, O'Callaghan C. Analysis of ciliary beat pattern and beat frequency using digital high speed imaging: comparison with the photomultiplier and photodiode methods. Thorax. 2000;55:314–7.

59. Sanderson MJ. High-speed digital microscopy. Methods. 2000;21(4):325–34.

60. Chilvers MA, Rutman A, O'Callaghan C. Ciliary beat pattern is associated with specific ultrastructural defects in primary ciliary dyskinesia. J Allergy Clin Immunol. 2003;112(3):518–24.

61. Schwabe GC, Hoffmann K, Loges NT, Birker D, Rossier C, de Santi MM, et al. Primary ciliary dyskinesia associated with normal axoneme ultrastructure is caused by DNAH11 mutations. Hum Mutat. 2008;29(2):289–98.

62. Stannard WA, Chilvers MA, Rutman AR, Williams CD, O'Callaghan C. Diagnostic testing of patients suspected of primary ciliary dyskinesia. Am J Respir Crit Care Med. 2010;181(4): 307–14.

63. Thomas B, Rutman A, O'Callaghan C. Disrupted ciliated epithelium shows slower ciliary beat frequency and increased dyskinesia. Eur Respir J. 2009;34(2):401–4.

64. Chilvers MA, McKean M, Rutman A, Myint BS, Silverman M, O'Callaghan C. The effects of coronavirus on human nasal ciliated respiratory epithelium. Eur Respir J. 2001;18(6):965–70.

65. Smith CM, Hirst RA, Bankart MJ, Jones DW, Easton AJ, Andrew PW, O'Callaghan C. Cooling of cilia allows functional analysis of the beat pattern for diagnostic testing. Chest. 2011;140(1):186–90. Epub 2010 Dec 30.

66. Jackson CL, Goggin PM, Lucas JS. Ciliary beat pattern analysis below 37 °C may increase risk of primary ciliary dyskinesia misdiagnosis. Chest. 2012;142(2):543–4.

67. Papon JF, Bassinet L, Cariou-Patron G, Zerah-Lancner F, Vojtek AM, Blanchon S, et al. Quantitative analysis of ciliary beating in primary ciliary dyskinesia: a pilot study. Orphanet J Rare Dis. 2012;7(1):78.

68. Bertrand B, Collet S, Eloy P, Rombaux P. Secondary ciliary dyskinesia in upper respiratory tract. Acta Otorhinolaryngol Belg. 2000;54(3):309–16.

69. Hirst RA, Rutman A, Williams G, O'Callaghan C. Ciliated air-liquid cultures as an aid to diagnostic testing of primary ciliary dyskinesia. Chest. 2010;138(6):1441–7. doi:10.1378/ chest.10-0175. Epub 2010 Jul 8.

70. Jorissen M, Willems T, Van der Schueren B, Verbeken E. Secondary ciliary dyskinesia is absent after ciliogenesis in culture. Acta Otorhinolaryngol Belg. 2000;54(3):333–42.

71. Jorissen M, Willems T, Van der Schueren B, Verbeken E, De Boeck K. Ultrastructural expression of primary ciliary dyskinesia after ciliogenesis in culture. Acta Otorhinolaryngol Belg. 2000;54(3):343–56.

72. Jorissen M, Willems T, Van der Schueren B. Ciliary function analysis for the diagnosis of primary ciliary dyskinesia: advantages of ciliogenesis in culture. Acta Otolaryngol. 2000;120(2):291–5.

Chapter 5
Functional Evaluation of Cystic Fibrosis Transmembrane Conductance Regulator

George M. Solomon and Steven M. Rowe

Abstract Cystic fibrosis is caused by mutations in the cystic fibrosis transmembrane regulator (CFTR) gene which encodes an epithelial anion channel and regulatory protein. Derangements of CFTR protein function result in thickened, viscous mucus in the airways, GI tract, pancreas, sweat gland, and reproductive tract. The diagnosis and prognosis of CF is facilitated by demonstrating functional decrements of CFTR activity, and is a cornerstone of the diagnostic criteria. This chapter details the conduct and interpretation of the two most widely available diagnostic tests for CFTR functional analysis: sweat chloride testing and nasal potential difference (NPD). Details regarding the methods for conduct of these tests, sources of error, and emerging results supporting their interpretation are discussed.

Keywords Sweat chloride • Nasal potential difference • Sweat rate • CFTR • Diagnosis • Prognosis • Ion transport • ENaC • Chloride • Sodium

Introduction

Cystic fibrosis (CF) is an autosomal recessive genetic disease caused by mutations in the epithelial anion channel, cystic fibrosis transmembrane regulator (CFTR) [1]. CF is the most common genetic disease in Caucasians occurring in 1 in 2,500–3,500 live births, and 1 in 25 Caucasians are carriers for gene mutations [2]. There have been descriptions of abnormally high sweat salinity in children associated with premature death for centuries, but the first comprehensive description of CF as a distinct clinical entity was published in 1938 by Anderson [3]. The onset of an extreme heat wave in the Northeastern United States in the summer of 1948 led di Sant'Agnese to describe high-salt concentrations in the sweat of infants with CF and introduce the concept linking inadequate ion trafficking with the clinical features of the disease [4]. Hence functional decrements in CFTR manifested in the

G.M. Solomon, M.D. • S.M. Rowe, M.D., M.S.P.H. (✉)
Division of Pulmonary Allergy and Critical Care Medicine, Department of Medicine,
University of Alabama at Birmingham, MCLM 706, 1918 University Blvd,
Birmingham, AL 35294-0005, USA
e-mail: msolomon@uab.edu; smrowe@uab.edu

© Springer Science+Business Media New York 2015
S.D. Davis et al. (eds.), *Diagnostic Tests in Pediatric Pulmonology*,
Respiratory Medicine, DOI 10.1007/978-1-4939-1801-0_5

sweat gland were among the first characteristics recognized with the disorder, and remain a cornerstone underlying the diagnosis today.

Before the discovery of the CFTR gene and description of the CFTR protein in 1989 [5–7], early observations based on di Sant'Agnese's work led to postulation of a derangement of a chloride anion channel as central to disease pathogenesis. Observations by Quinton that the sweat gland is impervious to chloride in CF patients [8, 9] as well as various contributions from studies of nasal epithelium and subsequent membrane patch-clamp analysis of epithelial cells from the airways of patients with CF [10–13] provided conclusive evidence of a defect in chloride permeability of plasma membranes in the lung. These findings helped set the stage for the seminal description of the CFTR protein after the gene was sequenced in 1989.

Derangements of CFTR, an anion channel of chloride and bicarbonate, result in epithelial dysfunction, predominantly affecting the lungs, pancreas, gastrointestinal system, and reproductive tract. Disease manifestations include pancreatic insufficiency; newborn bowel obstruction (meconium ileus); recurrent sinopulmonary infections and bronchiectasis; abnormal sweat electrolytes that may produce profound electrolyte derangements; male infertility (bilateral absence of the vas deferens); and biliary obstruction and cirrhosis [1, 14–16]. While the functional derangements are diffuse, sweat testing and nasal potential difference (NPD) remain the primary functional assays used to quantify CFTR activity as a diagnostic aid, and are also supplemented by alternative functional tests, such as intestinal current measurements [17–21] and sweat rate [22, 23], although the latter is primary a research tool at present.

Functional Assays of CFTR Are Important for Confirmation of Diagnosis

The diagnosis of CF is ultimately based on clinical suspicion of the disease. A growing role for early detection is leading to earlier recognition of illness before the clinical characteristics become apparent. The first organized CF newborn screening programs (NBS) were developed in the 1980s and first implemented in Colorado in 1987 and in Australia and Europe in the 1980s [24] after early retrospective trials demonstrated improved mortality and clinical outcomes in the 1970s [25]. The number of programs in the USA and abroad has increased exponentially in the last decade, and all US states have implemented NBS programs largely after the Center for Disease Controls and Cystic Fibrosis Foundation Consensus statement in 2004 recommended that CF NBS should be considered by all states [26] invoking prospective data that screening and subsequent early interventions in CF-diagnosed newborns improved nutritional, gastrointestinal, respiratory, and cognitive functioning [27–30]. Assessment of CFTR function plays a prominent role in the diagnostic evaluation of CF, even prior to the onset of clinical manifestations. Hence appropriate conduct and interpretation of results are imperative to provide an appropriate diagnosis and treatment plan.

The diagnosis of CF is based on a positive NBS or suspicious clinical characteristics in patients from infancy and into adulthood. In 2008, the Cystic Fibrosis Foundation published comprehensive diagnostic guidelines for infants and adults with suspected CF [31]; a similar approach was adopted in the European CF Society's 2006 guidelines (Fig. 5.1). The guidelines were similar and primarily differed only in the timing of CFTR mutation analysis and cutoffs for quantitative sweat chloride testing [32]. In addition, as compared to the European diagnostic guideline, the US guideline deemphasizes NPD because of lack of standardization, although NPD is recommended as an alternative diagnostic modality. Nevertheless, comparison of these approaches on a prospective basis demonstrates good concordance between the methodology and accuracy for both diagnostic algorithms [33].

A common feature in both algorithms is the central role of quantitative sweat chloride testing to confirm the diagnosis in the presence of a positive NBS or compatible clinical characteristics. Functional assays include quantitative sweat chloride as the initial test of choice, and NPD testing as an acceptable alternative in cases of inconclusive sweat chloride values or inadequate genetic analysis. Because of the central role of these CFTR functional assays, it is imperative that the basic methodology, interpretation, and limitations be understood to determine the role of these functional assays in diagnosing CF. Moreover, it is increasingly recognized that CFTR-related disorders represent a spectrum of disease, with pancreatic insufficient CF as the most severe form. It is notable that functional assessments of CFTR reflect this diversity, although the precise relationship between genotype and CFTR functional decrements can vary. CFTR biomarkers demonstrate the ability to distinguish these various phenotypes whereby increasingly severe phenotypes of clinical disease are reflected by more severe reductions in CFTR function by sweat chloride or NPD, although considerable overlap exists likely due to both biologic and environmental causes [34].

Sweat Chloride Testing

Early descriptions of derangements of CF as a salt-losing syndrome in the sweat prompted development of sweat electrolyte analysis in the 1950s [35]. Gibson and Cooke described the pilocarpine iontophoresis method in 1959 paired with a sweat pad collection system to analyze sweat electrolytes [36]. Other refinements in the test have been made since making sweat chloride analysis the most reliable method for confirming the diagnosis of CF in a positive NBS or suspected clinical syndrome [37]. Because changes in sweat chloride have been highly sensitive to use of efficacious CFTR modulators under development [38–40], sweat testing has also been frequently used as a biomarker of CFTR activity in the context of clinical trials, although data continue to emerge regarding its tissue proclivity, particularly in the context of multi-agent therapy.

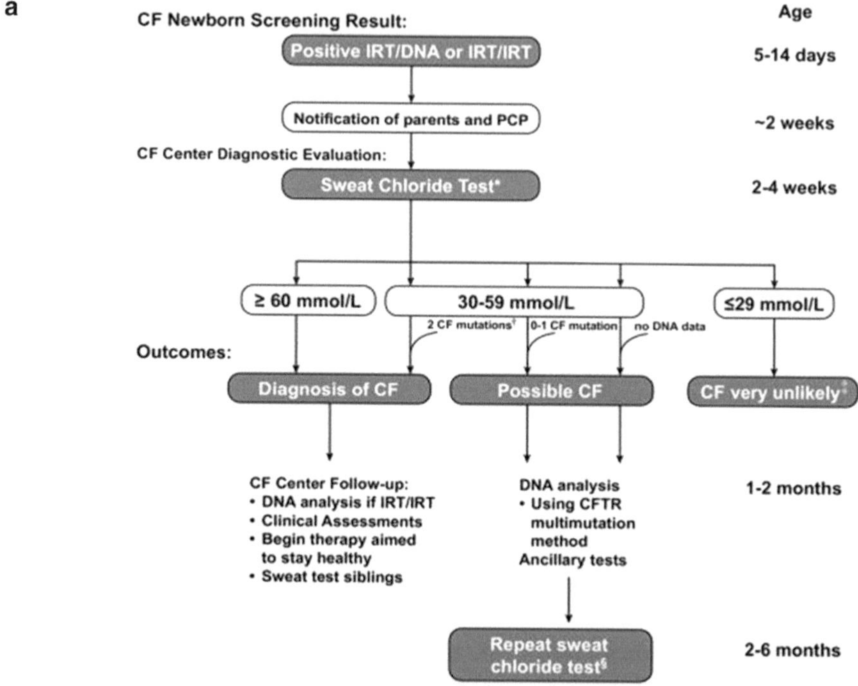

Fig. 5.1 CF diagnostic algorithms. (**a**) North American CF diagnostic algorithm emphasizes clinical suspicion and the importance of newborn screening in the diagnostic process. Reprinted with permission from Farrell, P.M., et al., *Guidelines for diagnosis of cystic fibrosis in newborns through older adults: Cystic Fibrosis Foundation consensus report. J Pediatr,* 2008. **153**(2): p. S4–S14. (**b**). European Cystic Fibrosis Foundation Guidelines Algorithm for the diagnosis of cystic fibrosis emphasizes clinical suspicion of the disease and highlights the central role of sweat chloride testing in the diagnostic process. Reprinted with permission from De Boeck, K., et al., *Cystic fibrosis: terminology and diagnostic algorithms. Thorax,* 2006. **61**(7): p. 627–35

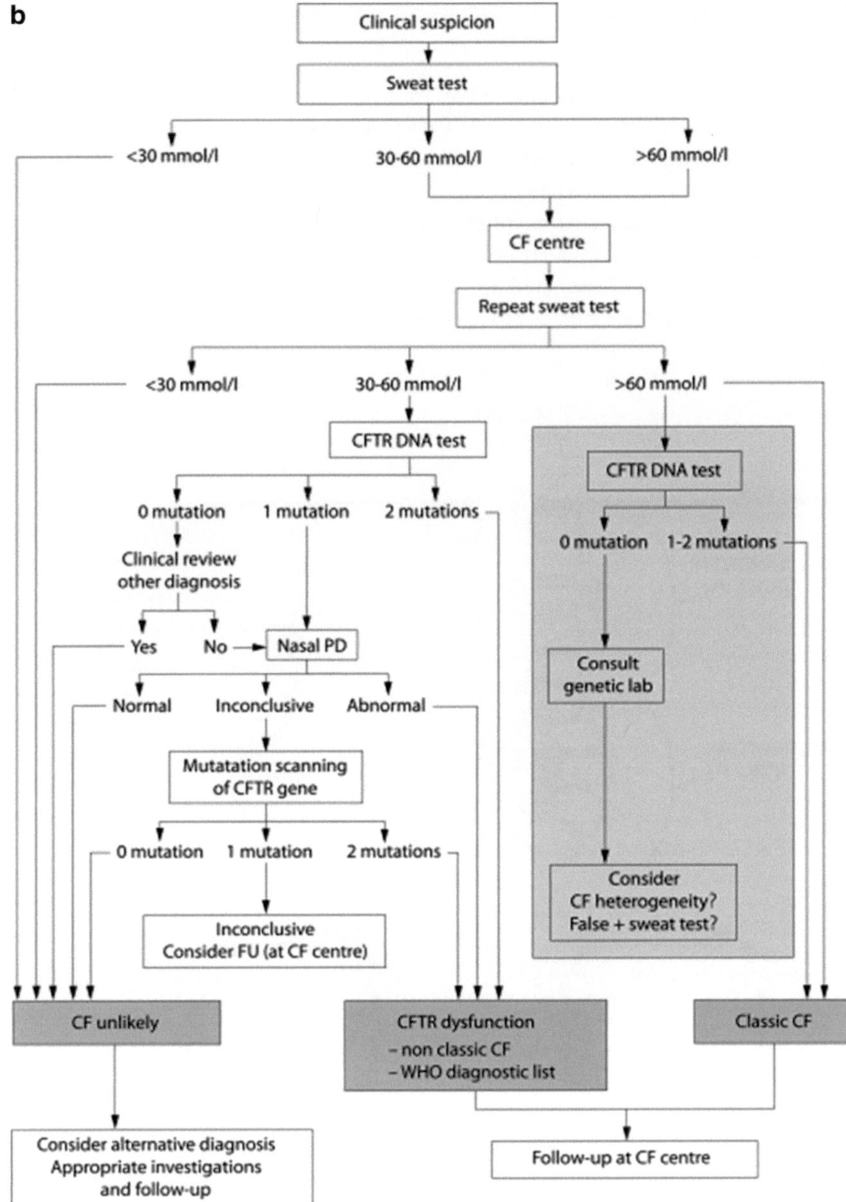

Fig. 5.1 (continued)

Sweat Gland Physiology

The human sweat gland is composed of two regions: the secretory coil and the reabsorptive duct [37]. As isotonic secretions first produced in the secretory coil travel out the gland through the reabsorptive duct, sodium and chloride are selectively reabsorbed in the water-impermeable environment resulting in the elaboration of hypotonic sweat on the skin surface of normal subjects. In CF, the reduced function of CFTR is accompanied by downregulation of the epithelial sodium channel (ENaC), which results in diminished absorptive capacity for both sodium and chloride in the sweat gland (see Fig. 5.2) [1]. Absent or reduced function of CFTR has

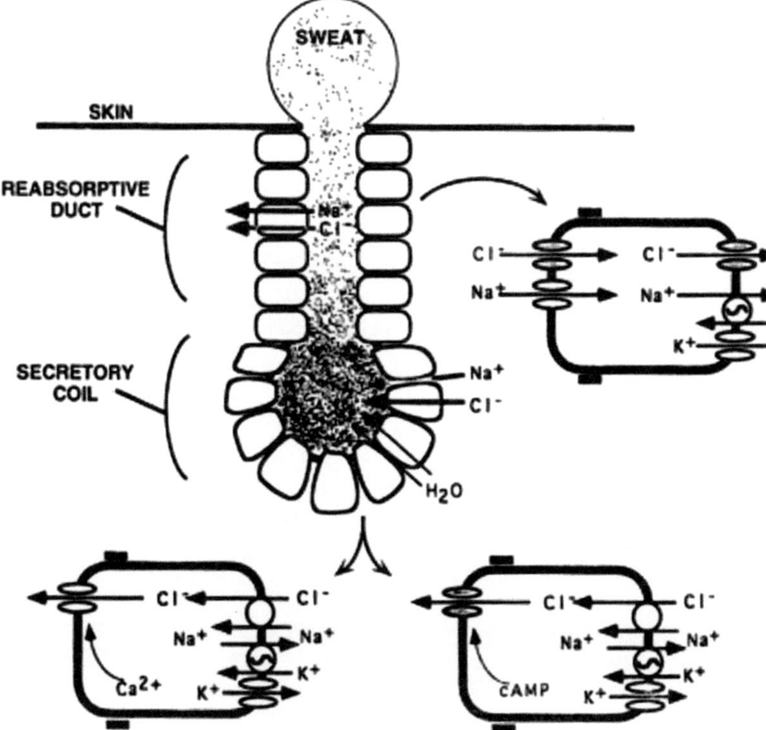

Fig. 5.2 Schematic representation of sweat production and electrolyte transport by the sweat gland. This figure shows the reabsorptive and secretory duct. The CFTR chloride channel is indicated by *shading*; all other channels, transporters, and pumps are indicated by *open symbols*. Sodium (Na+) absorption in the sweat duct occurs by sodium entry into the cell across the apical membrane driven by a favorable electrochemical gradient. Sodium then exits across the basolateral membrane in exchange for potassium (K+) on the Na+/K+-ATPase transporters, which maintains a low intracellular Na+ concentration. These processes are the same in normal and CF sweat gland ducts. Na+ transport establishes the ion concentration and voltage gradients that drive passive chloride absorption. When CFTR is defective, chloride fails to follow Na+ absorption; preventing the sodium and chloride absorption increases their concentrations in the sweat. This figure is reproduced from Welsh MJ, Ramsay BW, Accurso F, Cutting GR. Cystic Fibrosis. In: Scriver ABC, Sly WS, Valle D, editors. The Molecular and Metabolic Basis of Inherited Disease. New York: McGraw-Hill; 2001. p. 5150; with permission from The McGraw-Hill Companies

been linked to the chloride resorptive activity. In addition, reduced sodium transport is enhanced by diminished co-anion delivery that helps to drive low absorption. As a consequence, the sweat sodium and chloride values are elevated in CF patients compared to normal individuals. Inherent advantages of the test are its simplicity and safety, in addition to the fact that the sweat gland is not altered by CF pathophysiology, providing a reliable indicator of CFTR activity not affected by end-organ dysfunction.

Principles Underlying the Sweat Chloride Test

An understanding of sweat gland physiology provides the basic premise underlying sweat chloride testing. Sufficient CFTR function allows for coordinated regulation of the CFTR, alternative chloride channels, and ENaC to produce hypotonic sweat. This electrolyte composition results in a low sweat chloride content. In deficient or absent CFTR function states, muscarinic stimulation of the apocrine sweat gland causes excessive chloride and other electrolytes to extrude on the skin surface because of deficient reclamation in the reabsorptive duct. Because sweat rate acts as a covariate to total ionic absorptive capacity, the extremes of sweat rate can also alter chloride values, and can be assessed independently with emerging techniques [22].

General Methods

Sweat chloride testing should be performed at accredited centers using accepted methods to avoid technical problems frequently encountered prior to wide standardization of the technique. The methods for sweat testing are described in the current standard operating procedures (available upon request from the CFF Thereapeutics Development Network) which involve three technical portions: sweat stimulation, collection, and analysis. Current methodology employs the Gibson and Cooke method of pilocarpine iontophoresis [41] which conforms to European and Australian standards [42, 43]. The preferred site for stimulation and collection is the middle portion of the extensor surface of the forearm, but successful stimulation has been achieved in other sites including the upper arm, calf, and thigh [37]. After the skin is inspected for the presence of lesions, inflammation, breaks, or abnormalities, the appropriately selected site is prepped and washed. Duplicate measurement on the contralateral forearm should be performed simultaneously when possible to ensure repeatability. After the skin is prepped, the electrodes are affixed to the skin surface with a pilocarpine-containing gel. Stimulation is achieved at a maximum of 4 mA current for 5 min, although most commercial systems are automated for stimulation. This current stimulation poses minimal risk although mild burn, urticaria, or skin irritation have been reported [44]. After stimulation, the electrodes are removed, the skin is prepped, and immediately a collection device such as the

Macroduct® (Wescor, Logan, UT) is placed. Sweat is collected in this fashion for 30 min and chloride analysis conducted. In this fashion, samples can be stored at −70 °C until analyzed. An alternative method is the application of prespecified gauze to the area followed by evaluation of sweat weight and analysis of electrolyte content. Chloride concentration should be performed at a reference laboratory according to Clinical Laboratory Standards Institute guidelines. Approved methods for sweat chloride analysis include colorimetric titration (chloridimeter) and manual titration using the Schales and Schales mercuric nitrate procedure, or by automated analyzers using ion-selective electrodes [45].

Sources of Error

Successful sweat collection depends on appropriate patient selection and reducing errors in the collection process which result in the majority of errors [37]. Assuring that adequate sweat is collected and avoidance of evaporation are mandatory. Under current international guidelines which recommend use of the Macroduct® system, adequate sweat volume is achieved if ≥ 15 µL of sweat is collected within the 30-min collection period. The use of this system helps to minimize errors from evaporation, contamination, and loss of sweat volume, and is therefore regarded as the gold standard method of collection as it alleviates many of these sources of error. These errors are more inherent in the gauze collection method as accurate sweat rate of 1 g/m²/min is difficult to quantify by this method in order to ensure that an acceptable sweat amount is collected for analysis. In addition, because of air exposure, this method is prone to evaporative losses leading to inadequate sweat amount defined as 75 mg of sweat collected in 30 min.

Several medical conditions are associated with false-positive and -negative values for sweat chloride testing. Conditions which cause false-positive values include atopic eczema, untreated Addison's disease, ectodermal dysplasia, glycogen storage diseases, and untreated hypothyroidism [44, 45]. False negatives from medical confounding conditions most often arise from peripheral or limb edema or, less commonly, from mineralocorticoid administration.

Because variable expression among tissues affects an important minority of CFTR mutations, sweat chloride can provide misleading information regarding diagnosis or prognosis. For example, patients with the R117H mutation can exhibit relatively preserved sweat chloride (particularly when accompanied with 7T or 9T intronic thymidine sequences), but still manifest sinopulmonary disease that is CFTR related [46]. Alternatively, splicing mutants can exhibit tissue-specific expression that impairs sweat chloride as a readout of pulmonary physiology [15, 47]. In these cases, secondary functional assessments such as NPD or intestinal current measurements have an important role to assess diagnosis and severity of functional CFTR decrements in the organ of interest.

Age at collection can affect the sweat chloride. Sweat chloride tests are falsely elevated in the first 24 h after birth, but rapidly decline thereafter [48] allowing for adequate sweat chloride collection after the first 2 weeks of infancy as a general rule.

African American infants may demonstrate reduced sweat rates in the first 2 weeks of life [41, 44]. Other studies have determined that sweat values may be accurate at 48 h after birth if adequate sweat is obtained. Population studies in NBS programs from Colorado demonstrate that adequate sweat is obtained for accurate diagnosis of CF after positive newborn screen at a mean of 6 weeks after birth [49]. Advanced age may be associated with errors in the measurement of sweat chloride; a small number of studies to date have identified a trend toward increasing sweat chloride values in adolescence and adulthood that should be considered during evaluation of older individuals [50, 51]. Altered sodium metabolism can also be a confounding factor.

Diagnostic Ranges

Sweat chloride values are variable on a continuum from the lower limit of detection (10 mmol/L) to the upper limit of detection (160 mmol/L). Some controversy exists about diagnostic cutoffs as discussed in brief in the previous section, especially the "normal" cutoff value for infants, established as <30 mmol/L [52]. Generally accepted ranges for US, European, and Australian diagnostic guidelines for CF are sweat chloride values greater than 60 mmol/L and negative tests are defined as <40 mmol/L, with values from 40 to 60 mmol/L as indeterminate or borderline. These accepted intervals and interpretation are summarized in Table 5.1. These reference intervals are based on very few standardized studies to determine reference ranges [50]. Farrell and Koscik evaluated 707 subjects over a broad age range; all subjects had CFTR sequencing and clinical characteristics documented and sweat chloride testing was performed using pilocarpine iontophoresis and acceptable collection and analysis methods. A cutoff of <40 mmol/L for sweat chloride established infants as "normal," which represented a mean plus three standard deviations. An important methodological flaw in this study was that subjects who were CFTR mutation carriers were included among normal children ($n=128$), which can minimally affect sweat chloride. Other studies did not address carrier status or were performed before 1989 when the CFTR gene was sequenced [50, 53–58]. A recent infant study performed on infants 5–6 weeks of age indicates that a cutoff of $\geq$30 mmol/L may establish concerns for a CF diagnosis [52], and has been adopted in diagnostic algorithms for this age group. In these cases, sweat chloride is

Table 5.1 Diagnostic ranges for sweat chloride values

	Children-adult (ages >6 months)	Infants (age ≤6 months)
Consistent with diagnosis of CF	>60 mmol/L	>60 mmol/L
Borderline/indeterminate	40–60 mmol/L	40–60 mmol/L; note that values of 31–40 have been shown to be borderline/indeterminate and require further investigation in this group (see text)
Negative	<40 mmol/L	<40 mmol/L: see note above

frequently monitored over the first year of life to assess whether sweat chloride abnormalities persist during development.

There exists a spectrum of CFTR-related illnesses from carrier status, CFTR-related disorders to CF with or without pancreatic insufficiency. The spectrum of these disorders is inadequately assessed by newborn screening or genetic analysis alone [59]. A continuum of sweat chloride values (from borderline to very high values) can be observed among various forms of disease caused by dysfunctional CFTR, from classic pancreatic insufficient CF to pancreatic sufficient CF to individuals with CFTR-related disorders and asymptomatic carriers [60, 61]. Although the ranges are broad, the differences in mean sweat chloride among these groups correlate to severity of illness and degree of CFTR dysfunction. Nevertheless, some studies demonstrate that the degree of CFTR dysfunction detected by worsening sweat chloride does not correlate to lung function severity [62], a reminder of the heterogeneity of these measurements with respect to both genetic and environmental factors and their inherent limitations.

Emerging Methods of Sweat Metabolism

Recent efforts have built upon prior assessments of sweat rate as a diagnostic tool for CF, which were originally reported in 1984 [23]. The assay takes advantage of CFTR-dependent sweating that is stimulated by β-adrenergic stimuli, as opposed to cholinergic sweating that is independent of CFTR. Evaluation of β-adrenergic sweat rate using evaporimetry has recently been introduced, and, as opposed to sweat chloride, establishes a clear decrement in obligate carriers [22]. How this test can be used to supplement CF diagnostic information will continue to emerge with additional studies.

Nasal Potential Difference

The measurement of nasal potential difference (NPD) provides a direct evaluation of sodium and chloride transport in secretory epithelial cells via assessment of transepithelial bioelectric properties [63–65]. This serves as a diagnostic aid in difficult cases where abnormal CFTR function is suspected [31, 32] or where tissue proclivity makes assessment of the airway informative. In addition, since chloride and sodium transport can be distinguished, disorders of sodium metabolism can also be assessed and reliably distinguished. NPD has been used as an important endpoint in clinical trials evaluating therapeutic agents intended to replace dysfunctional CFTR with wild-type CFTR complementary DNA (including viral and nonviral gene transfer [66–68]), restore mutant CFTR function [69–74], or address other abnormalities in CF ion transport such as novel high-affinity ENaC blockers, channel-activating protease inhibitors, or activators of alternate Cl⁻ channels [1, 75–78].

Principles Underlying Nasal Potential Difference Measurements

The premise behind NPD measurements is that the bioelectric abnormality of the CF nasal airway reflects transport abnormalities observed in the lower airways of CF patients. In normal subjects, the bioelectric potential is maintained by a balance of sodium absorption and chloride transport, resulting in the tight regulation of the airway surface liquid volume, ionic content, and pH, which are important for maintaining mucociliary clearance and airway defense. The nasal cavity is accessible which makes it a good site to examine the ion transport characteristics of airway epithelia. Because respiratory epithelia form a tight monolayer harboring a stable and sufficient transepithelial resistance, the active secretion or absorption of charged salts such as sodium (Na^+) and chloride (Cl^-) ions induces a potential difference, measured as a voltage across the epithelial surface [79]. The bioelectric potential can be measured by using a high-impedance voltmeter between two electrodes, with one in continuity with each side of the epithelial surface (Fig. 5.3). The electrode on the airway surface (the exploring electrode) rests against the surface of the nasal

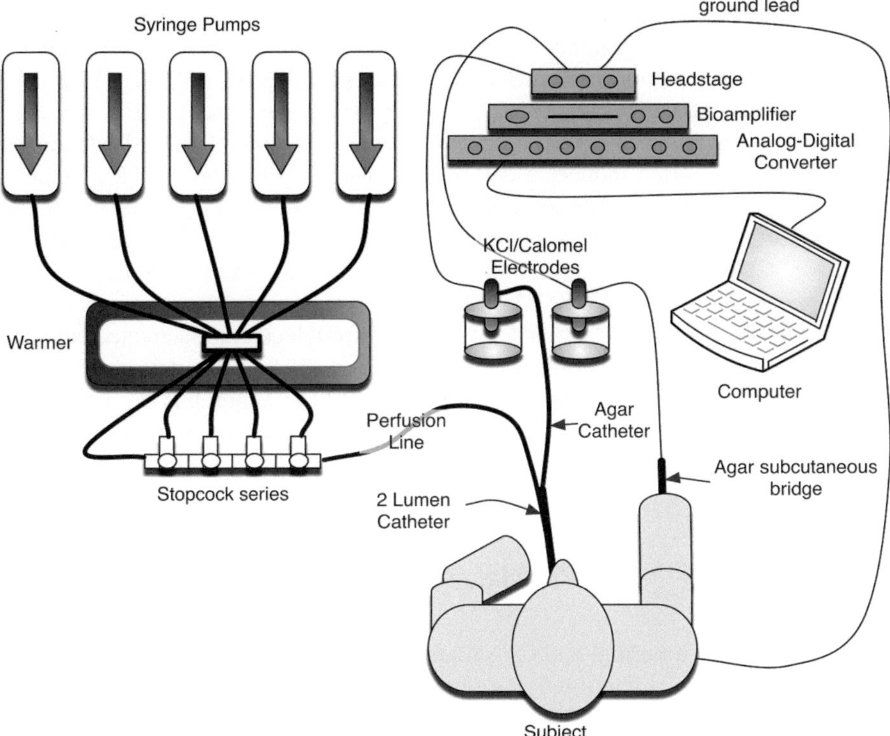

Fig. 5.3 Schematic of the nasal potential difference apparatus

epithelium. The internal electrode (the reference electrode) can theoretically be placed in any interstitial compartment of the body, although generally the subcutaneous tissue of the forearm is used. Subsequently, various solutions are perfused to isolate sodium transport, CFTR-dependent chloride transport, and CFTR-independent chloride transport. Due to the importance of appropriate placement within the nasal cavity and the need for an electrically quiet environment, some training and experience are required to achieve accuracy and reproducibility with the method, and are often supported by research centers within CF clinical trial networks.

General Methodology

Less than a centimeter into the nose, the squamous ("skin type") epithelium becomes ciliated pseudocolumnar epithelium under the inferior turbinate, sharing many characteristics with the more distal airways [80–82]. Under basal conditions Na^+ absorption is the primary ion transport activity in normal airway epithelia [63]. The resulting (or basal) PD is negative or polarized (viewed from the epithelial surface) and in normal subjects is usually between −15 and −25 mV. The measurement continues by the sequential perfusion of compounds that block inwardly directed sodium transport through inhibition of ENaC (amiloride), followed by augmentation of chloride transport through CFTR. During perfusion of amiloride, the potential difference depolarizes as ENaC transport is reduced, and the PD typically approaches a low polarizing value (typically between 0 and −10 mV). Perfusion of a chloride-free solution induces a chloride diffusion PD through CFTR channels, resulting in a rapid and often large hyperpolarization of the PD. CFTR-mediated Cl^- transport is further enhanced pharmacologically by the addition of agents known to activate CFTR, such as isoproterenol (which increases intracellular cyclic AMP as a β2 receptor agonist) [83, 84]. It is not unusual to observe transient hyperpolarization that is believed to represent Cl^- transport through calcium-activated chloride channels (CaCC) during chloride-free perfusion (with or without isoproterenol). These transient polarizations typically resolve within 1–2 min, and are not CFTR dependent. Finally, ATP is perfused, which activates chloride secretion through alternative (non-CFTR) CaCCs and serves as a marker of epithelium integrity.

Healthy and CF Nasal PD Measurements

Example tracings in normal and CF subjects are shown in Fig. 5.4a, b. In CF, this ion transport profile is abnormal and the nasal PD measurement has a number of features that distinguish the PD signature. At the beginning of the measurement with buffered Ringer's, the basal PD in CF is much more negative due to increased ENaC activity although this is also explained by increased potential in the absence

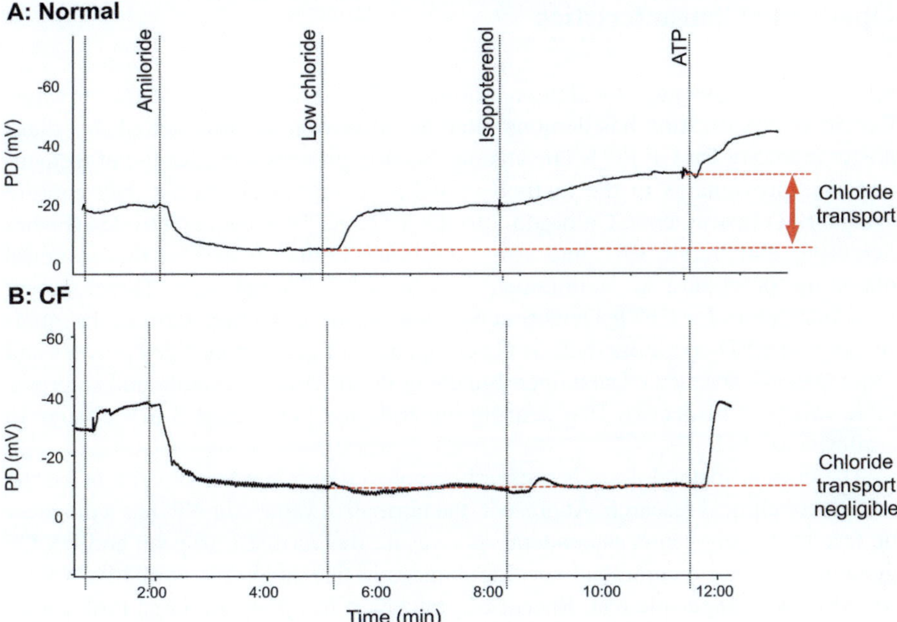

Fig. 5.4 Representative nasal potential difference (PD) tracings. (**a**) Perfusion tracing from a normal subject. The *x-axis* indicates time (min) and the *y-axis* represents the potential difference (mV, polarizing). Initiation of various perfusion solutions is designated by *arrows* (*bottom*). Sodium transport can be quantified by Ringer's perfusion (about 20 mV) or by a change after amiloride (100 μM) perfusion (ΔAmil). Chloride transport is quantified by the change in PD after zero chloride perfusion (Δ0Cl⁻), the change after isoproterenol (10 μM) or other cystic fibrosis transmembrane conductance regulator (CFTR) agonist (ΔIso), or the sum of these changes (total chloride secretion [TCS], shown in *red*). Both sodium and chloride transport can be captured in a single measure by the total change in PD (ΔPD, shown in *red*). (**b**) Perfusion tracing from a subject with CF. Compared with the tracing from a normal subject, the CF tracing has a relatively polarized PD in Ringer's, a large depolarization with amiloride, and no sustained repolarization with zero chloride and isoproterenol solutions. The large depolarization after ATP perfusion serves as a positive control

of CFTR [85]. The depolarizing response to amiloride is also enhanced. Although the sodium abnormality is usually readily apparent, the most consistent abnormality in CF is the absence of hyperpolarization following perfusion with chloride-free solution and isoproterenol. In CF, the addition of ATP (or other purines) leads to a large hyperpolarization, and occurs through non-CFTR-mediated chloride secretory pathways, including stimulation of P2Y2 receptors which activate CaCCs. In aggregate, the differences in Na and Cl transport are sufficient to discriminate CF from non-CF subjects, and also detect individuals with intermediate phenotypes [34, 86].

Operating Characteristics

NPD has the advantage of demonstrating CFTR abnormalities in the airways. Recent standardization has demonstrated an improved performance of this diagnostic modality for CF [87]. The standardization process includes the aforementioned improvements in the method including using an electronic data capture system (AD Instruments, Colorado Springs, CO), KCl calomel electrodes (Fisher Scientific, Pittsburgh, PA), and agar two-lumen human interface; this standard operating procedure is maintained by the CFF Therapeutics Development Network Center for CFTR Detection National Resource Center. Criteria for qualification of NPD operators include (1) completion of the standardized process and sequence, (2) absence of sustained breaks in the tracing, (3) stable and interpretable values at respective 10-s scoring interval, and (4) at least 3 mV change in amiloride or ATP.

The current methodology is presently employed at a number of centers for the conduct of clinical research. At present, the normative values for NPD as a diagnostic test are largely center dependent. As a result, the current European and US CF guidelines do not recommend specific diagnostic thresholds for normative values for NPD as a diagnostic test. Recent centralization has provided large multicenter databases which may provide normative values for normal and CF in the future. Other indices incorporating both sodium and chloride transport (e.g., the Wilshanski and Sermet scores) have been calculated with proposed diagnostic thresholds, although these are used only sporadically [88, 89].

Contraindications and Sources of Error

There are relatively few contraindications to nasal potential difference testing, although it does require a willing participant who can remain still for the duration of the procedure. Patients with severe mucosal disruption from prior nasal polyposis or sinus surgery may demonstrate errors in measurements due to abnormal turbinate epithelial properties. In addition, patients with allergic rhinitis may be intolerant of the nasal probe making testing difficult to complete. Rhinitis and acute viral upper respiratory infection may also directly alter the ion transport phenotype resulting in false-negative results. Cigarette smoking can also act as a confounder [90–92]. Because of concern for infection control, care should be taken in the evaluation of patients harboring *Burkholderia cepacia* or other virulent pathogens. Because NPD is technically challenging, the test is primarily available at research centers. Evaluation of infant and toddlers is particularly difficult, but can be performed if done with care [93].

Summary

CF is a systemic illness resulting from mutations in the CFTR gene leading to abrogated chloride channel and regulatory functions by the CFTR protein. This pathophysiology is responsible for many of the clinical manifestations of the disease, and its activity measured with diagnostic testing. The diagnosis of CF can be accurately established by demonstrating abnormal CFTR function in the sweat gland by sweat chloride analysis or by identification of abnormal CFTR function in the airways by the measurement of the transepithelial nasal potential difference. In the era of advancing genomics, an understanding of these important clinically available tests to establish a link between CFTR mutation and deranged protein function using these two measurements remains important and clinically relevant, and can provide prognostic information that guides therapeutic interventions.

References

1. Rowe SM, Miller S, Sorscher EJ. Cystic fibrosis. N Engl J Med. 2005;352(19):1992–2001.
2. Wilcken B, et al. Neonatal screening for cystic fibrosis: a comparison of two strategies for case detection in 1.2 million babies. J Pediatr. 1995;127(6):965–70.
3. Anderson D. Cystic fibrosis of the pancreas and its relationship to celiac disease: clinical and pathologic study. Am J Dis Child. 1938;56:344.
4. Di Sant'Agnese P, et al. Abnormal electrolyte composition of sweat in cystic fibrosis of the pancreas; clinical significance and relationship to the disease. Pediatrics. 1953;12:549–63.
5. Rommens JM, et al. Identification of the cystic fibrosis gene: chromosome walking and jumping. Science. 1989;245(4922):1059–65.
6. Kerem B, et al. Identification of the cystic fibrosis gene: genetic analysis. Science. 1989; 245(4922):1073–80.
7. Riordan JR, et al. Identification of the cystic fibrosis gene: cloning and characterization of complementary DNA. Science. 1989;245(4922):1066–73.
8. Quinton PM, Bijman J. Higher bioelectric potentials due to decreased chloride absorption in the sweat glands of patients with cystic fibrosis. N Engl J Med. 1983;308(20):1185–9.
9. Quinton PM. Chloride impermeability in cystic fibrosis. Nature. 1983;301(5899):421–2.
10. Knowles MR, et al. Abnormal ion permeation through cystic fibrosis respiratory epithelium. Science. 1983;221(4615):1067–70.
11. Knowles M, Gatzy J, Boucher R. Relative ion permeability of normal and cystic fibrosis nasal epithelium. J Clin Invest. 1983;71(5):1410–7.
12. Welsh MJ, Liedtke CM. Chloride and potassium channels in cystic fibrosis airway epithelia. Nature. 1986;322(6078):467–70.
13. Schoumacher RA, et al. Phosphorylation fails to activate chloride channels from cystic fibrosis airway cells. Nature. 1987;330(6150):752–4.
14. Cohn JA, et al. Relation between mutations of the cystic fibrosis gene and idiopathic pancreatitis. N Engl J Med. 1998;339(10):653–8.
15. Chillon M, et al. Mutations in the cystic fibrosis gene in patients with congenital absence of the vas deferens. N Engl J Med. 1995;332(22):1475–80.
16. Turcios NL. Cystic fibrosis: an overview. J Clin Gastroenterol. 2005;39(4):307–17.
17. Derichs N, et al. Intestinal current measurement for diagnostic classification of patients with questionable cystic fibrosis: validation and reference data. Thorax. 2010;65(7):594–9.

18. Clancy JP. Diagnosing cystic fibrosis in patients with non-diagnostic results: the case for intestinal current measurements. Thorax. 2010;65(7):575–6.
19. De Jonge HR, et al. Ex vivo CF diagnosis by intestinal current measurements (ICM) in small aperture, circulating Ussing chambers. J Cyst Fibros. 2004;3 Suppl 2:159–63.
20. Hug MJ, et al. Measurement of ion transport function in rectal biopsies. Methods Mol Biol. 2011;741:87–107.
21. Cohen-Cymberknoh M, et al. Evaluation of the intestinal current measurement method as a diagnostic test for cystic fibrosis. Pediatr Pulmonol. 2013;48(3):229–35.
22. Quinton P, et al. Beta-adrenergic sweat secretion as a diagnostic test for cystic fibrosis. Am J Respir Crit Care Med. 2012;186(8):732–9.
23. Sato K, Sato F. Defective beta adrenergic response of cystic fibrosis sweat glands in vivo and in vitro. J Clin Invest. 1984;73(6):1763–71.
24. Sharp JK, Rock MJ. Newborn screening for cystic fibrosis. Clin Rev Allergy Immunol. 2008; 35(3):107–15.
25. Shwachman H, Redmond A, Khaw KT. Studies in cystic fibrosis. Report of 130 patients diagnosed under 3 months of age over a 20-year period. Pediatrics. 1970;46(3):335–43.
26. Grosse SD, et al. Newborn screening for cystic fibrosis: evaluation of benefits and risks and recommendations for state newborn screening programs. MMWR Recomm Rep. 2004;53(RR-13):1–36.
27. Chatfield S, et al. Neonatal screening for cystic fibrosis in Wales and the West Midlands: clinical assessment after five years of screening. Arch Dis Child. 1991;66(1 Spec No):29–33.
28. Doull IJ, et al. Cystic fibrosis-related deaths in infancy and the effect of newborn screening. Pediatr Pulmonol. 2001;31(5):363–6.
29. Farrell PM, et al. Early diagnosis of cystic fibrosis through neonatal screening prevents severe malnutrition and improves long-term growth. Wisconsin Cystic Fibrosis Neonatal Screening Study Group. Pediatrics. 2001;107(1):1–13.
30. Farrell PM, et al. Bronchopulmonary disease in children with cystic fibrosis after early or delayed diagnosis. Am J Respir Crit Care Med. 2003;168(9):1100–8.
31. Farrell PM, et al. Guidelines for diagnosis of cystic fibrosis in newborns through older adults: Cystic Fibrosis Foundation consensus report. J Pediatr. 2008;153(2):S4–14.
32. De Boeck K, et al. Cystic fibrosis: terminology and diagnostic algorithms. Thorax. 2006;61(7): 627–35.
33. Ooi CY, et al. Comparing the American and European diagnostic guidelines for cystic fibrosis: same disease, different language? Thorax. 2012;67(7):618–24.
34. Wilschanski M, et al. Mutations in the cystic fibrosis transmembrane regulator gene and in vivo transepithelial potentials. Am J Respir Crit Care Med. 2006;174(7):787–94.
35. Gahm N, Shwachman H. Studies in cystic fibrosis of the pancreas; a simple test for the detection of excessive chloride on the skin. N Engl J Med. 1956;255(21):999–1001.
36. Gibson LE, Cooke RE. A test for concentration of electrolytes in sweat in cystic fibrosis of the pancreas utilizing pilocarpine by iontophoresis. Pediatrics. 1959;23(3):545–9.
37. Mishra A, Greaves R, Massie J. The relevance of sweat testing for the diagnosis of cystic fibrosis in the genomic era. Clin Biochem Rev. 2005;26(4):135–53.
38. Ramsey BW, et al. A CFTR potentiator in patients with cystic fibrosis and the G551D mutation. N Engl J Med. 2011;365(18):1663–72.
39. Accurso FJ, et al. Effect of VX-770 in persons with cystic fibrosis and the G551D-CFTR mutation. N Engl J Med. 2010;363(21):1991–2003.
40. Clancy JP, et al. Results of a phase IIa study of VX-809, an investigational CFTR corrector compound, in subjects with cystic fibrosis homozygous for the F508del-CFTR mutation. Thorax. 2012;67(1):12–8.
41. LeGrys VA, et al. Diagnostic sweat testing: the Cystic Fibrosis Foundation guidelines. J Pediatr. 2007;151(1):85–9.
42. Green A. Guidelines for the performance of the sweat test for the investigation of cystic fibrosis in the UK. UKNEQAS: Sheffield; 2003.

43. Coakley J, et al. Australian guidelines for the performance of the sweat test for the diagnosis of cystic fibrosis: report from the AACB Sweat Testing Working Party. Clin Biochem Rev. 2006;27(2):S1–7.
44. LeGrys VA. Sweat testing for the diagnosis of cystic fibrosis: practical considerations. J Pediatr. 1996;129(6):892–7.
45. National Committee for Clinical Laboratory Standards. Sweat testing: sample collection and quantitative analysis: approved guideline. NCCLS Document C34-A2. Wayne, PA: National Committee for Clinical Laboratory Standards; 2000.
46. de Nooijer RA, et al. Assessment of CFTR function in homozygous R117H-7T subjects. J Cyst Fibros. 2011;10(5):326–32.
47. Davis PB, Drumm M, Konstan MW. Cystic fibrosis. Am J Respir Crit Care Med. 1996;154(5):1229–56.
48. Hardy JD, et al. Sweat tests in the newborn period. Arch Dis Child. 1973;48(4):316–8.
49. Hammond KB, Turcios NL, Gibson LE. Clinical evaluation of the macroduct sweat collection system and conductivity analyzer in the diagnosis of cystic fibrosis. J Pediatr. 1994; 124(2):255–60.
50. Mishra A, Greaves R, Massie J. The limitations of sweat electrolyte reference intervals for the diagnosis of cystic fibrosis: a systematic review. Clin Biochem Rev. 2007;28(2):60–76.
51. Mishra A, et al. Diagnosis of cystic fibrosis by sweat testing: age-specific reference intervals. J Pediatr. 2008;153(6):758–63.
52. Jayaraj R, et al. A reference interval for sweat chloride in infants aged between five and six weeks of age. Ann Clin Biochem. 2009;46(Pt 1):73–8.
53. Shwachman H, Mahmoodian A, Neff RK. The sweat test: sodium and chloride values. J Pediatr. 1981;98(4):576–8.
54. Andrews BF, Bruton OC, Knoblock EC. Sweat chloride concentration in children with allergy and with cystic fibrosis of the pancreas. Pediatrics. 1962;29:204–8.
55. Davis PB, et al. Sweat chloride concentration in adults with pulmonary diseases. Am Rev Respir Dis. 1983;128(1):34–7.
56. Warwick WJ, Hansen L. Measurement of chloride in sweat with the chloride-selective electrode. Clin Chem. 1978;24(11):2050–3.
57. Warwick WJ, Hansen LG. Measurement of chloride in sweat by use of a selective electrode and strip-chart recorder. Clin Chem. 1978;24(2):381–2.
58. Gharib R, Joos HA, Hilty LB. Sweat chloride concentration; a comparative study in children with bronchial asthma and with cystic fibrosis. Am J Dis Child. 1965;109:66–8.
59. Mekus F, et al. Cystic-fibrosis-like disease unrelated to the cystic fibrosis transmembrane conductance regulator. Hum Genet. 1998;102(5):582–6.
60. Burgel PR, et al. Non-classic cystic fibrosis associated with D1152H CFTR mutation. Clin Genet. 2010;77(4):355–64.
61. Goubau C, et al. Phenotypic characterisation of patients with intermediate sweat chloride values: towards validation of the European diagnostic algorithm for cystic fibrosis. Thorax. 2009;64(8):683–91.
62. Davis PB, Schluchter MD, Konstan MW. Relation of sweat chloride concentration to severity of lung disease in cystic fibrosis. Pediatr Pulmonol. 2004;38(3):204–9.
63. Knowles M, Gatzy J, Boucher R. Increased bioelectric potential difference across respiratory epithelia in cystic fibrosis. N Engl J Med. 1981;305(25):1489–95.
64. Knowles MR, Paradiso AM, Boucher RC. In vivo nasal potential difference: techniques and protocols for assessing efficacy of gene transfer in cystic fibrosis. Hum Gene Ther. 1995; 6(4):445–55.
65. Middleton PG, Geddes DM, Alton EW. Protocols for in vivo measurement of the ion transport defects in cystic fibrosis nasal epithelium. Eur Respir J. 1994;7(11):2050–6.
66. Knowles MR, et al. A controlled study of adenoviral-vector-mediated gene transfer in the nasal epithelium of patients with cystic fibrosis. N Engl J Med. 1995;333(13):823–31.

67. Noone PG, et al. Safety and biological efficacy of a lipid-CFTR complex for gene transfer in the nasal epithelium of adult patients with cystic fibrosis. Mol Ther. 2000;1(1):105–14.
68. Middleton PG, et al. Nasal application of the cationic liposome DC-Chol:DOPE does not alter ion transport, lung function or bacterial growth. Eur Respir J. 1994;7(3):442–5.
69. McCarty NA, et al. A phase I randomized, multicenter trial of CPX in adult subjects with mild cystic fibrosis. Pediatr Pulmonol. 2002;33(2):90–8.
70. Wilschanski M, et al. Gentamicin-induced correction of CFTR function in patients with cystic fibrosis and CFTR stop mutations. N Engl J Med. 2003;349(15):1433–41.
71. Kerem E, et al. PTC124 induces time-dependent improvements in chloride conductance and clinical parameters in patients with nonsense-mutation-mediated cystic fibrosis. Pediatr Pulmonol. 2008;S31:294.
72. Clancy JP, et al. No detectable improvements in cystic fibrosis transmembrane conductance regulator by nasal aminoglycosides in patients with cystic fibrosis with stop mutations. Am J Respir Cell Mol Biol. 2007;37(1):57–66.
73. Accurso, FJ, et al. Effect of VX-770 in persons with cystic fibrosis and the G551D-CFTR mutation. N Engl J Med. 363(21):1991–2003.
74. Konstan MW, et al. Compacted DNA nanoparticles administered to the nasal mucosa of cystic fibrosis subjects are safe and demonstrate partial to complete cystic fibrosis transmembrane regulator reconstitution. Hum Gene Ther. 2004;15(12):1255–69.
75. Zeitlin PL, et al. A phase I trial of intranasal Moli 1901 for cystic fibrosis. Chest. 2004;125(1):143–9.
76. Rowe SM, Accurso F, Clancy JP. Detection of cystic fibrosis transmembrane conductance regulator activity in early-phase clinical trials. Proc Am Thorac Soc. 2007;4(4):387–98.
77. Rowe SM, et al. Correction of sodium transport with nasal administration of the prostasin inhibitor QAU145 in CF subjects. Pediatr Pulmonol. 2008;S31:A268.
78. Rowe SM, et al. Reduced sodium transport with nasal administration of the prostasin inhibitor Camostat in cystic fibrosis subjects. Chest. 2013;144(1):200–7.
79. Gatzy JT. Bioelectric properties of the isolated amphibian lung. Am J Physiol. 1967;213(2):425–31.
80. Knowles MR, et al. Measurements of nasal transepithelial electric potential differences in normal human subjects in vivo. Am Rev Respir Dis. 1981;124(4):484–90.
81. Knowles MR, et al. Measurements of transepithelial electric potential differences in the trachea and bronchi of human subjects in vivo. Am Rev Respir Dis. 1982;126(1):108–12.
82. Davies JC, et al. Potential difference measurements in the lower airway of children with and without cystic fibrosis. Am J Respir Crit Care Med. 2005;171(9):1015–9.
83. Anderson MP, et al. Demonstration that CFTR is a chloride channel by alteration of its anion selectivity. Science. 1991;253(5016):202–5.
84. Li C, Naren AP. Macromolecular complexes of cystic fibrosis transmembrane conductance regulator and its interacting partners. Pharmacol Ther. 2005;108(2):208–23.
85. Chen JH, et al. Loss of anion transport without increased sodium absorption characterizes newborn porcine cystic fibrosis airway epithelia. Cell. 2010;143(6):911–23.
86. Fajac I, et al. Nasal airway ion transport is linked to the cystic fibrosis phenotype in adult patients. Thorax. 2004;59(11):971–6.
87. Solomon GM, et al. An international randomized multicenter comparison of nasal potential difference techniques. Chest. 2010;138(4):919–28.
88. Wilschanski M, et al. Nasal potential difference measurements in patients with atypical cystic fibrosis. Eur Respir J. 2001;17(6):1208–15.
89. Sermet-Gaudelus I, et al. Clinical phenotype and genotype of children with borderline sweat test and abnormal nasal epithelial chloride transport. Am J Respir Crit Care Med. 2010;182(7):929–36.
90. Cantin AM, et al. Cystic fibrosis transmembrane conductance regulator function is suppressed in cigarette smokers. Am J Respir Crit Care Med. 2006;173(10):1139–44.

91. Clunes LA, et al. Cigarette smoke exposure induces CFTR internalization and insolubility, leading to airway surface liquid dehydration. FASEB J. 2012;26(2):533–45.
92. Sloane PA, et al. A pharmacologic approach to acquired cystic fibrosis transmembrane conductance regulator dysfunction in smoking related lung disease. PLoS One. 2012;7(6):e39809.
93. Southern KW, et al. A modified technique for measurement of nasal transepithelial potential difference in infants. J Pediatr. 2001;139(3):353–8.

Chapter 6
Allergic and Immunologic Testing in Children with Respiratory Disease

Carolina Z. Marcus and Clement L. Ren

Abstract Allergic and immunologic diseases frequently present with pulmonary manifestations; the pediatric pulmonologist is often confronted with the need to perform diagnostic testing for these conditions. In this chapter we review allergic and immunologic diseases that are commonly associated with pulmonary complications. We briefly discuss the clinical features of these diseases and appropriate diagnostic testing.

Keywords Allergy • Immunology • Autoimmunity • Hypersensitivity pneumonitis • Neutrophils

Evaluation of Allergy

Allergies are commonly found in patients with respiratory disease and can contribute to worsening of symptoms. Although many antigens can elicit an allergic response, aeroallergens, both perennial (dust mites, animal dander, molds) and seasonal, (tree, grass, and weed pollens) are of greatest relevance to respiratory disease. Allergies are immediate hypersensitivity reactions mediated by immunoglobulin E (IgE), and allergy testing identifies IgE directed at specific antigens. Allergy testing can be performed through skin testing or in vitro techniques.

Allergy skin testing is the quickest and most sensitive method for detection of allergic sensitization. Skin testing detects the presence of allergen-specific IgE on a patient's cutaneous mast cells. Binding of the allergen to membrane bound IgE on mast cells in the skin of the individual tested leads to mast cell activation and degranulation, producing a wheal and flare response. The wheal is the result of skin edema, and the flare represents the surrounding erythema. Not all sensitized patients develop clinical symptoms when exposed to the allergen that leads to a reaction on skin testing; therefore, results must be interpreted in the appropriate clinical

C.Z. Marcus, M.D. • C.L. Ren, M.D. (✉)
Department of Pediatrics, University of Rochester, Medical Center,
601 Elmwood Avenue, Rochester, NY 14642, USA
e-mail: clement_ren@urmc.rochester.edu

© Springer Science+Business Media New York 2015
S.D. Davis et al. (eds.), *Diagnostic Tests in Pediatric Pulmonology*,
Respiratory Medicine, DOI 10.1007/978-1-4939-1801-0_6

context. Thus, a positive skin test in the setting of allergic symptoms upon exposure to the allergen in question is usually sufficient to make the diagnosis.

Patients who are at high risk for an anaphylactic reaction to testing or have experienced anaphylaxis within the previous month, should not undergo skin testing. Relative contraindications to skin testing are poorly controlled asthma or a history of a severe allergic reaction to miniscule amounts of the allergen, as these individuals are at a higher risk of developing an anaphylactic reaction to skin testing. In the few weeks following anaphylaxis, the skin is often non-reactive, because during the episode there is a massive degranulation of cutaneous mast cells. Replenishment of this mast cell population can take up to 4 weeks or longer. To avoid false-negative test results, skin tests should be done at least 4 weeks after the anaphylactic episode. Certain skin conditions can pose a challenge to allergy skin testing, such as dermatographism or urticaria. Skin testing can be done on individuals with atopic dermatitis, provided it is performed on unaffected skin. A careful review of a patient's medications should be conducted prior to skin testing. In particular, histamine receptor 1 antagonists (e.g., loratidine or cetrizine) and other medications with anti-histamine properties can suppress skin tests and should be discontinued at least 1 week prior to testing.

The two major methods of allergy skin testing in current clinical practice involve the prick/puncture and intradermal testing techniques [1]. The prick/puncture method is usually carried out first. This form of testing is highly sensitive, but lacks specificity, and thus is useful in ruling out allergic sensitization. In other words, the negative predictive value of skin prick testing is very high. Prick/puncture testing involves placing droplets of single allergen extracts on the volar surface of the forearm or upper back, and then using a pin or other commercially available testing device to "prick" through each droplet. Histamine dichloride and saline are used as positive and negative controls, respectively. Measurements of the wheal and flare are then taken. A wheal diameter of larger than 3 mm is considered a positive test result. Biologically standardized skin testing extracts are commercially available for foods, insect venoms, environmental allergens (pollens, molds, animals, dust mites, cockroach), and penicillins. Though biologically standardized extracts for skin testing to natural rubber latex are currently available in Canada and Europe, these are not available in the USA.

Intradermal testing to a given allergen is done after prick/puncture testing to that allergen has been negative. This method involves the intradermal injection of 100- to 1,000-fold dilutions of allergen extracts, with a positive result having a wheal of 5 mm or larger. Saline is injected intradermally as a negative control, and histamine as a positive control. When testing for allergy to stinging insect venoms or medications, serial injections of gradually increasing concentrations are typically used. Though the overall rate of systemic reactions to allergy skin testing is quite low, higher rates of systemic reactions have been reported following intradermal injection of latex and food allergens. For this reason, intradermal testing with foods and/or latex is no longer recommended.

The overall rate of systemic reactions to allergy skin testing is low, though one recent prospective study found the rate of systemic reactions to reach 3.6 % [2].

The majority of systemic reactions in this study were triggered by intradermal testing, not prick/puncture, to inhalant allergens. In a prospective study of 5,908 children, the rate of systemic reactions to prick/puncture testing was 0.001 % [3]. Risk factors for systemic reactions in children included a history of asthma, active atopic dermatitis, and age less than 1 year [3]. Adverse reactions to allergy skin testing are almost always associated with intradermal testing in the absence of prior prick/puncture testing [4]. There is one reported case of fatal anaphylaxis to skin prick testing in an adult with food allergy and poorly controlled asthma who underwent testing with a very large panel of food allergens [4].

In the majority of cases, skin testing for IgE-mediated allergy is preferable to in vitro testing, as skin testing yields results quickly, is comparatively inexpensive, and has a higher sensitivity than in vitro tests. The overall sensitivity of skin prick/puncture testing is estimated to be greater than 90 %, whereas the specificity of this testing method is approximately 50 %, though these values vary within a narrow range, depending on the quality of the extract used as well as the degree of skin test positivity. A positive skin test only suggests the possibility of allergy, and thus the positive predictive value of the test is moderate and positive test results must be interpreted in clinical context. On the contrary, the negative predictive value of skin testing is high, and thus skin testing can exclude allergy with relative certainty. However, there are several situations in which in vitro testing is more appropriate than skin testing. In vitro testing poses no risk of an allergic reaction to the patient undergoing the testing. As such, in patients with significant cardiovascular disease or a history of severe anaphylaxis to small amounts of a given allergen, in vitro testing may be more appropriate. As opposed to skin testing, in vitro testing is not affected by concomitant medications. Moreover, in individuals with dermatologic conditions with diffuse cutaneous involvement, there may not be a clear area of skin in which to place skin tests, and thus in vitro testing is a reasonable alternative in this case. An anaphylactic episode can render the skin non-reactive for several weeks following the reaction, and thus skin testing is not reliable in this situation, whereas in vitro testing is an option.

The most commonly used in vitro tests are immunoassays. In the past, these tests were referred to as radioallergosorbent tests (RASTs), and involved the coupling of antibodies with radioactive tags. Since the late 1980s, most RAST tests have been replaced with more sensitive fluorescence enzyme-labeled assays, and thus today the term immunoassay is most appropriate. Currently, immunoassays are available for numerous foods, natural rubber latex, stinging insect venoms, environmental aeroallergens, certain antibiotics, and some occupational allergens. Enzyme-linked immunosorbent assays (ELISA) use enzyme-linked antibodies. When specific allergens are bound to a matrix (e.g., bead or other substrate), IgE antibodies bind to those allergens. Anti-IgE antibodies are then added to the antigen:IgE complex, such that the quantity of specific IgE to the allergen in question can be measured. Quantitative results are typically reported in kU/L, though some immunoassays report values in ng/mL. The conversion is 1 kU/L = 2.4 ng IgE/mL. Immunoassay results are arbitrarily divided into classes (usually I to IV). A higher class indicates a higher likelihood that the positive test is correlated with a clinical reaction.

There is a wide range of sensitivity and specificity of immunoassays, but on the whole, when standardized inhalant allergen extracts are utilized, allergy skin testing has a higher sensitivity and specificity than immunoassay testing. The overall sensitivity of immunoassays ranges from 60 to 95 %, and specificity from 30 to 95 %. As with skin tests, immunoassay results must be interpreted in the context of a clinical history of reaction(s) to the allergen(s) in question. Moreover, a negative immunoassay result to a particular allergen in an individual with a history that strongly suggests allergic reactions to that allergen does not rule out an allergy to that specific antigen. The presence of allergen-specific IgE reflects a person's sensitization to that particular allergen, but does not translate to clinical allergy. Commercial immunoassays are currently available for foods, insect venoms, environmental allergens (pollens, molds, animals, cockroach, and dust mites), natural rubber latex, a small number of beta-lactam drugs, and a small number of occupational allergens. Immunoassay systems that use well-characterized and standardized allergens, and have been validated according to the Clinical Laboratory Standards Institute, should be utilized when possible.

Immunologic Evaluation

The lung is constantly exposed to infectious agents, and immunodeficiency is commonly associated with pulmonary manifestations, such as lower respiratory tract infections, bronchiectasis, interstitial lung disease, opportunistic infections, and obstructive lung disease. Deficits in the adaptive immune system can be broadly divided into defects in humoral or cellular immunity.

Evaluation of Humoral Immunity

The production of antibodies or immunoglobulin (Ig) is the main function of the humoral immune system. B lymphocytes are the only cells known to produce antibody. Igs play a key role in the opsonization and clearance of encapsulated bacteria. Igs can further be divided into 5 isotypes: IgM, IgG, IgA, IgD, and IgE. The properties of the different Ig isotypes are summarized in Table 6.1. IgM is produced early in a humoral immune response and directs complement mediated destruction of infectious agents. IgG is the major circulating antibody, and it is the primary mediator of humoral immunity. IgG acts by opsonization—the process of antigen binding and clearance by the reticuloendothelial system, Maternal IgG crosses the placenta, and thus infants normally have maternal IgG protection until about 6 months of age. IgA is involved in mucosal immunity. IgD is present only in small amounts in the blood. It does not play a major direct role in humoral immunity, but is involved in regulation and activation of immune cells. IgE is the mediator of immediate hypersensitivity allergic reactions.

Table 6.1 Summary of immunoglobulin isotypes and their properties

Isotype	Location	Function
IgG	Free in blood plasma	Main immunoglobulin of acquired immunity; crosses placental barrier and provides passive immunity to fetus
IgA	Saliva, tears, breast milk; also found in GI, respiratory, and urogenital tract mucosa	Protects mucosal surfaces; prevents attachment of pathogens to epithelial cells
IgM	Surface of B cell; free in blood plasma	Forms part of the B cell receptor (BCR); first class of antibodies released by B cells during acquired immune response
IgE	Secreted by plasma cells in skin and GI and respiratory tract mucosa	Binds to basophils and mast cells to trigger release of histamine; involved in allergic and parasitic processes
IgD	Surface of B cell	Membrane immunoglobulin, part of cell surface receptor of B cell (BCR); important in activation of B cells

Deficits in humoral immunity can be either quantitative or functional [5]. Measurement of total IgG, IgA, and IgM levels is helpful as an initial screening tool to determine if there may be a defect in humoral immunity. Hypogammaglobulinemia is defined as an IgG level less than two standard deviations below the normal range, and agammaglobulinemia is defined by a total IgG level of <100 mg/dL. In IgG subclass deficiency, total IgG may be normal or low normal, but an IgG subclass may be markedly decreased. The best way to assess antibody function is to measure IgG titers to specific organisms that represent the two main types of antigens—proteins and polysaccharides. An easy way to do this is to measure antibody titers to routine vaccinations. Measurement of antibody titers to tetanus or diphtheria is useful to assess antibody function with regard to protein antigens. Since a low tetanus antibody titer may reflect waning postvaccination immunity, repeat titers should be obtained a month after revaccination. To assess response to polysaccharide antigens, measurement of titers before and after immunization with unconjugated pneumococcal vaccine can be performed. However, infants and young children normally have poor antibody responses to polysaccharide antigens, and the antibody response to vaccination can frequently be incomplete even in school age children. Therefore, the interpretation of immune responses to pneumococcal vaccination can be difficult and needs to be done in the overall clinical context of an individual patient.

The most severe form of antibody deficiency is X-linked agammaglobulinemia (XLA), also known as Bruton's agammaglobulinemia. The molecular defect in XLA is due to mutations in the Bruton's tyrosine kinase (BTK) gene. Absence of BTK results in a block in B cell maturation and as a result, there are no B cells present in patients with XLA. XLA is associated with near absent levels of all Ig isotypes. Flow cytometry shows an absence of circulating B cells.

Common variable immunodeficiency (CVID) is a heterogeneous disorder that is characterized by impaired B cell differentiation, leading to varying degrees of hypogammaglobulinemia and diminished antigen-specific responses. Patients with CVID usually have normal numbers of B cells, but the function of these cells is impaired, and quantification of antibody levels will typically reveal markedly reduced serum concentrations of IgG, in combination with low levels of IgA and/or IgM. There may be subtle defects in T cell function as well, but patients rarely develop opportunistic infections as a result. Individuals with CVID are at an increased risk of developing interstitial lung disease, as well as hematologic malignancy, particularly B-cell lymphomas. IgG subclass deficiency refers to a significant decrease in serum levels of one or more of the four subclasses of IgG, in a patient with a normal total IgG. This laboratory finding may not translate to clinical disease, as decreased levels of IgG subclasses are seen in the general population. However, some individuals with IgG subclass deficiency do present with recurrent sinopulmonary infections due to impaired antibody function. In particular, IgG2 deficiency is associated with recurrent respiratory infections with encapsulated organisms in children, and can be seen together with IgA deficiency. Selective IgA deficiency is one of the most common antibody deficiencies. Most individuals with IgA deficiency do not present with infections, since they have normal amounts of functioning IgG, but some do present with recurrent sinopulmonary and/or gastrointestinal infections. Rare cases have been reported of individuals with normal total IgG, IgA, IgM, and IgG subclass levels, but absent specific antibodies to polysaccharide antigens. These patients will demonstrate low titers of anti-pneumoccocal antibodies even after vaccination.

Evaluation of Cellular Immunity

Cellular immunity is mediated by T lymphocytes, and similar to the humoral immune system, defects in cellular immunity can be quantitative or functional [6]. The simplest test for quantitative T cell defects is the absolute lymphocyte number seen on a complete blood count (CBC). The absence of lymphocytes on a CBC should raise an immediate concern for a T cell immunodeficiency. However, in some cases enough circulating natural killer (NK) cells and B cells may be present, thereby leading to a lower normal peripheral blood lymphocyte number. In rare cases, engraftment of maternal T cells can raise the lymphocyte count in neonates. Ultimately flow cytometry is required to specifically quantify the number and types of T lymphocytes present. Table 6.2 summarizes the cell surface markers associated with different lymphocyte populations. Assessment of T cell function is performed by measuring the proliferation of peripheral blood mononuclear cells (which normally contain T cells) in response to a mitogen, such as phytohemagglutinin. The genetic basis for many T cell immunodeficiencies has been elucidated, and in some cases, testing for these specific gene mutations can be used for diagnosis.

Severe combined immunodeficiency (SCID) is characterized by near complete absence of T and B cells, and it represents the most severe form of cellular immunodeficiency. Most patients with SCID have severe lymphopenia, but as discussed

Table 6.2 Expression of cluster of differentiation (CD) cell surface markers on different immune cells

CD marker	Cell type
CD3	Expressed on all T cells
CD4	Helper T cells
CD8	Cytotoxic T cells (also expressed by some NK cells)
CD19 or CD20	Expressed on B cells
CD 16	Expressed on NK cells (not all)
CD 56	Expressed on the majority of NK cells
CD57	Expressed on the majority of NK cells; combinations of CD16/56/57 more reliably evaluate NK cell number than any individual marker
CD45RA	Naïve T cells
CD45RO	Memory T cells

NK natural killer cells (cytotoxic T lymphocytes involved in innate cellular immune responses)

above there may be rare cases where the lymphocyte count is low normal, so the diagnosis should be confirmed by flow cytometry. Because helper T cells are required to generate antibody responses, patients with SCID also lack Igs. The genetic basis of many forms of SCID has been identified. Although genetic testing is not usually used or required for diagnosis, this information may be helpful in identifying family members who are carriers or for future reproductive decision making by the parents of a child with SCID.

In addition to SCID, immunodeficiency can arise from other defects in cellular immunity. DiGeorge syndrome (DGS) results from errors in the formation of the third and fourth pharyngeal pouches during embryologic development. The majority (approximately 90 %) of patients with DGS have spontaneous heterozygous deletions in chromosome 22q11.2. The abnormality in embryologic development seen in DGS can lead to hypoplasia or complete absence of the thymus and adjacent parathyroid glands. Other midline structures, such as the heart and great vessels and craniofacial bones, may also be affected. There is a wide range in the degree of immunologic defect in children with DGS, from severe depression of T cell function in patients lacking a thymus, to normal or near normal function in children with mild thymic hypoplasia. Clinically, patients with DGSare classified as one of two subtypes, partial or complete DGS, based on the level of immunologic compromise. The majority of patients fall into the partial DGS classification. Complete DGS is considered a form of SCID, and this condition is fatal if not recognized early and treated with a thymic or bone marrow transplant. DGS can be diagnosed through clinical presentation and fluorescent in situ hybridization to detect microdeletions in chromosome 22q11.

Ataxia-telangiectasia (AT) is a complex multisystem autosomal recessive syndrome with associated abnormalities of the nervous system, endocrine system, skin, liver, and immune system. The defective gene in AT is located on chromosome 11q22.3, designated as the AT mutated gene (ATM). The ATM gene product is expressed in all tissues of the body, and is involved in detection of damaged DNA. The degree of immune dysfunction is variable in AT, but serum IgA and IgG subclasses can be low to absent, and may result in increased frequency of sinopulmonary infections with organisms such as *Streptococcus pneumoniae, Staphylococcus aureus, Haemophilus influenzae* and *Mycoplasma pneumoniae.* Various forms of chronic lung disease affect patients with AT. Aside from recurrent infections, patients can develop bronchiectasis, and also bronchiolitis obliterans and interstitial lung disease. Children with AT also have radiation-induced chromosomal fragility due to the inherent deficiency in DNA damage recognition and subsequent repair, and are at an increased risk for malignancy as a result. Thus, care should be taken to obtain the minimal amount of radiographic studies necessary to properly diagnose and/or monitor progression of disease. The diagnosis of AT is usually made clinically, but genetic testing for mutations in the ATM gene can also be performed.

Wiskott–Aldrich syndrome (WAS) is a rare X-linked disease characterized by eczema, thrombocytopenia, decreased Ig levels, and poor antibody responses. WAS is caused by mutations in the WAS protein (WASp). WASp plays an essential role in actin polymerization, which in turn is critical for T cell activation. Impaired T cell function then leads to the humoral immune abnormalities seen in WAS. WAS can be diagnosed by flow cytometric analysis of WASp expression in T cells, but definitive diagnosis is best made by analysis of WASp gene mutations.

Neutrophil Disorders

Polymorphonuclear neutrophils (PMNs) are the primary phagocytic cells of the immune system. They play a key role in eliminating opsonized bacterial and fungal pathogens through release of proteolytic enzymes and reactive oxidant species (ROS). This function may be impaired through abnormalities in cell adhesion, cell signaling, cell number, granule function or formation, and intracellular killing [7].

The most common PMN disorder is chronic granulomatous disease (CGD), with an estimated incidence of 1 in 200,000 in the USA. The primary defect in CGD is a loss of nicotinamide adenine dinucleotide phosphate-oxidase (NADPH) oxidase function. CGD exists in X-linked and autosomal recessive forms, depending on which gene coding for the NADPH oxidase complex is mutated; the X-linked form is more common. Loss of NADPH oxidase activity leads to a markedly reduced oxidative burst following phagocytosis. PMNs from patients with CGD can phagocytose bacteria, but cannot kill them, leading to the development of multiple large granulomas. Organisms that express catalase are particularly resistant to killing by PMNs from CGD patients, because catalase neutralizes any residual ROS produced by these patients by hydrolyzing superoxide to hydrogen peroxide. The most common catalase positive organisms that cause pulmonary infections in CGD are *Staphylococcus aureus* and *Aspergillus* species. *Burkholderia cepacia, Nocardia* species, and *Serratia marcescens* can also cause pulmonary infections in this group of patients.

Pneumonia caused by the aforementioned organisms is a common initial presentation in patients with CGD. Additional clinical features include atypical or unusually severe lymphadenitis, skin abscesses, and/or hepatomegaly. Less common initial presentations include intestinal lymphadenitis that can cause diarrhea and colitis and be mistaken for Crohn's disease. Pulmonary abscesses also occur frequently in patients with CGD. In a national CGD patient registry 16 % of patients had a lung abscess at some point in their course. Of those, the most common organism isolated was *Aspergillus* (23 %), although *Nocardia* species, *Burkholderia cepacia*, and *Staphylococcus* species can also cause abscesses.

The classic method to diagnose CGD is the nitroblue tetrazolium test (NBT), in which PMNs from the patient are incubated with beads impregnated with nitroblue tetrazolium dye. The PMNs naturally and spontaneously phagocytose the beads, and NADPH oxidation turns the dye blue. Performing a NBT is laborious, and the results can be subjective. For these reasons, the NBT has largely been supplanted by flow cytometry analysis of PMN oxidative burst activity. PMNs from the patient are loaded with an NADPH oxidative sensitive dye and then activated by incubation with phorbol ester and ionomycin [8]. Flow cytometry is then used to detect colorimetric changes induced by NADPH oxidase activity (Fig. 6.1).

Other PMN disorders include leukocyte adhesion molecule (LAM) deficiency, hyper-IgE syndrome, and Chediak–Higashi syndrome. LAM deficiency results from defects in expression of either integrin or selectin adhesion molecules on the surface of leukocytes. Without these adhesion molecules, PMNs cannot migrate to sites of infection. Delayed umbilical cord separation, marked leukocytosis, and chronic severe skin infections are common presenting signs. LAM deficiency can be diagnosed using flow cytometry staining for the specific adhesion molecules. Hyper-IgE syndrome (HIES) is a rare disorder of unknown etiology associated with impaired PMN function. Patients typically present with coarse facial features, recurrent skin infections, and extremely high serum IgE levels. Although some gene mutations have been linked to HIES, there is no specific diagnostic test at present, and the diagnosis is made clinically based on the appropriate clinical presentation and the exclusion of other conditions associated with high IgE levels (e.g., eczema or allergic bronchopulmonary aspergillosis). Chediak–Higashi syndrome (CHS) is an autosomal recessive disorder resulting from mutations in a lysosomal protein transport gene. Patients with CHS have multiple abnormalities, including reduced PMN phagocytosis and chemotaxis. In general, pulmonary complications in these disorders are very similar to those of CGD. Diagnosis of CHS is made by the characteristic appearance of the PMNs on microscopic examination. Mutations in the CHS-1 gene have also recently been identified as a cause for CHS.

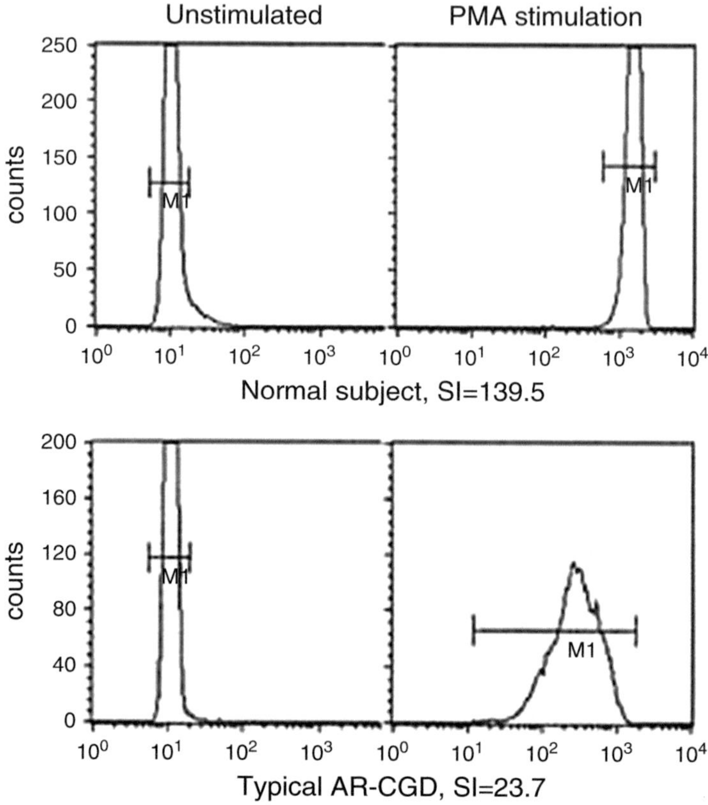

Fig. 6.1 Diagnosis of CGD by flow cytometry. Leukocytes were isolated from whole blood and incubated with dihydrorhodamine (DHR), an oxidase sensitive dye, and catalase. The cells were then stimulated with phorbol ester, which activates the neutrophils. In a normal control subject (panel **a**) there is a 2 log shift in DHR fluorescence with a signal intensity (SI) of 139.5, indicating an intact NADPH oxidase system. In contrast, neutrophils from a patient with X-linked CGD demonstrate no change in fluorescence after stimulation (panel **b**), and the SI is only 1.23. From Jirapongsananuruk et al. J Allergy Clin Immunol 2003;111:374–9

Hypersensitivity Pneumonitis

Hypersensitivity pneumonitis (HP), also known as extrinsic allergic alveolitis, represents a dysregulated pulmonary immune response to certain inhaled antigens [9]. A variety of animal and avian proteins, fungi, thermophilic bacteria, and small molecules have been implicated in triggering HP. In children, avian proteins account for the vast majority of identified triggers of HP (Fig. 6.2) [9].

The immunopathogenesis of HP involves both humoral (Gell and Coombs type III) and cell mediated (type IV) mechanisms. Recent animal and clinical studies have implicated type 1 helper T lymphocytes (TH1 cells) as playing a central role in

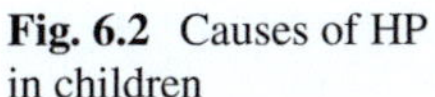
Fig. 6.2 Causes of HP in children

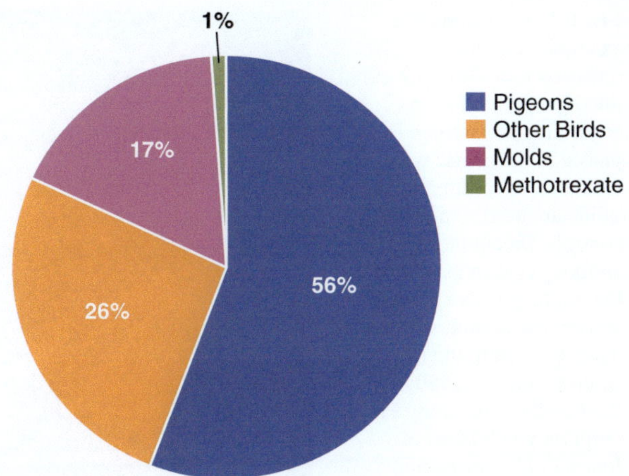

the pathogenesis of HP. In animal models of HP, high levels of interleukin 12 (IL-12), a cytokine produced preferentially by TH1 cells, are present. Conversely, inhibition of interferon gamma, another TH1 cytokine, protects animals against experimental HP. GATA-3 is a transcription factor that controls differentiation of T lymphocytes down the TH2 pathway, and transgenic mice that overexpress GATA-3 are protected from HP, because their T cells differentiate preferentially down the TH2 pathway Finally, adoptive transfer of TH1 cells from sensitized mice induce HP in naïve mice. Clinical evidence of the role of TH1 cells comes from bronchoalveolar lavage (BAL) studies, where elevated levels of IL-12 and CD4 positive TH1 cells have been seen.

There are three forms of HP: acute, subacute, and chronic. The acute form occurs within 1–2 days of antigen exposure and is accompanied by systemic signs of inflammation, such as fever and chills. Physical exam findings typically include diffuse crackles; pulmonary infiltrates are seen on chest radiograph. These acute symptoms resolve within a few days, providing there is no continued exposure to the offending antigen. The subacute form lasts from weeks to months, and is characterized by chronic cough and dyspnea. Chest radiographs at this stage will begin to show an interstitial inflammatory pattern. With continued antigen exposure, the disease transitions to a chronic form, with the development of pulmonary fibrosis.

Although the diagnosis of HP hinges primarily on a careful history and the appropriate clinical presentation, laboratory studies testing for antibodies against the offending agent can aid in the diagnosis. Most patients with HP demonstrate high titers of precipitating antibodies. These can be detected using gel diffusion, in which antigen in solution and the patient's serum are placed into wells in agar gel, along with appropriate controls (Fig. 6.3). As the antigen solution and serum diffuse into the agar, antigen–antibody immune complexes are formed, which precipitate out into the gel and form a visible line. A positive gel diffusion test demonstrates that the patient has been exposed to and developed an immune response against the offending agent. However, many individuals can develop antibody responses to HP

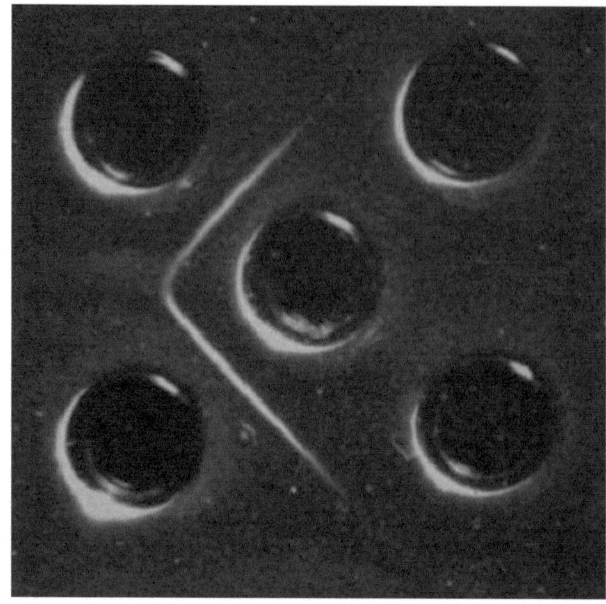

Fig. 6.3 Representative example of a positive gel diffusion test. Wells are cut into agar gel. Solution containing the antigen is placed in the center well. Nonreactive serum and saline are used as negative controls. Precipitating antibody is seen as a white line in the positive control and the test serum, while none are seen in the negative control wells. © 1959 Rockefeller University Press. Originally published in Journal of Experimental Medicine. 109:94–114

antigens without developing disease. Conversely, antibody tests can be falsely negative if the correct antigens are not used in the test. Therefore, HP ultimately is a clinical diagnosis, in which laboratory studies are supportive, but not diagnostic by themselves.

Allergic Bronchopulmonary Aspergillosis

Allergic bronchopulmonary aspergillosis (ABPA) is a hypersensitivity pneumonitis with allergic features triggered by exposure to *Aspergillus* mold [10]. Although ABPA can be triggered by a variety of *Aspergillus* species, by far the most common trigger is *Aspergillus fumigatus* (Af). The prevalence of ABPA is increased in patients with asthma and cystic fibrosis (CF). At some CF Centers, the prevalence of ABPA is reported to be as high as 15 %, although the overall national prevalence is estimated at 2 %. The pathogenesis of ABPA is thought to arise from a TH2 driven hypersensitivity immune response. TH2 cells secrete IL-4, IL-5, and IL-13, which promote recruitment of eosinophils to the lung and production of anti-Af IgE.

The diagnostics of ABPA can often be difficult because the clinical features of ABPA overlap with other conditions and clinicians have used varying diagnostic criteria. The most commonly used diagnostic criteria are shown in Table 6.3 [10]. The presence of 6 or more major criteria is usually accepted as diagnostic of ABPA, but patients with fewer than 6 major criteria can still be considered to have ABPA based on the clinician's judgment. ABPA can be further subdivided into seropositive ABPA (ABPA-S) and ABPA with central bronchiectasis (ABPA-CB). The minimal diagnostic criteria for ABPA-S and ABPA-CB are shown in Table 6.4. It should be emphasized

Table 6.3 Diagnostic criteria for ABPA

Major criteria
• Asthma
• Pulmonary infiltrates on chest radiograph
• Immediate skin test reactivity to Af (or equivalent positive serum test)
• Eosinophilia
• Precipitating antibodies (IgG) to Af
• Elevated total serum IgE >1,000 IU/mL
• Central bronchiectasis
• Elevated specific serum IgE and IgG to Af
Minor criteria
• Presence of Aspergillus in sputum
• Expectoration of brownish black mucus plugs
• Delayed skin reaction to Aspergillus antigen

Table 6.4 Minimal diagnostic criteria for ABPA-S and ABPA-C

ABPA-S
• Asthma
• Immediate cutaneous hyperreactivity to Aspergillus antigens
• Transient pulmonary infiltrates on chest radiograph
• Elevated IgE
Raised *A f*-specific IgG and IgE
ABPA-CB
• Asthma
• Immediate cutaneous hyperreactivity to Aspergillus antigens
• Central bronchiectasis
• Elevated IgE
• Raised *A f*-specific IgG and IgE

that these diagnostic criteria were developed for adult patients, but in the absence of similar criteria for children, they are usually applied to the pediatric population as well. Patients with CF present an additional diagnostic challenge, since bronchiectasis is a normal feature of the disease and Af can frequently be present in the sputum in the absence of ABPA. The CF Foundation (CFF) recently held a consensus conference to develop diagnostic criteria for ABPA in CF patients, which resulted in definitions of classic cases of ABPA and minimal diagnostic criteria (Table 6.5) [11].

As can be seen from the diagnostic criteria, laboratory studies play a key role in the diagnosis of ABPA [10, 11]. Since an elevated IgE is a feature of any form of ABPA, total IgE is the recommended screening test for ABPA. The CFF consensus conference recommends doing this test annually in CF patients. In CF patients, an IgE >500 IU/mL is considered suspicious for ABPA, and levels of 200–500 IU/mL should be repeated. In non-CF patients, the cutoff is >1,000 IU/mL. It is important to note that some laboratories report IgE as ng/ml and 1 IU=2.4 ng. Therefore, attention should always be paid to the units on the laboratory report. If a patient's

Table 6.5 CF Foundation Consensus Conference criteria for classic ABPA diagnosis and minimal diagnosis of ABPA

Classic case
• Acute or subacute clinical deterioration not attributable to another etiology
• Serum total IgE concentration of >1,000 IU/mL[a]
• Immediate cutaneous reactivity to Af or equivalent positive serum test
• Precipitating antibodies or serum IgG antibodies to Af
• New or recent abnormalities on chest radiograph or CT that have not cleared with antibiotics and standard physiotherapy
Minimal diagnostic criteria
• Acute or subacute clinical deterioration not attributable to another etiology
• Total serum IgE concentration of >500 IU/mL[b]
• Immediate cutaneous reactivity to Af or in vitro demonstration of IgE antibody to Af
• One of the following:
– Precipitins to Af or in vitro demonstration of IgG antibody *to Af*
– New or recent abnormalities on chest radiograph or chest CT that have not cleared with antibiotics and standard physiotherapy

[a]Unless patient is receiving systemic corticosteroids (if so, retest when steroid treatment is discontinued)

[b]If ABPA is suspected and the total IgE level is 200–500 IU/mL, repeat testing in 1–3 months is recommended. If patient is taking steroids, repeat when steroid treatment is discontinued

screening IgE raises concern for ABPA, the next step is to look for evidence of anti-Af IgE and IgG. The former can be detected either by prick skin testing with Af antigen or an in vitro serum test of anti-Af IgE, such as RAST testing. Anti-Af IgG can be detected using a precipitating antibody test. Other diagnostic tests used in research only include assays of lymphocyte responses to Af or IgE and IgG responses to recombinant Af allergens or peptides . In addition to its role as a screening test for ABPA, measurement of total IgE can also be used as a way to track treatment response, remission, and relapse of ABPA.

Autoimmune Pulmonary Disease

The lung can be involved in a variety of autoimmune diseases [12, 13]. Although much more common in adults, these diseases can present in childhood. Pulmonary hemorrhage can be seen in systemic lupus erythematosis (SLE), Henoch–Schonlein purpura (HSP), and Goodpasture's syndrome. SLE is diagnosed through a combination of clinical features and positive anti-nuclear antibodies. There are no serologic diagnostic tests for HSP; it is usually diagnosed clinically, although immunofluorescence staining of the kidney will demonstrate IgA deposition. Goodpasture's syndrome is caused by antibodies directed against glomerular basement membrane (GBM) proteins, some of which cross react with similar proteins in the lung. The diagnosis can be made through measurement of serum anti-GBM antibodies. Idiopathic pulmonary hemorrhage (IPH) is a rare condition of recurrent hemoptysis for which no underlying etiology can be determined. IPH is thought to be immune-mediated and is often treated with immunosuppressive therapy. Some cases of IPH have been reported to be associated with positive precipitating antibodies to milk protein, although the causative role of milk protein is controversial. Nonetheless, many clinicians will evaluate patients with IPH for milk precipitins and if they are positive limit milk protein from the patient's diet.

There are several vasculitides that can affect both the upper airway and the lungs. These diseases are extremely rare in the pediatric population [13]. The diagnosis of pulmonary vasculitides is based on the clinical presentation and laboratory markers. Measurement of anti-neutrophil cytoplasmic antibodies (ANCAs) is an important element of the diagnostic workup of patients with suspected vasculitis. Three different ANCA staining patterns have been described: cytoplasmic (c-ANCA), perinuclear (p-ANCA), and atypical (a-ANCA). C-ANCAs bind to proteinase-3, a serine protease contained in neutrophil granules. They are most commonly associated with granulomatosis with polyangitis (formerly known as Wegener's disease), a multisystem disorder characterized by erosive sinusitis, obstructive airway disease, pulmonary nodules, alveolar hemorrhage, and gloumerulonephritis. C-ANCAs are both sensitive and specific for this condition. In general p-ANCAs are directed against myeloperoxidase, and the perinuclear staining pattern is an artifact resulting ethanol fixation of the microscope slide. P-ANCAs are elevated in Churg–Strauss Syndrome (CSS), which is characterized by asthma, eosinophilia, and neuropathy. However, p-ANCAs can also be elevated in a number of other autoimmune diseases, so an elevated p-ANCA titer is not necessarily diagnostic of CSS. A-ANCAs demonstrate a staining pattern that does not fit either a perinuclear or cytoplasmic pattern. They also tend to be nonspecifically associated with a variety of autoimmune diseases. Table 6.6 lists some of the autoimmune diseases with prominent respiratory tract involvement, some of their clinical features, and associated laboratory findings.

Table 6.6 Autoimmune diseases with pulmonary involvement

Disease	Pulmonary manifestations	Serologic findings
Systemic lupus erythematosis	Pulmonary hemorrhage/hemoptysis	+ANA
Henoch–Schonlein purpura	Pulmonary hemorrhage/hemoptysis	None
Idiopathic pulmonary hemosiderosis	Pulmonary hemorrhage/hemoptysis	+ Precipitating antibodies to milk protein[a]
Goodpasture's syndrome	Pulmonary hemorrhage/hemoptysis	+ Anti-GBM antibodies
Granulomatosis with polyangitis (formerly known as Wegener's disease)	Upper airway disease (sinusitis, mastoiditis)	+c- ANCA (cytoplasmic staining pattern)
	Pulmonary nodules, granulomas, and infiltrates	
	Pulmonary hemorrhage	
Churg–Strauss syndrome	Asthma	+p-ANCA
	Pulmonary infiltrates	

ANA antinuclear antibodies, *GBM* glomerular basement membrane, *c-ANCA* anti-neutrophil cytoplasmic antibodies with a cytoplasmic staining pattern, *p-ANCA* anti-neutrophil cytoplasmic antibodies with a perinuclear staining pattern
[a]In some cases

References

1. Bernstein IL, Li JT, Bernstein DI, Hamilton R, Spector SL, Tan R, et al. Allergy diagnostic testing: an updated practice parameter. Ann Allergy Asthma Immunol. 2008;100(3):S1–148.
2. Bagg A, Chacko T, Lockey R. Reactions to prick and intradermal skin tests. Ann Allergy Asthma Immunol. 2009;102(5):400–2. Epub 2009/06/06.
3. Norrman G, Falth-Magnusson K. Adverse reactions to skin prick testing in children – prevalence and possible risk factors. Pediatr Allergy Immunol. 2009;20(3):273–8. Epub 2009/02/18.
4. Bernstein DI, Wanner M, Borish L, Liss GM. Twelve-year survey of fatal reactions to allergen injections and skin testing: 1990–2001. J Allergy Clin Immunol. 2004;113(6):1129–36. Epub 2004/06/23.
5. Ballow M. Primary immunodeficiency disorders: antibody deficiency. J Allergy Clin Immunol. 2002;109(4):581–91. Epub 2002/04/10.
6. Buckley RH. Primary cellular immunodeficiencies. J Allergy Clin Immunol. 2002;109(5): 747–57. Epub 2002/05/08.
7. Lekstrom-Himes JA, Gallin JI. Immunodeficiency diseases caused by defects in phagocytes. N Engl J Med. 2000;343(23):1703–14.
8. Jirapongsananuruk O, Malech HL, Kuhns DB, Niemela JE, Brown MR, Anderson-Cohen M, et al. Diagnostic paradigm for evaluation of male patients with chronic granulomatous disease, based on the dihydrorhodamine 123 assay. J Allergy Clin Immunol. 2003;111(2):374–9.
9. Fan LL. Hypersensitivity pneumonitis in children. Curr Opin Pediatr. 2002;14(3):323–6.
10. Agarwal R. Allergic bronchopulmonary aspergillosis. Chest. 2009;135(3):805–26. Epub 2009/03/07.
11. Stevens DA, Moss RB, Kurup VP, Knutsen AP, Greenberger P, Judson MA, et al. Allergic bronchopulmonary aspergillosis in cystic fibrosis – state of the art: Cystic Fibrosis Foundation Consensus Conference. Clin Infect Dis. 2003;37 Suppl 3:S225–64.
12. Frankel SK, Schwarz MI. The pulmonary vasculitides. Am J Respir Crit Care Med. 2012;186(3):216–24.
13. Godfrey S. Pulmonary hemorrhage/hemoptysis in children. Pediatr Pulmonol. 2004;37(6): 476–84.

Chapter 7
Interpretation of Pulmonary Function Tests in Clinical Practice

Anastassios C. Koumbourlis

Abstract Pulmonary function tests (PFTs) are diagnostic modalities that evaluate qualitatively and quantitatively the size and function of the lungs. The most common areas of evaluation in clinical practice are: (a) the measurement of the lung volume, (b) the assessment and measurement of the airway function (upper and lower), and (c) the ability of the lung to diffuse oxygen. Several other tests can be performed to evaluate specific aspects of the lung function such as lung or respiratory system compliance and resistance, airway hyperreactivity/hyperresponsiveness, airway inflammation. This chapter focuses on the principles of interpretation (and its pitfalls) of the most commonly used tests that are commercially available for use in children and adolescents in an inpatient or outpatient setting.

Keywords Pulmonary function tests • Lung volume • Airway function • Airway hyperreactivity/hyperresponsiveness • Airway inflammation

Indications

PFTs are not pathognomonic of a specific disease but they can be highly specific of the type of the disease process (e.g., obstructive vs. restrictive lung disease) and most importantly of which component of the lung function is affected. In general, obtaining PFTs should be considered in the following situations: (a) to determine the specific nature of an unknown disease process (e.g., obstructive vs. restrictive lung defects); (b) to study the progression of a known condition (e.g., changes in lung function in a patient with cystic fibrosis); (c) to evaluate the effect of a particular therapy (e.g., reversibility of lower airway obstruction after treatment with bronchodilator); (d) to establish a baseline in patients whose lung function may be

A.C. Koumbourlis, M.D., M.P.H. (✉)
Division of Pulmonary and Sleep Medicine, Children's National Medical Center/George Washington University, School of Medicine and Health Sciences, Washington, DC, USA

Children's National Medical Center, 111 Michigan Avenue, N.W., Washington, DC 20010, USA
e-mail: akoumbou@childrensnational.org

© Springer Science+Business Media New York 2015
S.D. Davis et al. (eds.), *Diagnostic Tests in Pediatric Pulmonology*,
Respiratory Medicine, DOI 10.1007/978-1-4939-1801-0_7

affected in various often unpredictable ways either by a disease process and/or by its treatment (e.g., a patient with malignancy who is about to start treatment with radiation and chemotherapy).

Evaluation of Lung Volumes

Background

Volume is the amount of space taken up by an object, whereas capacity is the amount of a substance that can be held by an object. If the object has a fixed volume, its capacity will depend on the substance that is filling it (e.g., air vs. liquid). In the case of the respiratory system, lung volume is the space the lungs occupy inside the thoracic cavity and lung capacity is the amount of air the lungs can hold. The lung volume and the corresponding capacity are not fixed, but they change as the lungs inflate and deflate.

The evaluation of lung volumes consists of measurements at different phases of the respiratory cycle. The total lung capacity (TLC) is the maximum amount of air that the lungs can hold (Fig. 7.1). Functional residual capacity (FRC) is the amount of air that fills the lungs in between breaths, and it is at that level where the actual breathing occurs. The tidal volume (VT) (the amount of air taken into the lungs with a regular breath), inflates the lungs above the level of FRC. The amount of air that can fill the lungs from FRC to TLC is the inspiratory capacity (IC), whereas, the maximal amount of air that can be emptied from FRC with a maximal exhalation is the expiratory reserve volume (ERV). The amount of air that remains inside the

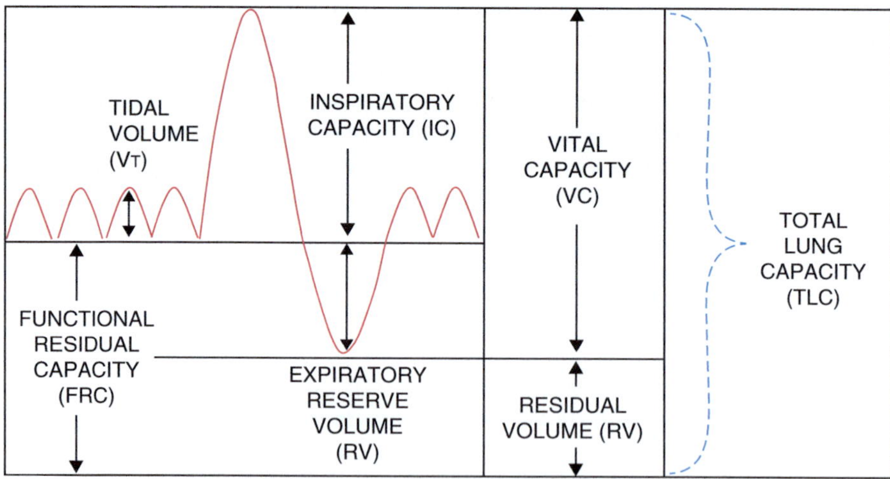

Fig. 7.1 Schematic representation of the total lung capacity and its various subdivisions (for explanation of the abbreviations, see text)

Table 7.1 Relationships between lung volumes and capacities

Index	Relationship to TLC	Relationship to each other
FVC (or SVC)	FVC/TLC: ~75 %	
FRC	FRC/TLC: ~50 %	
IC	IC/TLC: ~50 %	IC/FVC: ~66 %
RV	RV/TLC: ~25 %	RV/FRC: ~50 %
ERV	ERV/TLC: ~25 %	ERV/FRC: ~50 %
IRV	IRV/TLC: ~40 %	IRV/IC: ~80 %

lungs after a maximal exhalation is the residual volume (RV). The amount of air that can inflate the lungs from RV to TLC is the slow (or inspiratory) vital capacity (SVC), whereas the amount of air that can be exhaled during a forced exhalation from TLC to RV is the forced vital capacity (FVC).

The TLC, RV, and FRC are "static" lung volumes (also referred to as "absolute" volumes), whereas all the others are "dynamic." The static lung volumes depend on the interactions between the compliance and elastic recoil of the lung and of the chest wall, as well as on the strength of the respiratory muscles. Diseases and conditions affecting the lung parenchyma such as fibrosis, interstitial lung disease, pulmonary edema, atelectasis, etc. are characterized by low lung compliance that limits the distensibility of the lungs, and thus the TLC. The same is true for conditions limiting the expansion of the chest wall, either due to chest wall deformity (severe kyphoscoliosis, asphyxiating thoracic dystrophy, etc.), and/or due to respiratory muscle weakness (e.g., spinal muscular atrophy). The FRC depends on the balance between the elastic recoil of the lungs and of the chest wall. The RV depends on the expiratory muscle strength, the elastic recoil of the lung and of the chest wall, and on the airway closure. Thus, elevated RV can occur both due to premature airway closure as in obstructive lung diseases, but also due to thoracic cage abnormalities or expiratory muscle weakness that prevent the chest wall from returning to its neutral position. In a normal healthy lung the various measured volumes and capacities are in a specific and pretty consistent relationship to each other, that changes relatively little throughout life (Table 7.1).

Lung volumes can be measured with three basic methods. It is beyond the scope of this chapter to explain in detail the theory behind and the technical aspects of each method. However, it is important to know and understand their basic differences because they often have a direct impact on the interpretation of the results. The first method is based on gas dilution. Its two most common applications are the Helium dilution and the Nitrogen washout. In the Helium dilution technique, the patient is breathing a tracer gas (Helium) from a container with known volume. When steady state is achieved, the Helium is equilibrated between the lungs and the container. The difference in the volume of the container before and after the equilibrium has been achieved is assumed to represent the FRC. In the Nitrogen washout, the patient is breathing 100 % oxygen that "washes" the nitrogen out of the lungs. Since the nitrogen exists in a fixed concentration in the lungs and it is not diffused into the blood stream like the oxygen, the measured amount that is washed out can be used to calculate the FRC. Both techniques are performed while the patient breathes with regular tidal breaths and thus they require minimal cooperation from the patient.

The second method is the body plethysmography that measures the compressible thoracic volume during a panting maneuver. The technique is sensitive, reproducible and accurate. However, it requires a certain level of cooperation from the patient that cannot be achieved by young children. Body plethysmography measures the air in the thoracic cavity (TGV), not just in the lungs. The third method is the estimation of lung volume from standard chest radiographs (or from computed tomography) based on mathematical formulas that measure the volume within the perimeter of the thoracic cage and the diaphragm (minus the volume of the mediastinum). This technique is very rarely used in clinical practice especially in pediatrics.

In a healthy normal individual there is very little difference between the measurements made by the gas dilution techniques compared with those obtained by body plethysmography. However, significant differences do exist when measurements are made in patients with obstructive lung disease. This is because the gas dilution techniques are measuring the communicating gas volume whereas the body plethysmography measures the compressible gas volume in the thoracic cavity. Thus, in cases of severe air-trapping or of non-communicating air-filled cystic lesions, the gas dilution techniques tend to underestimate the lung volume. On the other hand body plethysmography may overestimate the lung volume because it may take into account even air that is not in the thoracic cavity (e.g., abdominal "bloating," or large oropharyngeal cavity). Therefore, when comparing results it is important to know what technique was used for each of the measurements. Ideally, both techniques should be used. In such case, the difference between the TGV and the FRC is assumed to represent the true air-trapping.

Interpretation

The critical parameter for the interpretation of lung volumes is the TLC. If it is below the predicted normal values then there is loss of lung volume. An increased TLC can be found either in cases of generalized hyperinflation or in individuals with large lungs (fairly commonly seen in athletes). What determines the type of a disease process (i.e., restrictive or obstructive) is the relationship of the TLC to its subdivisions. Thus, in a healthy individual the TLC and all of its subdivisions are within the normal range and proportional to each other as outlined in Table 7.1. Similarly, in restrictive lung defects, the TLC and all of its subdivisions are proportionately decreased, so the ratios of the various subdivisions to TLC remain the same as in a healthy lung. In contrast, in obstructive lung diseases the TLC can be normal, increased (in case of generalized hyperinflation) or even decreased (in case of a mixed defect). However, regardless of the actual value of TLC, the ratios of RV/TLC, FRC/TLC are increased and as a result the VC and the IC are going to be decreased.

There are very limited data on lung volumes for non-Caucasians. Blacks are supposed to have smaller lung volumes than whites by approximately 15 %. In some PFT laboratories, the software automatically subtracts 15 % of the predicted normal values for whites but in others this has to be done manually, otherwise all black patients will appear to have a "restrictive lung disease." Thus, when interpreting a test that was performed in an outside laboratory, it is very important to determine what predicted normal values the laboratory is using. There is very little information on lung volumes for other racial groups (although Hispanics tend to have values that are more similar to whites than blacks).

Evaluation of the Airway Function

Background

The respiratory tract is essentially a continuum that starts from the nose and ends in the alveoli. For purposes of convenience the different segments of the respiratory tree are classified as into "upper" airways, that consist of the nose, pharynx, larynx and the extrathoracic part of the trachea, and the "lower" airways, that include the intrathoracic trachea, and all generations of the bronchii. The intrathoracic airways are further divided into the large or "central" airways (main stem, lobar and segmental bronchii) and the small or "peripheral" airways. These distinctions are useful because different diseases processes and conditions affect primarily or selectively some but not all (or at least not to the same degree) of these groups.

The evaluation of the airway function essentially refers to the direct or indirect measurement of the resistance to airflow posed by the airways. Although direct measurements of the airway resistance can be made, the most commonly used evaluation in clinical practice is the spirometry/maximal expiratory flow–volume curve (MEFVC) (Fig. 7.2). The test is performed with a forced exhalation from TLC to RV, the latter being the point when there is no more flow. The exhaled volume is

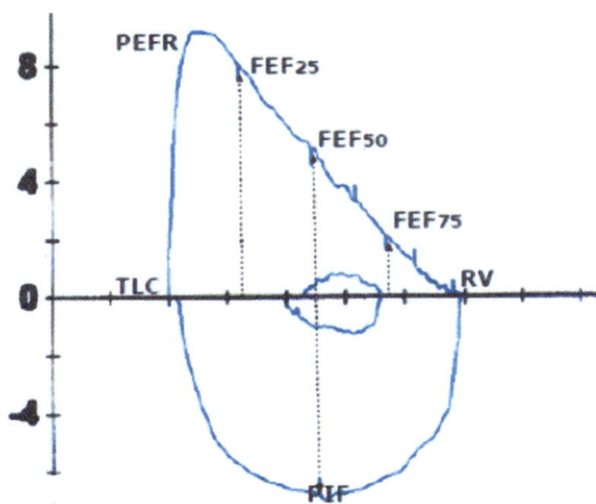

Fig. 7.2 Normal maximal expiratory and inspiratory flow–volume curve depicting the various indices of lung function. Note the difference in the shape of the expiratory and inspiratory curves as well as the small size of the tidal breath relative to FVC

plotted against time, thus allowing its extrapolation into flow rate. Measurements are being made either on volumes exhaled in a particular unit of time (e.g., FEV_1 is the volume exhaled during the first second of exhalation) or in terms of flow rate at specific levels of lung deflation. Although measurements can be made at any level, the standard measurements usually include the maximal expiratory flow (FEFmax), and the forced expiratory flow rates when 25 %, 50 % and 75 % (FEF_{25}, FEF_{50} and FEF_{75}) of the FVC has been exhaled. The average flow rate between 20 and 75 % of FVC (FEF_{25-75}) is also calculated.

The rationale for and clinical significance of these measurements is based on the fact that the volume of exhaled air and the flow rates measured in the beginning of exhalation (roughly during the first 25 % of the vital capacity) reflect primarily the resistance to airflow posed by the large airways, whereas the flow rates measured towards the end exhalation (generally after 50 % of the vital capacity has been exhaled), reflect primarily the resistance of the small peripheral airways. Thus, the test provides not only a quantitative assessment of the obstruction but it can also specify which part of the tracheobronchial tree is primarily affected. More specifically, the proximal portion of the MEFV curve (approximately between 100 and 75 % of the FVC) reflects the function of the large airways (distal trachea, main stem bronchii, segmental bronchii) and is represented primarily by the PEFR, FEF_{25} and in part by the FEV_1. The middle portion of the curve (reflected by the FEF_{25}, FEF_{50}, and in part by the FEV_1 and the FEF_{25-75}) represents the function of the medium sized central airways. The distal portion of the curve (represented by the FEF_{75} and in part by the FEF_{25-75}) reflects the function of the small peripheral airways.

One of the major advantages of the MEFVCs is that they are in part "effort independent." The beginning of the forced exhalation (that includes the FEFmax, the FEV_1, and the FEF_{25}), depends primarily on the strength of the expiratory muscles and on the overall understanding and cooperation of the patient and therefore it is "effort dependent." In contrast, the later part of the exhalation depends entirely on the elastic recoil of the lungs, and thus it is "effort independent." Figure 7.3a, b illustrates this point. Figure 7.3a shows three superimposed curves with the same vital capacity but with different degree of effort during exhalation. Although the FEFmax, the FEF_{25}, and the FEF_{50} vary significantly between the different curves, the flows at the distal end are virtually identical. Similarly, in Fig. 7.3b there are several superimposed MEFV curves produced with the same amount of effort but from different volumes. The curves are very different in their proximal (effort dependent) limb, but they are virtually identical in their distal end that consists of the effort independent portion. As a result measurements made in the effort dependent portion of the MEFV curve should be interpreted with caution especially if there is doubt about the amount of effort the patient made.

The function of the upper airways can be evaluated with the performance of maximal inspiratory flow–volume (MIFV) curves produced with a maximal breath from RV to TLC. In contrast with the triangular shape of the MEFV curve, the MIFV curve of a person with normal extrathoracic airways has a semicircular shape (Fig. 7.2). As a result, the maximal inspiratory flow occurs at approximately 50 %

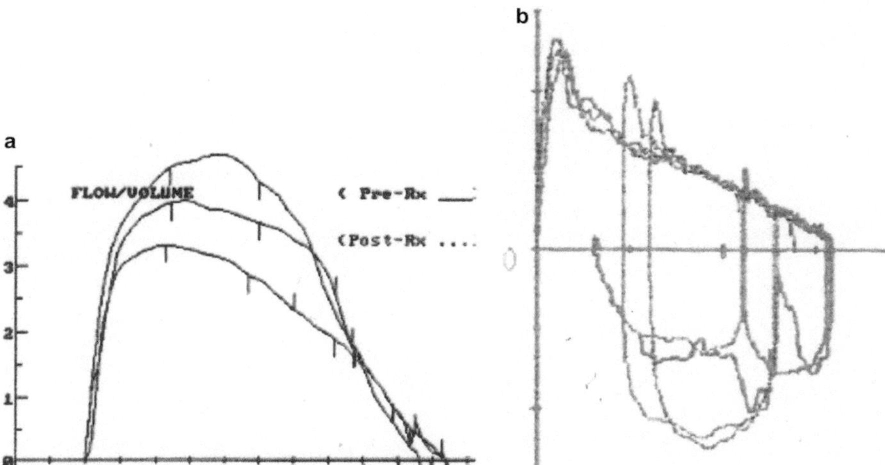

Fig. 7.3 (**a**) Three superimposed expiratory flow–volume curves with virtually the same FVC, but produced with different effort. As a result there is significant difference in the measured FEFmax and FEF$_{25}$. However, there are no differences in the distal end of the MEFVC that is the effort-independent portion. (**b**) Multiple MEFVCs with different volume but produced with the same amount of effort. The MEFVCs differ in the FVC but their distal (effort independent) portion is superimposable

of the VC, thus corresponding with the FEF$_{50}$ and not with the FEFmax that is measured in the very beginning of forced exhalation. In a healthy lung with normal airways the ratio of FEF$_{50}$/FIFmax is approximately 1.

Interpretation of Maximal Expiratory Flow–Volume Curves

Disease processes affect not only the values of measured parameters but the overall shape of the MFVCs as well. Thus, a fairly accurate qualitative assessment of the nature of the problem can be often made by the visual inspection of the curves. The following patterns can be identified.

- "Normal" (Fig. 7.2): The expiratory curve that has the shape of a "right triangle," with a sharp peak and a straight (and occasionally convex) descending limb (in reality, the angle between the ascending limb and the horizontal axis is less than 90°). The inspiratory MFV curve has a very different configuration resembling "half-circle."
- "Obstructive" (Fig. 7.4): The MEFV curve of a patient with obstructive lung disease has a characteristic concave appearance. The degree of concavity varies and it may involve only part or the entire length of the expiratory limb. The small, peripheral airways are the first and more severely affected, whereas the larger airways can be relatively spared. It is not uncommon, to have significant (even severe) decrease in FEF$_{25-75}$ but "normal" FEV$_1$ and FEFmax. It is important to note that the inspiratory MFVC is usually not affected in obstructive lung defects.

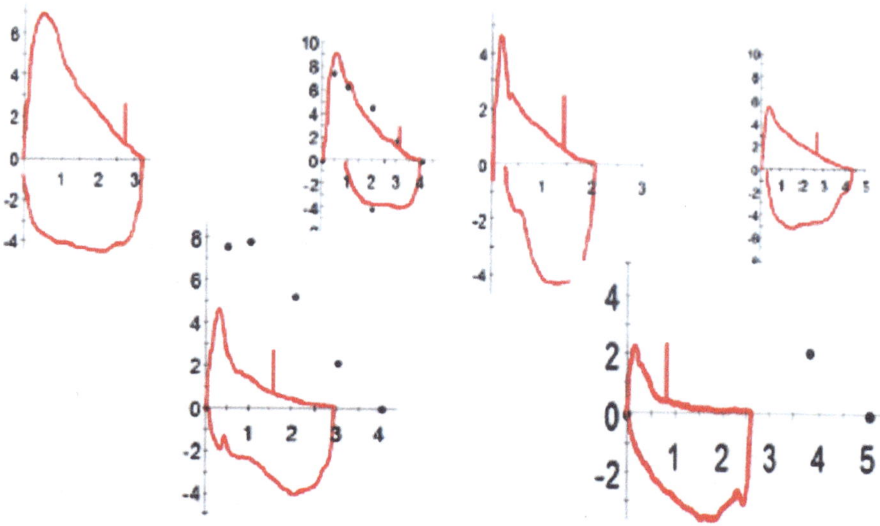

Fig. 7.4 Different variations of lower airway obstruction. All MEFVCs show concavity in their distal end indicating small airway obstruction but only some show significant involvement of the large airways. Note that in all of them the degree of lower airway obstruction has minimal or no effect on the inspiratory flows

- "Restrictive" pattern (Fig. 7.5): The MFEV curve in restrictive lung defects may look like a "miniature" normal. However, because they are usually associated with conditions that cause an increase in the elastic recoil of the lungs, the produced expiratory flow rates are higher than normal and the MEFVC has a very tall and narrow shape, almost resembling an "isosceles triangle." In such cases, the inspiratory MIFV curve may be a "mirror image" of the MEFV curve.
- "Variable intrathoracic soft tissue obstruction" (Fig. 7.6): Conditions such as tracheobronchomalacia that affect the large and central airways, produce a characteristic flattening of the proximal portion of the MEFVC. In such cases the maximal inspiratory flow–volume curve is usually normal.
- "Variable extrathoracic soft tissue obstruction" (Fig. 7.7): Affected patients have a very characteristic flattening of the inspiratory portion of the MFVC, whereas the expiratory portion remains unaffected. A ratio of $FEF_{50}/FIFmax > 1.2$ is highly suggestive of variable extrathoracic soft tissue obstruction.
- "Fixed airway obstruction" (Fig. 7.8): A fixed airway obstruction produces a very characteristic flattening of the inspiratory and expiratory portions of the MFVC (Fig. 7.8a). In such cases the obstruction is in the large intrathoracic airways (e.g., vocal cords, subglottic space, mid-trachea). Affected patients present with a biphasic (inspiratory/expiratory) sound that is a mixture of "harsh wheeze" and "muffled stridor." The noise will be worse with activity and diminishes during sleep due to the shallow breathing. Although fixed airway obstruction is usually due to a structural abnormality, it can be also caused by functional

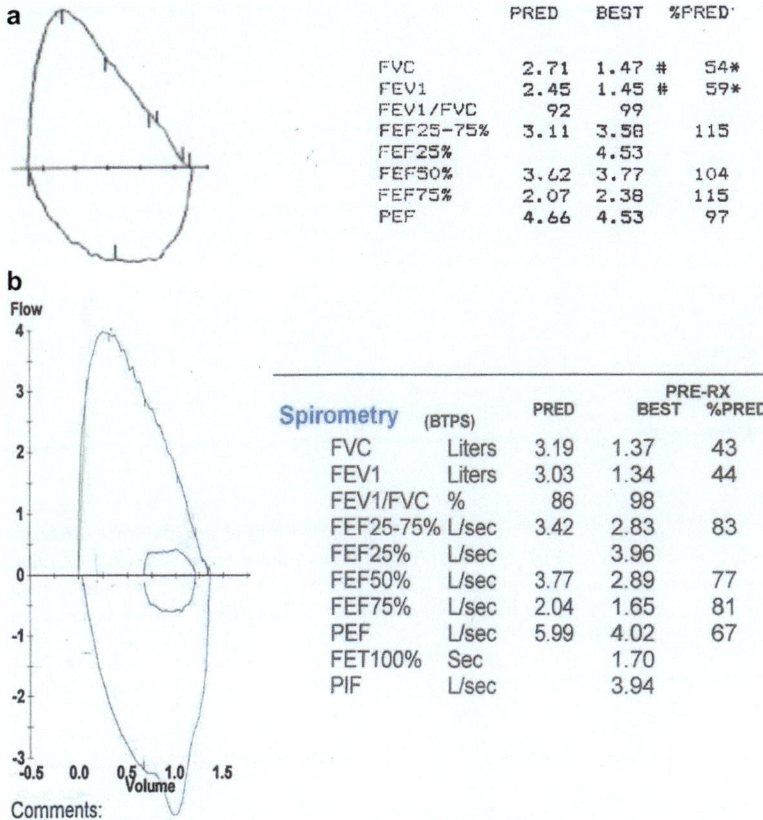

Fig. 7.5 (**a**) The MEFVC in patients with restrictive lung defect often resembles a "miniature" of a normal MEFVC. (**b**) Severe restrictive lung defects (often seen in patients with chest wall muscle weakness) present with a characteristic tall and narrow flow–volume curve, in which the inspiratory curve appears like a "mirror-image" of the expiratory curve

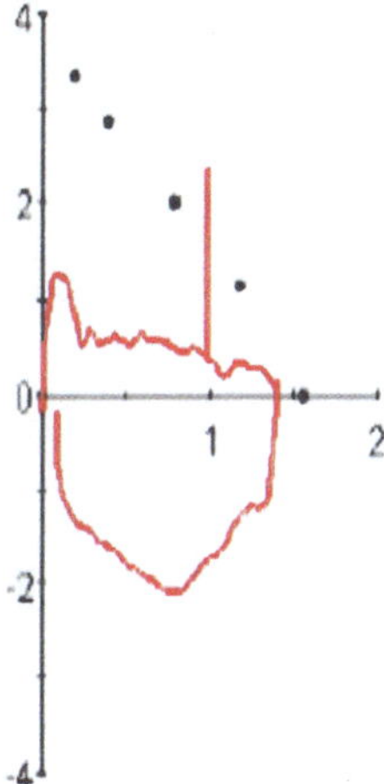

Fig. 7.6 Patient with severe tracheobronchomalacia following repair of tracheoesophageal fistula at birth. The airway closes almost immediately after the beginning of exhalation limiting all the measured expiratory flow rates. However, there is virtually no effect on the inspiratory flows

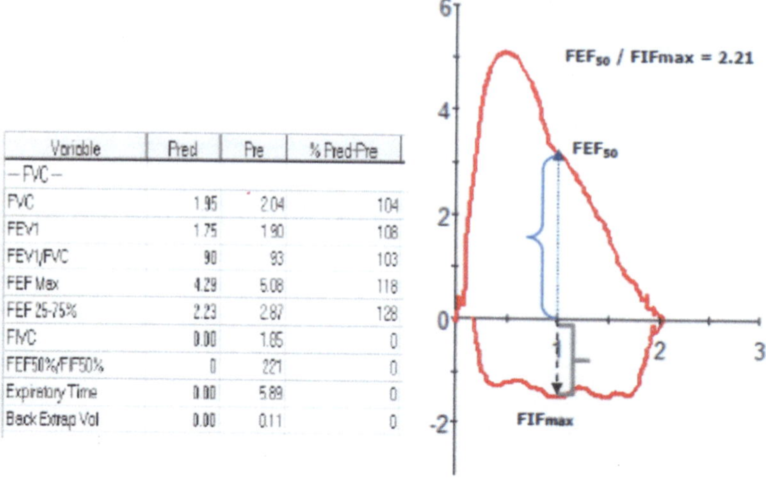

Fig. 7.7 The inspiratory flow–volume curve is flattened limiting the maximal inspiratory flow (FIF$_{50}$) to less than half of the FEF$_{50}$. The expiratory flow–volume curve is normal. Similar picture can be seen in a healthy normal individual due to closure of the vocal cords during inspiration. Thus, it is imperative to document that the flattening of the inspiratory flow–volume curve occurs consistently in all the efforts

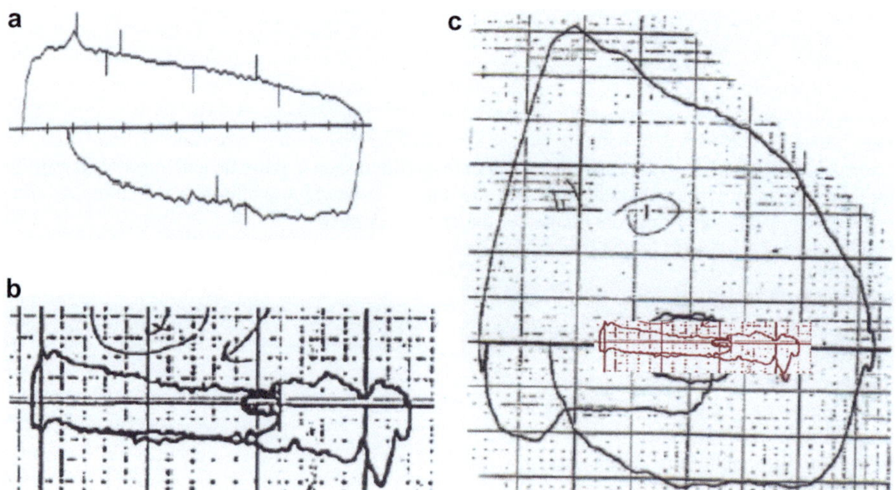

Fig. 7.8 (**a**) Acquired tracheal stenosis secondary to radiation therapy for lymphoma. The fact that both the expiratory and inspiratory flow–volume curves are flattened to the same degree indicates that the obstruction is very high up in the tracheobronchial tree (mid-trachea). (**b**) The test shows very severe fixed airway obstruction. The patient had audible inspiratory and expiratory wheezing but no hypoxemia. (**c**) Repeat effort a few minutes later produced a normal flow–volume curve. The patient had received no medication but she had been distracted through conversation. This is characteristic of vocal cord dysfunction

disorders such as vocal cord dysfunction (Fig. 7.8b). The patient may present with severe inspiratory/expiratory wheezing, not responding to any treatment and they are usually anxious or panicky. If they can perform spirometry they produce a picture of very severe fixed airway obstruction that resolves spontaneously as soon as the patient relaxes (Fig. 7.8c).

Pitfalls in the Interpretation of MEFVCs

There are several potential pitfalls in the performance of MFVCs that may affect their interpretation. The most common ones, especially among young children are due to poor technique/effort.

1. "Incomplete" (Fig. 7.9): the patient stopped the exhalation prematurely, before it reached the point of RV. This is reflected in the abrupt termination of the

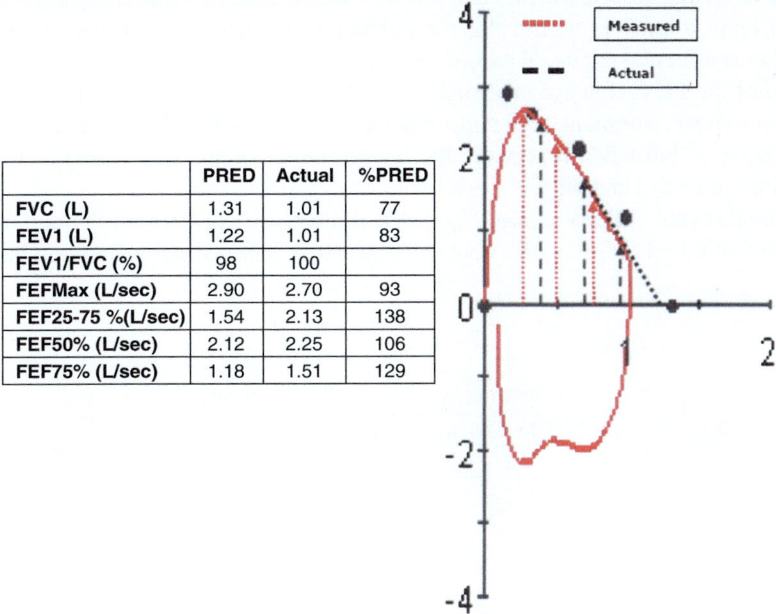

	PRED	Actual	%PRED
FVC (L)	1.31	1.01	77
FEV1 (L)	1.22	1.01	83
FEV1/FVC (%)	98	100	
FEFMax (L/sec)	2.90	2.70	93
FEF25-75 %(L/sec)	1.54	2.13	138
FEF50% (L/sec)	2.12	2.25	106
FEF75% (L/sec)	1.18	1.51	129

Fig. 7.9 The patient interrupted the exhalation prematurely as indicated by the vertical drop of the descending limb. As a result, the FVC is underestimated and the expiratory flow rates (*red dotted arrows*) overestimated. The *black dashed arrows* and *line* represent what the true flows and FVC would have probably been had the patient exhaled completely. Although most of the measured values are erroneous, one can still infer that the lower airway function is probably within the normal range because the flow–volume curve is convex, the FEV_1 and the FEFmax (that are not affected by the premature inspiration) are within the normal range, and even the FVC although underestimated is borderline normal. It should be noted that interpretation of the test without examining the flow–volume curve would have led to the erroneous conclusion of a mild restrictive defect based on the borderline "low" FVC and the disproportionately increased FEFs

expiratory flow (vertical drop) and it is a common problem with young children and/or with patients who cannot exhale for several seconds. When this occurs, the computer software, "assigns" the point of the cessation of flow as the RV, thus underestimating the value of the true FVC and overestimating the values of the FEFs. This combination of decreased FVC and increased expiratory flow rates can be easily misinterpreted as "restrictive lung defect" when in fact the lung function may be normal or obstructive. Thus, it is imperative to verify whether the measured parameters correlate with the shape of the MEFVC.

Although an incomplete MEFVC is not considered valid for interpretation it often contains useful and clinical information. Specifically, presence of lower airway obstruction can be reliably assumed (a) when the MEFVC has a clear concave pattern, (b) when the FEV_1 and the measured expiratory flows are disproportionately low relative to the FVC despite the fact that they are overestimated. In addition, a reasonably valid assessment can be made about the lung volume. Specifically, if the value of the measured FVC is close to or within the normal range despite the fact that it is underestimated, one can safely assume that the lung volume is within the normal range. Finally, because the incomplete effort is affecting the distal part of the MEFV curve, it does not affect the FEFmax and/or the FEV_1 that are measured in the beginning of exhalation. It is up to the interpreter's judgment to decide whether an incomplete MEFV curve can be interpreted but when it is made the interpretation should be explicit as to what values are valid and why.

2. "Submaximal" MEFV curve (Fig. 7.10) is the result of (a) a submaximal inhalation that failed to inflate the lungs to TLC, (b) a submaximal exhalation because

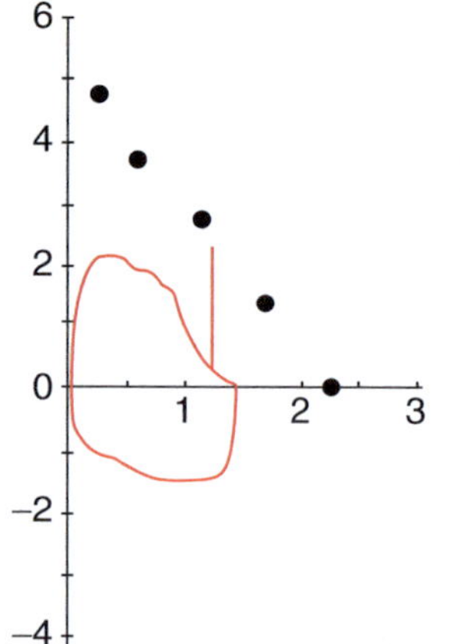

	Pred	Pre BD	%Pred-Pre
FVC (L)	2.25	1.45	64
FEV1 (L)	2.11	1.24	59
FEV1/FVC (%)	85	85	100
FEF Max (L/sec)	4.77	2.20	46
FEF 25-75% (L/sec)	2.74	1.49	54
FEF 50% (L/sec)	2.81	1.79	64
FEF 75% (L/sec)	1.42	0.66	47
FIVC (L)		1.50	
FIF 50% (L/sec)		1.39	
FIF Max (L/sec)	2.82	1.47	52
SVC (L)	2.25	1.46	65
IC (L)	1.51	1.23	82
ERV (L)	0.70	0.20	29

Fig. 7.10 A submaximal effort can be easily misinterpreted as "restrictive lung defect" (proportionate decrease in FVC, FEV_1, and all expiratory flow rates)

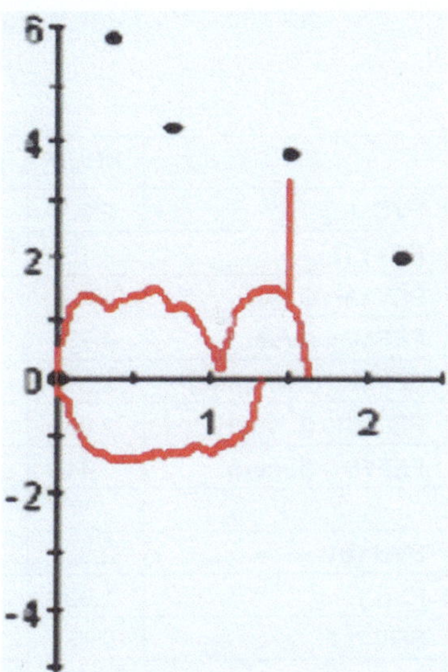

Fig. 7.11 This is a non-interpretable test because it does not have a recognizable pattern, it has a submaximal start, artifacts, and premature termination of the exhalation

the patient did not exhale with maximal force, (c) submaximal effort only in the beginning of the exhalation. The latter is probably the most common among young children who seem to have trouble understanding the concept of blowing-out "fast and hard." In the first two cases all measured parameters are going reduced, but the proportions among them remain the same. In the third case, the parameter that is mostly (or exclusively) affected is the FEFmax and to a lesser extent the FEF_{25} and the FEV_1. Thus, their percent predicted value is going to be considerably higher than that of the FEFmax.

3. "Non-interpretable" (Fig. 7.11): the curve does not have any recognizable pattern, usually due to excessive cough, very premature inspiratory efforts (occurring at <50 % of the FVC), leak around the mouthpiece, etc. In such case, no interpretation can or should be given.
4. Evaluation of lung volume. The MEFVCs can provide a basic quantitative assessment of lung volume with the measurement of the FVC. A normal FVC usually corresponds with a normal total lung capacity (i.e., TLC). An increased FVC suggests the presence of large lungs (commonly seen among athletes) or some degree of generalized hyperinflation. A decrease in FVC can be seen when there is actual loss of lung volume, but it can be also the result of air-trapping. Thus, a decrease in FVC should be further evaluated by measurements of lung volumes in order to determine whether the decrease is due to loss of lung volume or due to air-trapping. This is particularly important when the MEFVC does not have a definite pattern of obstructive or restrictive lung disease (Fig. 7.12).

	PRED	Actual	%PRED
FVC (L)	2.33	1.33	57
FEV1 (L)	2.15	1.21	56
FEV1/FVC (%)	85	91	107
FEFMax (L/sec)	4.75	1.50	74
FEF25-75 %(L/sec)	2.59	1.83	68
FEF50% (L/sec)	2.83	2.13	75
FEF75% (L/sec)	1.41	0.88	62
SVC (L)	2.33	1.61	65
IC (L)	1.60	1.28	80
ERV (L)	0.75	0.25	33
TGV (L)	1.30	1.81	124
RVpleth (L)	0.70	1.28	184
TLCpleth (L)	2.88	2.90	101
RV/TLCpleth(%)	25	44	178

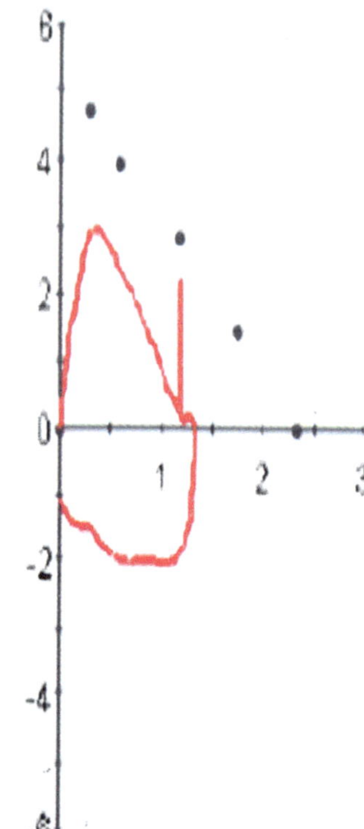

Fig. 7.12 Interpreting only the spirometric part of this test would lead into the conclusion that the patient has a mild restrictive lung defect (decreased FVC with the FEV_1 and all expiratory flow rates being increased relative to FVC). However, measurement of the lung volumes reveals that the total lung capacity is completely normal and that the SVC (and FVC) are actually decreased because of significant air-trapping

Evaluation of Hyperreactivity and (Hyper) responsiveness

Background

The terms airway/bronchial hyperreactivity (or simply reactivity) and airway/bronchial hyperresponsiveness (or responsiveness) are often used interchangeably to describe bronchoconstriction and/or bronchodilation. In this chapter, the term hyperreactivity refers to bronchoconstriction, whereas hyperresponsiveness refers to bronchodilation.

The presence of airway hyperreactivity can be assessed with the performance of a bronchoprovocation challenge. In such studies, the patient performs MEFV curves before and after exposure (usually by inhalation) to substances capable of causing bronchoconstriction. The most common direct challenge is by meth choline that is being inhaled in increasing concentrations until a predetermined drop in one or more of the measured indices occurs (most commonly, a 20 % decrease from baseline in the FEV_1). MEFV curves are performed after each concentration (Fig. 7.13a, b). If the decrease in FEV_1 occurs with a concentration of ≤ 1 mg/ml, the test is

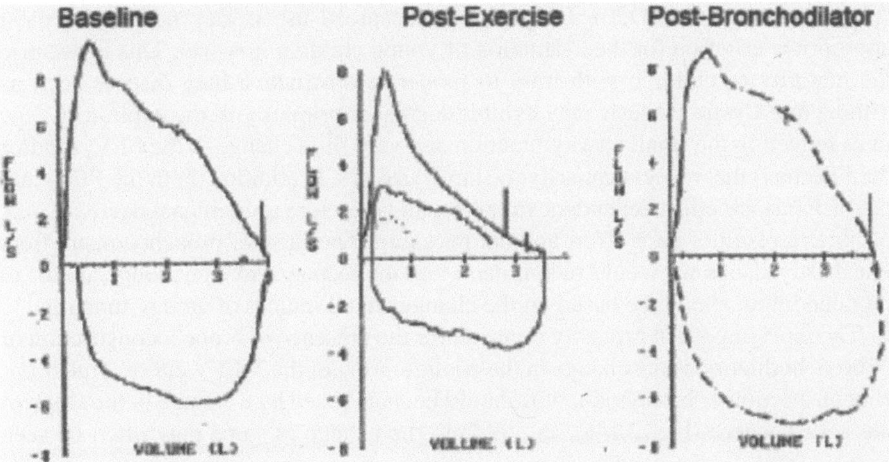

	Baseline	Post-exercise	%decreasefrom baseline	Post-bronchodilator
FVC (%pred)	117	102	-13	119
FEV1 (%pred)	133	97	-27	133
PEFR (%pred)	184	154	-16	168
FEF25-75 (%pred)	147	62	-58	146

Fig. 7.13 Exercise challenge test. Baseline spirometry was normal. Post-exercise spirometry showed significant decrease in all indices and change in the shape of the flow–volume curve from convex to concave. Post-bronchodilator spirometry showed that all values had returned to their baseline levels

considered "positive," and the likelihood of asthma is high. If there is no significant decrease with concentrations of ≥ 16 mg/ml, asthma is effectively ruled out. Histamine can be also used instead of methacholine under the same criteria.

Challenges can also be performed with nonspecific substances such as hypertonic saline, mannitol, adenosine monophosphate or even with exposure to a suspected allergen. Non-pharmacologic challenges include exercise (Fig. 7.13), and eucapneic hyperventilation. Which test should be performed depends on what question the test aims to answer. Direct challenges (e.g., methacholine) are very sensitive but not specific, and therefore they are best in ruling out airway hyperreactivity. Indirect challenges such as exercise challenge are very specific but not as sensitive, and therefore they are very good in confirming presence of airway hyperreactivity (e.g., exercise induced asthma). The presence of airway hyperresponsiveness is usually assessed by the performance of spirometry/MEFV curves before and after the administration of bronchodilators.

Interpretation

The most commonly used criterion for the presence of hyperreactivity is the decrease in FEV_1 by 20 % from baseline and the dose that causes such decrease is termed "provocative dose" (PD20). Despite its widespread use it may not be the most appropriate criterion for the evaluation of young children however. This is because the majority of children with mild to moderate obstructive lung disease such as asthma and Cystic Fibrosis may exhibit decreases primarily in the expiratory flow rates reflecting the small airway function and very little change in the FEV_1 (and/or the FEFmax) that reflect primarily the large airways. In addition, both the FEV_1 and the FEFmax are effort dependent variables, and therefore a significant decrease may occur as a result of poor effort and not necessarily because of bronchoconstriction. For these reasons we would recommend that the response to a challenge and/or to bronchodilator should be based on the changes in all indices of airway function.

The most important probably criterion for the presence of bronchoconstriction or of bronchodilation is the change in the configuration of the MEFV curve. True bronchoconstriction or bronchodilation should be manifested by a change in the slope of the MEFV curve (Fig. 7.14a). In children, the change in slope may often be seen

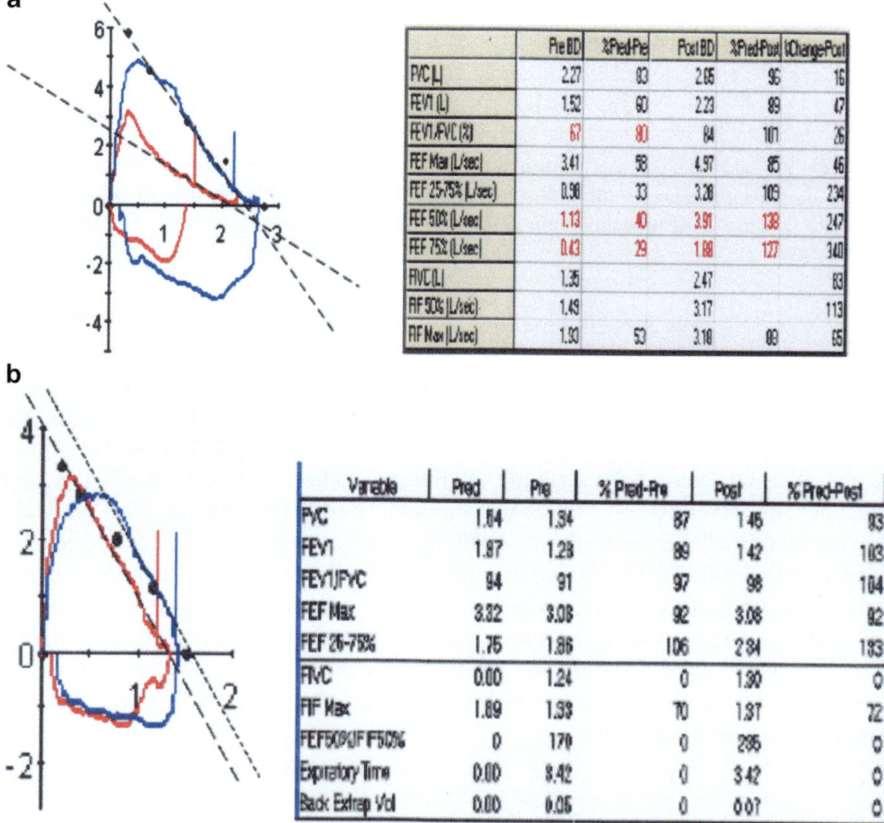

a

	Pre BD	%Pred-Pre	Post BD	%Pred-Post	%Change-Post
FVC (L)	2.27	83	2.65	95	16
FEV1 (L)	1.52	60	2.23	89	47
FEV1/FVC (%)	67	80	84	107	26
FEF Max (L/sec)	3.41	58	4.97	85	46
FEF 25-75% (L/sec)	0.96	33	3.20	109	234
FEF 50% (L/sec)	1.13	40	3.91	138	247
FEF 75% (L/sec)	0.43	29	1.88	127	340
FIVC (L)	1.35		2.47		83
FIF 50% (L/sec)	1.49		3.17		113
FIF Max (L/sec)	1.93	53	3.18	89	65

b

Variable	Pred	Pre	% Pred-Pre	Post	% Pred-Post
FVC	1.54	1.34	87	1.45	93
FEV1	1.87	1.23	89	1.42	103
FEV1/FVC	94	91	97	98	104
FEF Max	3.32	3.08	92	3.08	92
FEF 25-75%	1.75	1.86	106	2.34	133
FIVC	0.00	1.24	0	1.30	0
FIF Max	1.89	1.33	70	1.37	72
FEF50%/FIF F50%	0	170	0	285	0
Expiratory Time	0.00	8.42	0	3.42	0
Back Extrap Vol	0.00	0.05	0	0.07	0

Fig. 7.14 (**a**) True response to bronchodilator is indicated by significant increase in the measured indices and by change in the slope of the flow–volume curve. (**b**) An increase in the measured indices without change in the slope of the flow–volume curve could be due to a better inspiratory/ expiratory effort. However, it does not rule out presence of hyperresponsiveness

only in the effort independent portion. A change only in the FEFmax and in FEV_1 is probably due to effort (Fig. 7.14b). What percentage change is clinically significant is still rather undetermined. We recommend the following: $FVC \geq 10$ % from baseline; $FEV_1 \geq 12$ %; $FEFmax \geq 25$ % and $FEF_{25-75} \geq 25$ %. What is very important for every laboratory and for every professional who interprets the tests is to be consistent in the criteria they use.

Evaluation of the Diffusing Capacity

Background

The measurement of the diffusing capacity (DL) is a commonly used test that evaluates the ability of carbon monoxide (CO) to pass from the alveolar space into the capillary circulation. The DL is defined as the rate at which the CO enters the blood, divided by the difference in partial pressure between the alveoli and the pulmonary capillaries that is the driving force for the diffusion. The measurement of the diffusing capacity of CO is used as surrogate of the diffusion of oxygen. The reason for the use of the CO is based on the fact that its affinity for hemoglobin is 200 times greater than that of oxygen and therefore it is bound to Hb very rapidly, and because under normal circumstances its partial pressure in the blood is close to zero.

The most commonly used technique for the measurement of DLCO is the single breath technique (DL_{SB}), in which the patient exhales to RV and then rapidly inspires to TLC a mixture of gas that contains a small amount of CO (0.3 or 0.5 %), as well as an inert gas (usually Helium or methane). The patient is instructed to hold his/her breathe for a period of 10 s, during which the CO is diffused through the alveolar membrane into the blood stream and it is combined with Hb. After 10 s the patient exhales. The difference in CO between the inspired air and the expired air is assumed to be due to the combined with Hb CO and it allows for the calculation of the rate of the diffusion.

The resistance to diffusion by the alveolar membrane (Dm) depends on multiple factors including the overall gas exchange area, the thickness of the alveolar membrane, the affinity to hemoglobin, the amount of available Hb, and the pulmonary capillary blood volume. Conditions that alter any or all of these factors will affect the diffusing capacity as well. Such conditions include absolute loss of lung volume (e.g., decrease in TLC due to significant scoliosis); loss of gas exchange surface area regardless of changes in TLC (e.g., destruction of alveoli in emphysema); loss of alveolar space (e.g., filling of the alveoli with material other than air as in the case of alveolar proteinosis); thickening of the alveolar membrane (e.g., fibrosis); severe anemia (e.g., sickle cell crisis); decreased perfusion of the lung (e.g., severe pulmonary hypertension); increased partial pressure of CO in the capillaries that prevents the diffusion (e.g., heavy smokers may develop carboxyhemoglobin in excess of 10 %).

The DLCO is dependent on the lung volume. This means that a larger lung is going to diffuse more CO than a smaller lung even if they are both normal. To adjust for these differences, the DLCO is corrected for the alveolar volume (DLCO/VA). This ratio is known as "diffusion constant" and it a measure of efficiency of the functioning units of the lungs.

Interpretation

In a healthy lung, the diffusing capacity and the diffusion constant are pretty proportional. Both restrictive and obstructive lung diseases can affect the DLCO and its decrease in absolute terms is proportional to the lung volume (e.g., if hypothetically a healthy lung diffuses 100 molecules of CO, a 50 % decrease in TLC will result in the diffusion of only 50 molecules). However, the diffusion constant will be still normal. In certain conditions, when the decrease in DLCO is due to vascular reasons (e.g., sickle cell disease, pulmonary hypertension) the body has certain compensatory mechanisms (e.g., increase in the heart rate and decrease in transit times of the red cells through the capillaries) that increase the "efficiency" of the ventilated and perfused areas. Thus, although the absolute value of the DLCO will be low, the DLCO/VA will be normal or even increased compared with the normal.

In cases of pulmonary hemorrhage the measurement of DLCO can be of great importance both diagnostically and for the monitoring of the condition. Pulmonary hemorrhage generally decreases the TLC because of the flooding of the alveoli with blood. This normally would result in decreased DLCO. However, the red cells that are in the alveolar spaces bind the molecules of CO before it even gets diffused into the capillaries and as a result the measured DLCO is abnormally high especially in relation to the decreased lung volume. As the pulmonary hemorrhage resolves and the alveolar spaces gradually empty from the red cells, the measured DLCO decreases (Fig. 7.15).

Special Issues

"Normal" Versus "Within the Normal Range"

The absolute values of the various indices of lung function differ significantly among different individuals depending on their age, race, gender and size (primarily the height). Thus, the absolute value of any of the indices of lung function does not convey by itself the degree of normalcy, i.e., the same value may be completely normal for an individual and completely abnormal for another. Thus, the measured indices are usually presented as percentage of the predicted normal ("%pred") values derived from measurements made in asymptomatic healthy individuals of same age, gender, race and height. Values within 2 standard deviations above or below the

% pred	November	August	September
TLC	86	63	55
SVC	92	55	43
RV	71	80	83
RV/TLC	20	32	156
FVC	93	55	41
FEV$_1$	89	56	41
FEF$_1$/FVC	82	87	85
FEF$_{25-75}$	72	61	39
DLCO	86	112	48
DLCO/V$_A$	101	192	109

Fig. 7.15 Serial PFTs in a patient who had undergone bone marrow transplant. In the first column the TLC and the DLCO are within the normal range and proportional to each other (in terms of their %predicted values). In the second column there has been a significant decrease in TLC whereas the DLCO actually increased that is a typical finding in cases of pulmonary hemorrhage. The hemorrhage was confirmed by bronchoscopy. The third column shows a decrease in the DLCO to levels proportional to the TLC reflecting the clearing of the blood from the alveolar spaces

mean are considered to represent the "normal range." This system is easily understood by patients and doctors alike and it allows for easy comparisons between patients and/or between testing periods on the same patient.

It is very important to emphasize that having a value within the "normal range" is not synonymous to being "normal." To be interpreted as normal a test requires that each of the measured indices is within the normal range but also that they are proportional to each other. This is because the "range of normal" for virtually all indices is pretty wide (e.g., it ranges from approximately 90–110 % for the FVC to almost 60–140 % for the FEF$_{25-75}$). For example, the MEFVC in Fig. 7.16a as well as the ratio FEV$_1$/FVC show a clear obstructive pattern, although both the FVC and the FEV$_1$ are within their respective normal range. The same degree of obstruction can be seen in Fig. 7.16b although both the FVC and the FEV$_1$ are well below the lower level of normal. On the other hand, in Fig. 7.16c, the decrease in both the FVC and the FEV$_1$ is proportional and therefore the airway function (although not the lung volume) is normal.

Despite their usefulness, the various series of predicted normal values have also a number of inherent problems. This is mainly because they have not been derived from repeated longitudinal measurements on the same cohort of individuals but

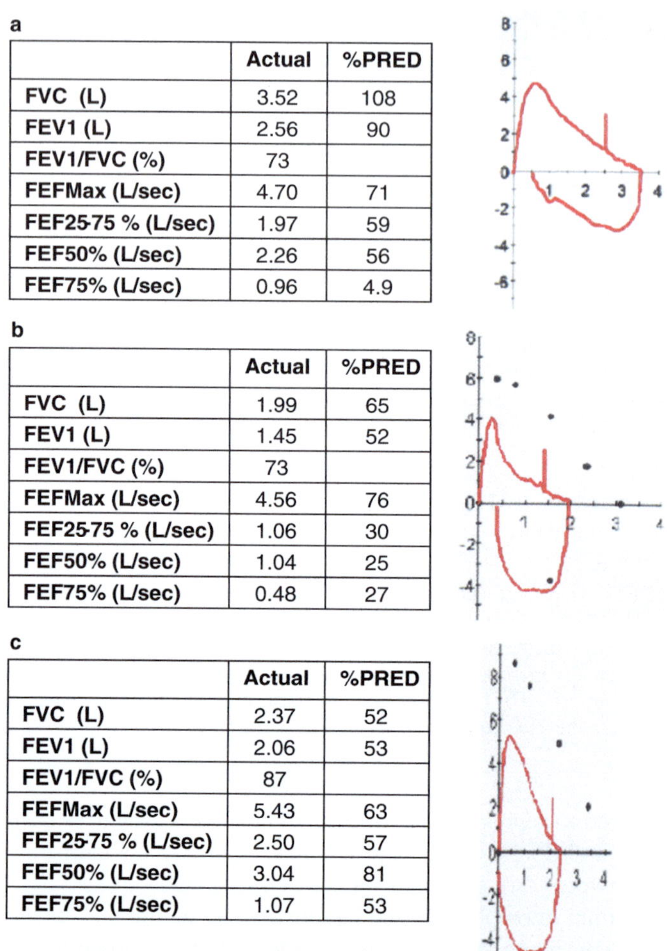

a

	Actual	%PRED
FVC (L)	3.52	108
FEV1 (L)	2.56	90
FEV1/FVC (%)	73	
FEFMax (L/sec)	4.70	71
FEF25-75 % (L/sec)	1.97	59
FEF50% (L/sec)	2.26	56
FEF75% (L/sec)	0.96	4.9

b

	Actual	%PRED
FVC (L)	1.99	65
FEV1 (L)	1.45	52
FEV1/FVC (%)	73	
FEFMax (L/sec)	4.56	76
FEF25-75 % (L/sec)	1.06	30
FEF50% (L/sec)	1.04	25
FEF75% (L/sec)	0.48	27

c

	Actual	%PRED
FVC (L)	2.37	52
FEV1 (L)	2.06	53
FEV1/FVC (%)	87	
FEFMax (L/sec)	5.43	63
FEF25-75 % (L/sec)	2.50	57
FEF50% (L/sec)	3.04	81
FEF75% (L/sec)	1.07	53

Fig. 7.16 The ratio FEV_1/FVC does not depend on how normal or abnormal the values of its components are. (**a**) The ratio FEV_1/FVC is low although both the FVC and the FEV_1 are within the normal range. (**b**) The ratio FEV_1/FVC is the same with the one from (**a**) although the FVC and the FEV1 are below the lower normal levels. (**c**) The ratio FEV_1/FVC is above the predicted normal although both the FVC and the FEV_1 are abnormally low

from different cohorts that varied from each other. Values for non-Caucasians are much less accurate and often based on gross and inaccurate generalizations (for example, series on predicted normal values from Mexican-Americans had been used for a long-time for all patients classified as "Hispanics" despite the often obvious differences between them).

In order to minimize these problems an effort has been undertaken to compile databases with the contribution of data from many parts of the world. The product of this effort is the Global Lung Function Initiative (GLI) Reference Equations for

Spirometry. Its advantage over the older series is that it is based on approximately 75,000 measurements performed on healthy males and females, ages 3–95 years of age in more than 70 counties worldwide. A second change in the new equations is the departure from the traditional "percent of the predicted normal" and the introduction of the z-scores as the means of presenting and correcting the values. The z-score is a statistical method that describes how far from the normal range a value is. The method is based on the fact that, 95 % of normally distributed values fall within ± 2 z-scores. Although the GLI equations and the z-scores offer advantages especially for research purposes, they do not completely eliminate the drawbacks of the currently used series of predicted normal values especially considering that they are currently limited to spirometry and they are heavily derived from Caucasian populations. Furthermore, they are conceptually much less understood by patients and doctors alike. Thus, for the remaining of this chapter we refer to the traditional system of "percent predicted."

Many clinicians (and even clinical researchers) in adult medicine often use a "cutoff" value to separate normal from abnormal values. Although this is a quick and easy way to define "normalcy" it is bound to overestimate or underestimate the lung function of many patients. Cutoff values are particularly unsuitable for pediatric patients because the definition of "normal" varies significantly among the various age groups (for example a ratio of FEV_1/FVC of 85 % would be completely normal for an older teenager but very abnormal for a 6 year-old).

The Acceptability of the Tests

Because pulmonary function tests require from the patient a certain level of cooperation and effort, it is important for those who interpret the test to know that it represents the patient's maximal effort. For this, one has to rely to a large extend on the observation of the respiratory technician who is performing the test. Certain criteria for the acceptability of a test were developed for adult patients but they are not applicable to children. More recent criteria are more suitable but still not optimal for children (Table 7.2). As a study in young children showed (Table 7.3) most of the young children have difficulty meeting the criterion of the back extrapolated volume of <0.05 (an indicator of how hard and fast a patient breathes out) and many of them fully exhale in less than 3 s. A second criterion of acceptability is the reproducibility of the test (at least three reproducible efforts for adults and older children

Table 7.2 ATS/ERS criteria of acceptability of spirometry

Adults	Preschool children
Free of artifacts	Free of artifacts
Vextr <5 % of FVC (or <150 ml)	Vextr (VBE): <12.5 % FVC (or <80 ml)
Exhalation: ≥ 6 s	Exhalation: ≥ 3 s
3 curves with FVC, FEV1 within 150 ml from highest	2 curves with FVC, FEV_1 within 100 ml from highest or 10 % of highest

Table 7.3 Percentage of children who meet the ATS/ERS criteria for spirometry

Age (N)	4 years ($N=68$)	5 years ($N=231$)	6 years ($N=342$)	7 years ($N=343$)
Extrapolated volume (V_{ext})				
V_{ext} <5 %	72 %	76 %	83 %	86 %
Expiratory time				
≤1 s	34 %	20 %	12 %	5 %
1.1–2.9 s	62 %	64 %	57 %	40 %
3–5.9 s	4 %	13 %	28 %	42 %
≥6 s	0 %	3 %	3 %	13 %

and two for younger children). However, it is not unusual for younger children to master only one effort. It is our opinion, that in clinical practice reproducibility is desirable but not absolutely necessary and that even one technically acceptable effort could and should be accepted for interpretation (for a detailed discussion on the subject see references [9, 10]). After all, the concern about non-reproducible suboptimal efforts is that they can make the results look worse than they really are. However, there are no technically acceptable efforts that can make the results look better than they really are (erroneously high flows are measured only when the patient terminates the exhalation prematurely). This should be obvious in the visual inspection of the MEFVC and the numerical values should not be used. However, be discarded but one can still derive useful information (see previous section on the interpretation of the MEFVCs). It is obvious that stricter criteria may be necessary for research purposes in order to assure the uniformity and quality of the data.

What Test to Use?

The fact that there are many different available tests of lung function does not mean that they should all be used on every patient, all the time. Like other diagnostic tests, the selection of the appropriate pulmonary function should be based on the question that the test is intended to answer (Is it an obstructive or a restrictive lung disease? Is the disease getting better or worse? Is the patient responding to a specific treatment? etc.) Table 7.4 presents some guidelines for the initial evaluation and for the follow-up of patients with a variety of different conditions.

How Often Should a Patient be Tested?

Like any other test, PFTs are not meant to replace the history taking and the physical examination of the patient, but to complement them because they can reveal changes in lung function that are not easily detectable by the physical examination and often

Table 7.4 Suggested pulmonary function tests for common clinical conditions

Clinical condition	Initial evaluation	Follow-up
Obstructive lung disease (e.g., asthma, cystic fibrosis)	1, 3 (6)[a]	2, (1, 3)[a]
Restrictive lung disease (e.g., interstitial lung disease)	1, 3, 4, (7)[a]	2, (3, 4)[a]
Dyspnea/chest pain of unknown origin	1, 3, 4, 7	
Chest wall abnormalities (e.g., pectus excavatum, scoliosis)	1, 3, 5, 7	2, 3, 5
Neuromuscular diseases (e.g., Duchenne muscular dystrophy)	1, 3, 5, (8, 9)[a]	2, 5, (8, 9)[a]
Hematologic disorders (e.g., sickle cell disease)	1, 3, 4	2, 4, (3)[a]
Cardiovascular diseases (e.g., congenital heart disease; pulmonary hypertension)	1, 3, 4, 7	2, 4 (3, 7)[a]
Chemotherapy/radiation therapy	1, 3, 4, (7)[a]	2, 4, (3)[a]
Types of pulmonary function tests		
1. Spirometry (pre/post bronchodilator)	4. Diffusing capacity	7. Cardiopulmonary exercise testing
2. Spirometry	5. Respiratory muscle strength	8. Capnometry
3. Lung volumes	6. Bronchoprovocation study	9. Peak cough flow

[a]Numbers in parentheses indicate optional tests to be performed as clinically indicated

not felt by the patient either. This is particularly true for slowly developing lower airway obstruction that may remain unnoticed by patients and doctors alike because the patients adapt to these changes and learn to adjust their breathing. Figure 7.17 illustrates this point in a patient with known asthma during four "routine" visits to the clinic. In all instances, the patient stated that he was feeling "fine" and the physical examination was pretty unremarkable. However, not only his baseline pulmonary function was markedly different in each visit but his response to bronchodilator therapy varied significantly as well. As a general rule we perform at least basic spirometry during every clinic visit even if the patient does not report any particular problems and of course when changes in the therapeutic regimen are made as well as in the beginning and at the end of hospitalization. In our institution, patients with Cystic Fibrosis are being tested once or twice/week during hospitalizations and the continuation of the intravenous antibiotics depends to a large extend on the improvement of the PFTs.

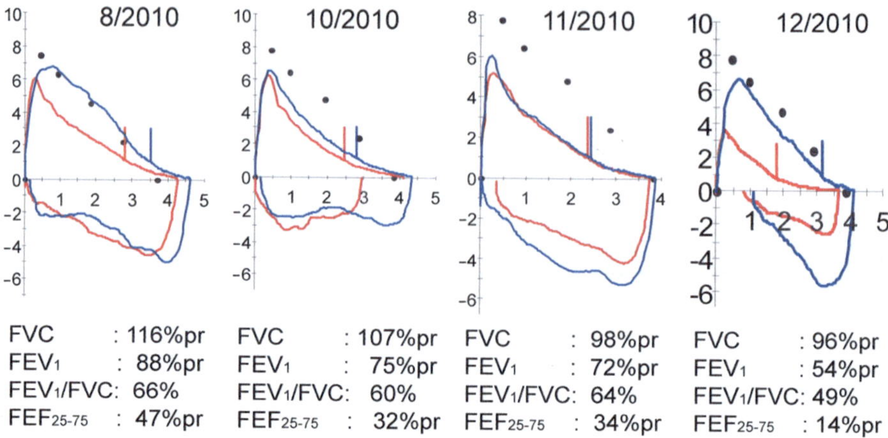

	8/2010		10/2010		11/2010		12/2010
FVC	: 116%pr	FVC	: 107%pr	FVC	: 98%pr	FVC	: 96%pr
FEV$_1$	: 88%pr	FEV$_1$	: 75%pr	FEV$_1$	: 72%pr	FEV$_1$	: 54%pr
FEV$_1$/FVC: 66%		FEV$_1$/FVC: 60%		FEV$_1$/FVC: 64%		FEV$_1$/FVC: 49%	
FEF$_{25\text{-}75}$	: 47%pr	FEF$_{25\text{-}75}$	: 32%pr	FEF$_{25\text{-}75}$	: 34%pr	FEF$_{25\text{-}75}$	: 14%pr

Fig. 7.17 Serial MEFVCs from the same patient at different time periods showing significant changes both in his baseline function as well as in his response to bronchodilators

Summary

Pulmonary function tests are noninvasive, easy to perform, relatively cheap, and usually accurate diagnostic tests of the lung function. The normalcy of a test should be based not only on the normalcy of the measured values but on the proportionality between them. Sudden changes in the PFTs of an individual that are not accompanied by relevant clinical changes should always raise the possibility of a "technical" error. The latter can be due to equipment malfunction or failure or more commonly due to the patients' suboptimal effort, lack of cooperation, etc. and often due to the use of inappropriate predicted normal values.

Guidelines for the Interpretation of Commonly Used Pulmonary Function Tests in Clinical Practice

Lung Volumes

Questions to be addressed: Is the TLC normal, increased, or decreased?

An increased TLC can be due to larger than average lungs (often seen in athletes), or due to nonspecific hyperinflation.

A decreased TLC is indicative of loss of lung volume.

- Are the various subdivisions proportionate to TLC (in terms of their %predicted value and/or in terms of their ratio to TLC)?

Based on the answers given to the above questions the possible interpretations are the following:

- *Normal lung volumes*: The TLC and all of its subdivisions are within the normal range and proportional to each other.
- *Restrictive lung defect*: The TLC and all of its subdivisions are proportionately decreased.
- *Obstructive lung disease*: The RV and FRC are increased relative to TLC (RV/TLC > 30 %; FRC/TLC > 60 %).
- *Mixed defect*: The TLC is decreased but the RV/TLC and FRC/TLC are increased.

Additional Points

- Because the TLC consists of the sum of VC and RV, when one of them increases the other one decreases (and vice versa). Thus, the SVC is disproportionately low relative to TLC when there is air-trapping (i.e., increased RV and RV/TLC). Conversely the SVC is disproportionately high relative to TLC when there is decreased RV (e.g., alveolar fibrosis as a result of chemotherapeutic agents).
- Increased RV can be present without increase in FRC (fairly common in patients with chest wall deformities that prevent the complete emptying of the lungs).

Maximal Expiratory Flow–Volume Curves/Spirometry

Visual Inspection

- Is the MEFVC technically acceptable (complete without artifacts)?
- What is the "shape" of the MEFVC (concave, convex, or tall and narrow)?
- Is the MIFVC a "mirror image" of the MEFVC?

Forced Vital Capacity (FVC)

Is the FVC within the normal range, increased, or decreased?

- A decreased FVC can be due to a restrictive lung defect causing loss of lung volume or due to an obstructive lung disease causing air-trapping. A decreased FVC should be further investigated with the measurements of lung volumes.

Forced Expiratory Volume in First Second (FEV$_1$)

- A decreased FEV$_1$ can be due to obstructive lung disease, due to a restrictive lung defect causing loss of lung volume or due to poor effort.

- The ratio of FEV_1/FVC is the major determinant of lower airway obstruction. However, a normal FEV_1/FVC ration does not preclude the presence of small/peripheral airway obstruction.

Ratio FEV_1/FVC

- The ratio FEV_1/FVC normal for age the normal values vary significantly according to the age of the patient; it is as high as 97 % for those less than 6 years of age and as low as the mid-80 % for older children.
- A proportional decrease in FVC and FEV_1 ($FEV_1/FVC > 90$ %) in an older child is suggestive of loss of lung volume (restrictive lung defect).
- A disproportionate decrease in FEV_1 relative to FVC ($FEV_1/FVC < 80$ %) is indicative of lower airway obstruction (LAO).

Maximal or Peak Expiratory Flow Rate (FEFmax or PEFR)

A decreased FEFmax can be due to:

- Obstructive lung disease. In such case the FEV_1 and the other expiratory flow rates indices should be equally or more affected;
- A restrictive lung defect causing loss of lung volume. In such case the FVC, FEV_1 and the other expiratory flow rates indices should be equally affected;
- Poor effort. This should be suspected when the %predicted value of the FEV_1 is much higher than the %predicted value of the FEFmax (e.g., FEFmax of 70 %predicted, FEV_1 90 %predicted).

Forced expiratory flow (FEF) at 25–75 %, 25 %, 50 %, 75 % of FVC:

- A disproportionate decrease in the FEFs in relation to FVC (e.g., FVC: 95 %predicted, FEFs: <60 %predicted) indicates lower airway obstruction.
- A ratio of FEF_{25-75} (%predicted)/FVC (%predicted) < 0.8 is highly suggestive of lower airway obstruction.
- A decrease in the FEFs that is proportionate to FVC (e.g., FVC 70 %predicted; FEF_{25-75}: 68 %predicted) is suggestive of a restrictive defect.
- An increase in the FEFs relative to FVC (e.g., FVC: 85 %predicted; FEF_{25-75}: 110 %predicted) suggests increased elastic recoil of the lung. This is normal in infants and very young children (usually less than 6 years of age) but abnormal in older ones and suggestive of a restrictive lung disease.

Inspiratory Flow–Volume Curves

- A flattened inspiratory curve suggests variable extrathoracic soft tissue obstruction if it is consistent. If it is intermittent it is usually due to vocal closure.
- A ratio $FEF_{50}/FIF_{50} > 1.2$ is also suggestive of variable extrathoracic obstruction.
- Flattening of the inspiratory and expiratory flow–volume curves indicates fixed airway obstruction.

Diffusing Capacity

- Is the DLCO normal or decreased?
- Is the DLCO proportional to the lung volume (TLC or FVC)?
- Is the DLCO/VA proportional or increased?

Bibliography

1. ATS/ERS Task Force Standardisation of Lung Function Testing: General considerations for lung function testing. 2005. http://www.thoracic.org/statements/resources/pfet/PFT1.pdf.
2. ATS/ERS Task Force Standardisation of Lung Function Testing: Interpretative strategies for lung function tests. 2005. http://www.thoracic.org/statements/resources/pfet/pft5.pdf.
3. ATS/ERS Task Force Standardisation of Lung Function Testing: Standardization of the measurement of lung volumes. 2005. http://www.thoracic.org/statements/resources/pfet/pft3.pdf.
4. ATS/ERS Task Force Standardization of Lung Function Testing: Standardization of the single-breath determination of carbon monoxide uptake in the lung. 2005. http://www.thoracic.org/statements/resources/pfet/pft4.pdf.
5. ATS/ERS Task Force Standardization of Lung Function Testing: Standardization of spirometry. 2005. http://www.thoracic.org/statements/resources/pfet/PFT2.pdf.
6. Hankinson JL, Odencrantz JR, Fedan KB. Spirometric reference values from a sample of the general US population. Am J Respir Crit Care Med. 1999;159(1):179–87.
7. Cockcroft D, Davis B. Direct and indirect challenges in the clinical assessment of asthma. Ann Allergy Asthma Immunol. 2009;103(5):363–9.
8. Quanjer PH, Stanojevic S, Cole TJ, Baur X, Hall GL, Culver BH, Enright PL, Hankinson JL, Ip MS, Zheng J, et al. Multi-ethnic reference values for spirometry for the 3–95-yr age range: the global lung function 2012 equations. Eur Respir J. 2012;40(6):1324–43.
9. Seed L, Wilson D, Coates AL. Children should not be treated like little adults in the PFT lab. Respir Care. 2012;57(1):61–70.
10. Stocks J, Kirkby J, Lum S. How to avoid misinterpreting lung function tests in children: a few practical tips. Paediatr Respir Rev. 2014. pii: S1526-0542(14)00025-6.

Chapter 8
Infant and Preschool Pulmonary Function Tests

Janet Stocks

Abstract Heightened awareness of the relevance of early lung development on subsequent lung health and the need to identify lung disease before changes become irreversible, has resulted in increased efforts to monitor lung function from birth and throughout the preschool years. International collaborative efforts to adapt techniques and develop standardized protocols, together with increased availability of appropriate commercial devices mean that it is now possible to perform a wide range of pulmonary function tests (PFTs) in infants and preschool children less than 6 years of age. The aims of this chapter are to (a) briefly describe which PFTs can be performed in spontaneously breathing sleeping infants and awake preschool children using commercially available equipment, (b) discuss how to interpret PFTs in children under 5 years, and (c) consider the extent to which these tests might contribute to clinical management of infants and preschool children.

Keywords Respiratory function tests • Infant • Children • Child • preschool • Normal values • Lung function • Spirometry • Lung volumes • Airways resistance • Repeatability of results

Abbreviations

ATS/ERS	American Thoracic Society/European Respiratory Society
BDR	Bronchodilator responsiveness
BPD	Bronchopulmonary dysplasia
CF	Cystic fibrosis
Crs	Respiratory compliance
FEFV	Forced expiratory flow volume
$FEV_{0.5}$	Forced expired volume in 0.5 s

J. Stocks, Ph.D. (✉)
Respiratory, Critical Care and Anaesthesia Section, UCL, Institute of Child Health,
30 Guilford St, London WC1N 1EH, UK
e-mail: j.stocks@ucl.ac.uk

© Springer Science+Business Media New York 2015
S.D. Davis et al. (eds.), *Diagnostic Tests in Pediatric Pulmonology*,
Respiratory Medicine, DOI 10.1007/978-1-4939-1801-0_8

FRC	Functional residual capacity
FVC	Forced vital capacity
LCI	Lung clearance index
LLN	Lower limit of normal
MBW	Multiple breath washout
PFT	Pulmonary function test
QC	Quality control
Rint	Interrupter resistance
RR	Respiratory rate
Rrs	Respiratory resistance
SDS	Standard deviation score (also known as Z-score)
SOT	Single occlusion technique
sRaw	Specific airways resistance
tPTEF/tE	Time to reach peak tidal expiratory flow as a ratio of expiratory time
ULN	Upper limit of normal
VT	Tidal volume

Introduction

Pulmonary function tests (PFTs) are an integral component of clinical management in school-aged children and adults with lung disease. By contrast, the lack of suitable equipment and difficulties in undertaking such measurements in small, potentially uncooperative subjects meant that, until recently, assessments of pulmonary function in those less than 5 years of age was restricted to specialized research establishments. The realization that insults to the developing lung may have lifelong effects, with much of the burden of respiratory disease in later life having its origins prenatally or during the first years of life, has focused attention on the need to develop sensitive methods of assessing respiratory function in infants and preschool children. Assessment of respiratory function in the very young is relevant not only to our understanding of respiratory health and disease, during childhood, but also throughout later life. Such tests can provide objective outcome measures to identify early determinants of respiratory function, distinguish changes due to disease from those related to growth and development, and be used to evaluate the effects of new therapeutic advances as part of well-designed research studies. However, their role in clinical management or as a diagnostic tool remains limited, as discussed below.

The aims of this chapter are to:

- Briefly describe which PFTs can be performed in spontaneously breathing sleeping infants (birth to ~2 years) and awake preschool children (3–5 years of age) using commercially available equipment.
- Discuss how to interpret PFTs in children under 5 years.
- Consider the extent to which these tests may contribute to clinical management of infants and preschool children.

This chapter focuses on commonly used tests for which commercially available equipment is available. It will not cover the use of forced oscillation techniques or the multiple breath washout technique which are covered elsewhere in this book (Chap. 10), nor the application of PFTs in ventilated infants or young children. Due to the enormous increase in literature in this field during recent years, references cited are generally limited to those published in the past 5 years, the bibliographies of which would inform the interested reader regarding prior relevant literature.

Methods of Assessing Pulmonary Function in Infants and Young Children

Although assessment of lung size, compliance, and gas-exchanging surface area may be valuable when assessing the impact of congenital cardiac defects or disruption of alveolar development in survivors of bronchopulmonary dysplasia [1–8], most respiratory problems beyond the neonatal period are characterized by some form of central or peripheral airway obstruction. Consequently, the most frequently used PFTs in early life are those designed to assess airway function by measuring either airways resistance or forced expiratory flows and volumes. There is, however, increasing awareness that airway obstruction may be determined not only by the caliber of the airways but also by the compliance of the airway wall and the elastic recoil of the surrounding parenchyma, leading to the search for suitable outcomes that will reflect these characteristics and hence improve the interpretation of results. Furthermore, as discussed in Chap. 10, there is increasing evidence that conventional measures of airway function such as forced expiratory maneuvers, that focus on the conducting airways, may be insensitive to early lung disease in conditions such as cystic fibrosis (CF), which commences in the lung periphery, and which are therefore better evaluated by measuring ventilation inhomogeneity [9–12].

An ideal lung function test for infants and young children would be one that is:

- Simple and involves no risk
- Acceptable to both the child and the parents
- Independent of subject cooperation
- Applicable to any age and arousal state
- Reproducible
- Sensitive enough to distinguish between health and disease
- Able to reflect the clinical situation or provide accurate and specific information about lung structure and function
- Cheap and measurable using commercially available equipment, built to internationally approved standards, allowing standardized data collection and interpretation and for which
- Appropriate reference ranges from healthy children, derived over a wide age span during infancy or early childhood, have been developed

Although no such test currently exists, there are a number of techniques that have been shown to be safe and feasible in sleeping infants and toddlers (generally below 2 years of age) and preschool children and which are now commercially available [13].

Special Consideration When Testing Infants

In addition to the marked developmental changes in respiratory physiology that occur during the first years of life which affect both the measurement and interpretation of results [14], the major differences in undertaking infant PFTs relate to sleep state, sedation, ethical issues, posture, and the need to miniaturize and adapt equipment for measurements in small subjects, who tend to be preferential nose breathers and who cannot be asked to undertake special breathing maneuvers [14]. Although attempts have been made to assess lung function in awake infants, measurements are normally made during sleep. A representative and stable end-expiratory level is essential for reproducible measures of tidal breathing, resting lung volume (functional residual capacity or FRC), respiratory mechanics (resistance and compliance), or partial forced expiratory flow-volume (FEFV) maneuvers. This can normally only be achieved if the child is in quiet, rather than rapid eye movement, sleep.

Unless clinically indicated, sedation is generally contraindicated for PFTs in newborn infants. Successful measurements using a full range of tests can usually be achieved during natural sleep after a feed in all infants up to at least 44 weeks postmenstrual age. Tests based on tidal breathing recordings may be applicable in the unsedated infant up to 4 months postnatal life [15, 16], whereas forced expiratory maneuvers and whole body plethysmography generally require sedation, certainly beyond 3 months of age. For all studies involving infants, strict safety precautions must be followed. In addition to adherence to local infection control procedures, resuscitation equipment, including suction, must be available, and two skilled operators, fully trained in basic life support, one of whom has prime responsibility for monitoring the well-being of the infant, must be in attendance throughout testing. Pulse oximetry is used for continuous monitoring throughout the testing session. Given the rapid rate of somatic growth during infancy and early childhood, accurate measurements of height and weight using a calibrated stadiometer and scales are essential.

Which Tests Can Be Performed in Infants and Toddlers?

Commercially available equipment is now available to assess a wide range of PFTs in sleeping infants and young children <2 years of age, including that used to assess

- Tidal breathing [15–17]
- Passive respiratory mechanics (i.e., compliance and resistance; usually based on the single breath occlusion (SOT) technique) [1, 2, 18, 19]
- Plethysmographic lung volumes (Fig. 8.1) [2, 8, 20–24]

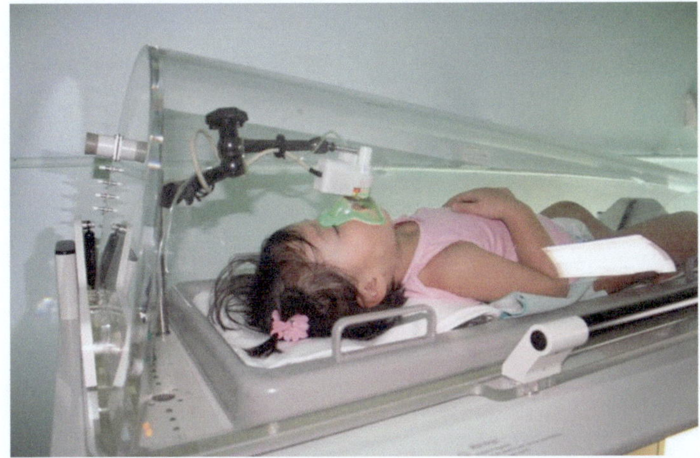

Fig. 8.1 Infant whole body plethysmography for assessment of functional residual capacity. Photo courtesy of Janet Stocks. (NB: Parental permission has been obtained to reproduce all photographs in this chapter. Copyright for all illustrations has been retained by Janet Stocks)

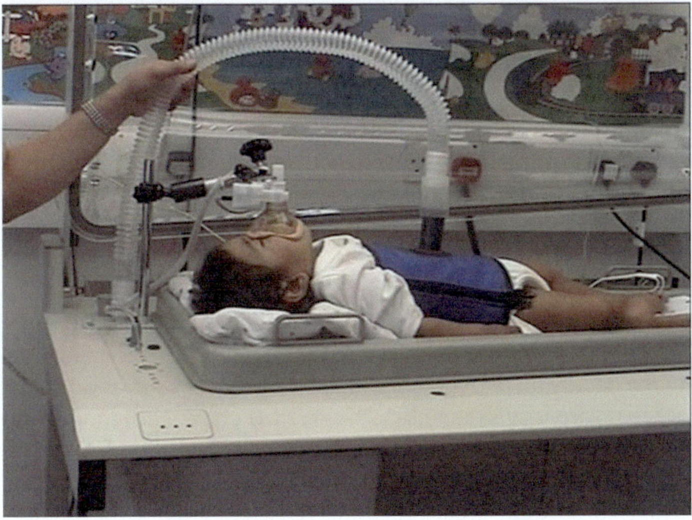

Fig. 8.2 The rapid thoraco-abdominal compression technique. Photo courtesy of Janet Stocks

- Functional residual capacity (FRC) and indices of ventilation inhomogeneity (such as the Lung Clearance Index or LCI) using multiple breath inert gas washout (MBW) techniques [15, 25–27] (see Chap. 10) and
- Forced expiratory flow-volume (FEFV) maneuvers, using the tidal or raised volume rapid thoraco-abdominal compression technique (Figs. 8.2 and 8.3) [8, 23, 24, 28–37]

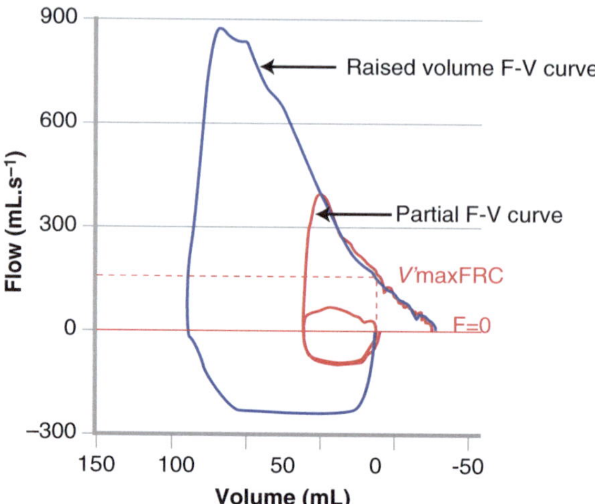

Fig. 8.3 Forced expiratory flow–volume curves obtained during tidal breathing (partial *F–V* curve) and after inflating the lungs to 30 cmH$_2$O (2.94 kPa) (raised volume *F–V* curve). Courtesy of Janet Stocks

Details of how to undertake these tests have been published elsewhere [14, 34, 38–45] and will only be summarized briefly here. Regrettably, although some groups have published results using this technique, valid measurements of plethysmographic airways resistance are not feasible using currently available commercial equipment [46, 47].

The choice of which test(s) to use in which infant, and the order in which they are performed, needs to be informed by the underlying reason for performing the test, the underlying assumptions of each test, the likely total duration of sleep (and hence testing session) and the level of expertise required for accurate measurements, rather than simple availability of equipment. Although recording of tidal breathing and respiratory mechanics using the occlusion technique appear simple, their validity can easily be compromised by leaks around the face mask, lack of quiet regular breathing or, in the case of single occlusion technique, violation of the theoretical assumptions underlying the measurements due to lack of complete relaxation during the occlusion and throughout the subsequent expiration and/or inability to represent the respiratory system by a single time constant in the presence of lung disease [14, 19, 43]. Strict quality control indicates that these conditions are frequently not met leading to a failure rate of at least 30 % [23]. Generally speaking, assessments based on quiet tidal breathing (e.g., respiratory mechanics using the occlusion technique, multiple breath washout or plethysmography) should be undertaken before those entailing forced expiratory maneuvers.

Which Tests Can Be Performed in Preschool Children?

Up until the last decade, it was commonly stated that assessment of lung function in preschool children (2–5 years) was virtually impossible, since they lacked the necessary coordination, comprehension and cooperation to participate, this period being dubbed the "dark ages" of pediatric pulmonology. Although this view is still held by many, there is now a considerable body of evidence that a wide range of lung function measurements are indeed feasible in the majority of children above 3 years of age, provided the techniques and quality control criteria are suitably adapted, and the tests are performed in a child-friendly environment by operators with suitable expertise and aptitude [9, 10, 13, 14, 32, 46, 48–68]. Success rate increases with age [13, 67, 68], with high success rates feasible from around 3.5 years, unless the child has been born very prematurely or has any signs of developmental delay.

As for all PFTs, appropriate equipment and testing conditions, skilled and experienced personnel, and rigorous adherence to published guidelines are critical for ensuring high quality, reproducible data. When assessing preschool children, it is essential to try and minimize equipment dead-space, especially if adapting that used for measurements in older subjects. For certain tests, especially those requiring long periods of tidal breathing, the use of a suitably selected video to distract and entertain the child (without inducing laughter or conversation!) can be very useful. For such tests, a face mask may be preferable to that of a mouthpiece in order to reduce risk of leaks and improve cooperation. However, the potential effect of any added dead-space when using a mask must be considered. Most young children tolerate a nose clip and mouth piece satisfactorily for short measurements such as spirometry.

PFTs that are now commonly applied in this age group include

- Spirometry [3, 9, 10, 13, 14, 32, 52, 58, 64, 67, 69–71]
- Plethysmographic specific resistance (sRaw) [9, 10, 13, 14, 51, 52, 55, 72]

  - N.B. assessment of Plethysmographic FRC is also possible in specialist laboratories [48], but is generally poorly tolerated below 5–6 years of age

- Interrupter Technique for assessing respiratory resistance [57, 61, 66, 73–75]
- Multiple breath washout assessments of FRC and LCI [9–11, 13, 14, 51, 52] (see Chap. 10)
- Forced oscillation technique or impulse oscillometry for assessing respiratory impedance [13, 14, 49, 54, 55, 57, 60, 76–79] (see Chap. 10)

Assessments using the MBW and forced oscillations are considered in Chap. 10 and will therefore not be addressed further here except in general terms.

Preschool Spirometry (Fig. 8.4):

The use of carefully designed computerized incentives can be extremely helpful in gaining the young child's cooperation in effort-dependent tests such as spirometry, but must be selected carefully and used interactively. For example, while blowing candles out is a useful means of teaching the child to blow out fast, it will rarely encourage the child to continue to blow out until residual volume is reached, for which alternative incentives such as a bowling alley may be more useful. Similarly, the operator must select the desired threshold that the child needs to reach, for which availability of appropriate reference equations is essential, as well as an appreciation of the child's clinical condition. It is generally helpful to set targets

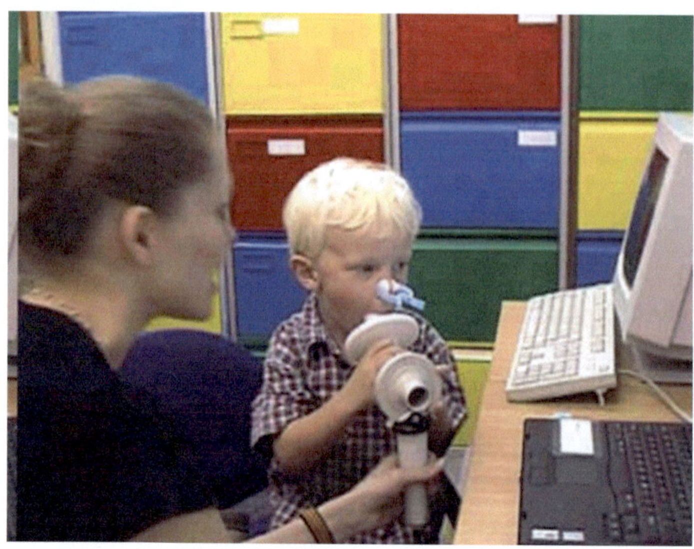

Fig. 8.4 Preschool spirometry. Photo courtesy of Janet Stocks

somewhat higher than that anticipated, to increase these further to encourage maximal effort if the child readily achieves the initial target, but to always allow the child to "win" by the end of the session in order to provide encouragement and a desire to return for future assessments!

Young children have a much shorter expiratory time constant (relatively large airway caliber in relation to lung volume) than older subjects and therefore empty their lungs rapidly during forced expiration. In healthy children <5 years of age, expiration may be completed in less than a second, such that FEV_1 cannot always be reported, $FEV_{0.75}$ providing a useful alternative [67, 68, 80]. If undertaking spirometry in preschool children, it is essential that Quality Control (QC) criteria are adapted accordingly; stipulation that a forced expired time of at least 6 s or even 3 s must be achieved is likely to be associated with a high failure rate. Conversely, applying adult criteria with respect to repeatability criteria will likely lead to acceptance of unduly variable results [67, 68, 80].

Current data suggest that while spirometry can be successfully performed in the majority of preschool children with CF, it is far less sensitive than the lung clearance index (LCI) from multiple breath washout, such that while early lung disease can sometimes be detected, the abnormalities are on average mild and highly variable [10, 58]. Given its sensitivity in older children with Bronchopulmonary Dysplasia (BPD) [3], spirometry could potentially provide a useful longitudinal measurement for young children with BPD, in whom both lung growth and airway obstruction may be significantly abnormal in early life [2, 26, 81]. Unfortunately there is a paucity of data on preschool spirometry in children with BPD, possibly associated with the difficulty of undertaking this technique in young children if there is reduced concentration span or coordination, such as may occur following extremely preterm delivery.

Spirometry is being increasingly used in children with recurrent wheezing, both to establish baseline lung function and document bronchodilator responsiveness (BDR) [14, 52, 62, 64, 82–84]. There are still limited data regarding the prevalence of BDR in normal preschool children and what constitutes a significant increase in forced expiratory volume after bronchodilator inhalation, but it has been suggested that a post-bronchodilator increase between 12 and 15 % in $FEV_{0.75}$ or FEV_1 is more commonly observed in preschool children with a clinical diagnosis of asthma than in healthy controls and exceeds the natural within-subject, between-test, within-occasion variability [52, 64, 67] . The use of FEF_{25-75} as an outcome to assess BDR is not recommended due to the high within and between-subject variability of this outcome [13]. Protocols for bronchial provocation and exercise testing in preschool children have been reported, but there is currently insufficient data to enable their use in clinical practice [13].

Plethysmographic Measurements of Specific Airway Resistance (sRaw)

sRaw is assessed while the child breathes tidally through a mouthpiece or modified facemask in a body plethysmograph (Figs. 8.5 and 8.6), without need for any special breathing maneuvers against an airway occlusion and is therefore well suited for preschool children. Since sRaw is the product of airway resistance (Raw) and FRC, both of which may increase in the presence of airway obstruction and hyperinflation, it is a potentially useful method for identifying obstructive lung disease in young children [14, 55, 72, 85]. sRaw has been found to be significantly elevated in preschool children with CF when compared with healthy controls, and appears to be

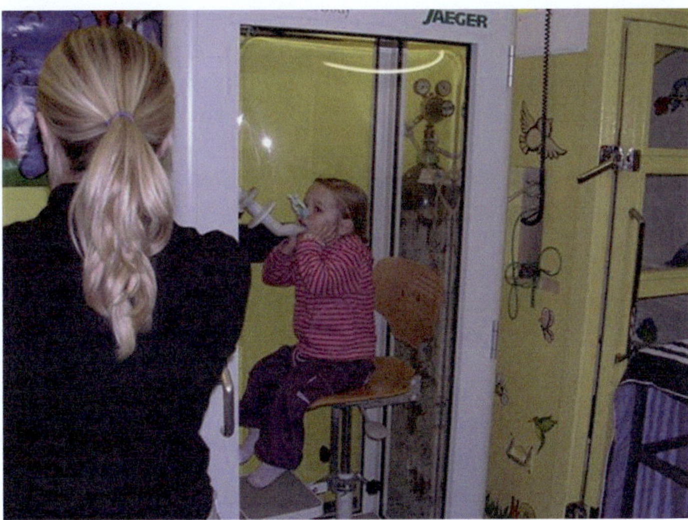

Fig. 8.5 Plethysmographic assessments of specific airways resistance in a preschool child. Photo courtesy of Janet Stocks

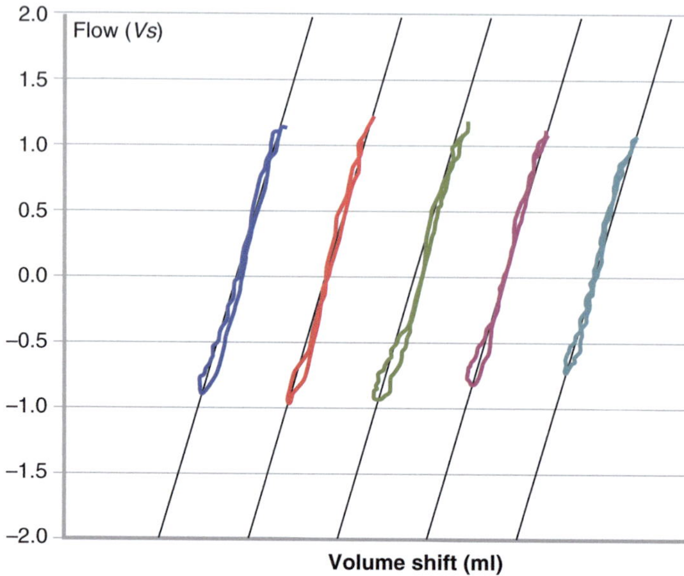

Fig. 8.6 Recording of plethysmographic pressure/flow loops for assessment of specific airway resistance. Courtesy of Janet Stocks

more discriminative than spirometry to early lung disease, though less so than the lung clearance index [9, 10, 86]. sRaw has been used in longitudinal birth cohort studies and been found to be higher in asthmatic children than in healthy controls. Although it has been suggested that bronchial hyper-responsiveness and BDR can be successfully determined using sRaw, with fair discrimination between healthy young children and those with asthma or wheeze [55, 72], the extent to which even healthy young children demonstrate significant bronchodilator responsiveness, means that a reduction in sRaw by at least 25 % is required before the change can be considered clinically significant. A recent study concluded that the capacity of sR_{aw} to discriminate between healthy young children and children with stable wheeze according to BDR is doubtful because of the large overlap in response between the two groups [52]. sRaw does not appear to have been used in children with prior BPD during the preschool years, possibly reflecting reduced concentration levels and delayed maturity in many of these children.

The Interrupter Technique

The interrupter resistance (Rint) technique is a quick, noninvasive measure of respiratory resistance that can be performed relatively easily in preschool children during tidal breathing. Rint is calculated from the ratio of pressure change to flow assessed at the airway opening during a brief (<100 ms) occlusion. Recent ATS/ERS guidelines recommend that occlusions for Rint occur during expiration. Although several studies have attempted to use Rint to assess lung function in preschool children with

CF, the lack of discrimination between healthy children and those with CF suggests that Rint will have limited clinical utility in this population. Higher values of Rint have been observed in preschool children with severe BPD when compared without BPD, but there is considerable overlap between groups [87]. As summarized in the recent ATS document on clinical utility of PFTs in young children [13], baseline Rint does not discriminate well between healthy children and those with recurrent wheeze due to the large inter-subject variability in Rint values in health. The main application of this test may be to assess BDR in wheezy children, although a reduction in Rint of at least 30 % is required before changes are considered to be of clinical significance [56, 73].

Challenges to Using Infant PFTs in Clinical Management

Despite numerous attempts to monitor changes in lung function as a means of identifying early onset of pulmonary disease during the first year of life, the natural course of pulmonary involvement in infants with respiratory disorders remains relatively poorly understood, for the following reasons

- Need for sedation
- Confounding by developmental changes in respiratory physiology [14]
- Lack of appropriate reference data
- Lack of information regarding within- and between-subject variability, especially in those with lung disease, without which it is impossible to interpret serial measurements or response to interventions including bronchodilators
- Difficulties in repeating measurements frequently enough to monitor change or long-term response to interventions accurately

Despite these significant challenges, among the 160 centers identified by a recent American Thoracic Society/European Respiratory Society (ATS/ERS) survey 37 (23 %) reported using infant PFTs purely for "clinical" applications and almost half of all respondents were using them to assess bronchodilator response (BDR). Given the time consuming nature of these tests (which may entail parents taking time off work), need for sedation and the considerable costs relating to equipment, consumables, and staffing costs for two specially trained and clinically qualified operators for each test [88], serious questions need to be asked regarding the clinical usefulness of results in any given child before undertaking or requesting infant PFTs "for clinical purposes."

Challenges to Using PFTs in Clinical Management of Preschool Children

The challenges to using PFTs in the clinical management of preschool children are similar, albeit not so difficult to address, as those encountered when dealing with infants. Anyone who has tested very young children will appreciate that, in addition to needing to adapt the technique, equipment and quality control criteria as discussed above, much more time needs to be allocated to obtaining technically satisfactory results in this age group, especially during their first few visits to the laboratory. Problems relating to lack of appropriate reference data and hence confidence in what constitutes an "unusual" or "abnormal" result for a preschool child are beginning to be resolved, thanks to international efforts to collate data from healthy young children [85, 89–92]. However, with the exception of recent multiethnic spirometry equations [91] such reference equations remain largely limited to children of non-Hispanic White European descent. Although there remains limited information regarding within-subject, within and between-occasion variability with which to assess the clinical significance of any observed acute response to a bronchodilator or longer term response to other interventions [66, 67, 74], several recent papers have begun to address these issues [13, 52, 64, 67].

As when assessing infants, the choice of techniques must reflect the underlying research or clinical question. While techniques such as forced oscillation and interrupter technique are often considered simpler to apply in this age range, they still require considerable quality control during data collection and analysis and the wide between-subject variability in health may limit the extent to which they can identify abnormal lung function in those with lung disease. While spirometry is perfectly feasible in preschool children it has been shown to be far less sensitive than the LCI in identifying early lung disease in young children with CF [9, 10] (Box 8.1).

> **Box 8.1. Which PFTs Should Be Used When Assessing Infants and Preschool Children?**
>
> - What is the research/clinical question?
> - What is the research/clinical question?
> - What is the underlying pathophysiology?
> - What is feasible in time available (duration of sleep in infants/concentration for young child)?
> - How much between-test variability may occur within any individual child?
> - Are valid reference equations available with which to interpret results?

Interpretation of Lung Function Results in Infants and Young Children and Their Role in Clinical Management

As in older subjects, the clinical usefulness of any lung function test within an individual infant or preschool child will always be enhanced if serial measures rather than a single assessment can be undertaken. However, during infancy the frequency with which PFTs can be repeated will be limited by need for sedation and the time consuming nature of the tests. When requesting such PFTs, it is essential that the choice of tests is based on the question to be answered, clinical reasoning, and a knowledge of the suspected underlying pathophysiology, rather than simply on the equipment that happens to be available in any given center [93]. Given the marked influence of factors such as preterm delivery, intrauterine growth retardation, sex, ethnic group, and maternal smoking during pregnancy, it is important to take a careful history from the parents when performing such tests in infants and young children with respiratory problems. It is also essential that such tests are only performed during periods of clinical stability, usually defined as being at least 2–3 weeks after any pulmonary exacerbation or upper respiratory tract infection. In addition to being potentially unethical due to the increased risk of sedation in a child who is acutely unwell or wheezing, attempts to assess efficacy of treatment by studying a child during the early phases of an exacerbation and then shortly after a course of antibiotics, corticosteroids, or bronchodilators, will at best reflect some natural improvement in lung function with time, but will provide minimal clinically useful information, unless part of a well-designed randomized trial with suitable placebo.

What Is Normal?

As discussed in more detail in Chap. 11, in order to identify the nature and severity of any underlying pathophysiology in an individual, it is essential to have a clear idea of the range of values to expect in a healthy child of similar age, sex, body size, and ethnicity. Reliable interpretation of pulmonary function results therefore relies on the availability of appropriate reference data to help distinguish between health and disease. The use of inappropriate reference equations and misinterpretation even when potentially appropriate equations are used, can lead to serious errors in both under and over-diagnosis, with its associated burden in terms of financial and human costs [94, 95]. It is important to remember that lung function results from healthy children and those with respiratory symptoms or disease often overlap to such an extent that a result within the normal range does not exclude disease. Similarly, while abnormal lung function results are often associated with symptoms and disease, they may simply be "atypical" and must always be interpreted in the light of all other clinically relevant information.

% Predicted or Z-Scores?

As discussed in Chap. 11, although clinicians in respiratory medicine are more familiar with the concept of expressing lung function as percent predicted, ([observed/predicted] $\times$ 100), a much better approach to interpreting lung function is to express results as Z-scores (or Standard Deviation Scores (SDS)) [94]. The Z-score is a mathematical combination of the percent predicted and the between-subject variability to give a single number that accounts for sex, age and height-related lung function variability expected within comparable healthy individuals (and, in certain cases also adjusts for ethnicity) [91]. The upper and lower limits of the normal range (ULN and LLN) are conventionally defined as Z-score of ± 1.64, a range that encompasses 90 % of healthy subjects. However, due to increased uncertainty regarding reliability of reference ranges for infants and young children and the fact that multiple PFTs are often used in the assessment, these limits should be set at ±1.96 Z-scores to encompass 95 % of the healthy population. An increasing number of clinical research studies are now reporting infant and preschool lung function as Z-scores [8, 10, 21, 23, 24, 33, 52, 64, 82, 96, 97]. Particular caution is required when interpreting results which lie close to the somewhat arbitrary "cutoffs" between the normal range seen in health and suspected disease, especially when results are limited to a single test occasion. As with all tests, PFTs should be seen as only one part of the whole clinical picture.

Reference Equations for Infant PFTs

Marked biases between predicted values can occur due to alterations in equipment and protocol, differences in population characteristics, the statistical methods applied or simply as a result of sampling error due to too few healthy subjects being studied. There is currently a dearth of appropriate reference equations for infant PFTs, many users relying on outdated values, based on too few subjects and collected with different equipment and software than is now available commercially. This can result in serious misdiagnosis and adversely affect interpretation of clinical research studies. The need for sedation and the time consuming nature of the testing procedure limits the number of healthy infants who can be studied at any one center. International collaborative efforts are urgently needed to address this problem before clinical studies in individual infants can be interpreted properly. As discussed in a recent editorial [98], issues surrounding the ethics of recruiting healthy infants for PFTs need to be addressed as an urgent priority, if we are to interpret results from those with lung disease with any confidence.

It has been shown that, whether using the tidal or Raised volume technique, serious mis-interpretation of forced expiratory maneuvers that are obtained with modern, commercially available equipment will occur if based on published reference equations derived from customized equipment developed within a different laboratory [99]. While a temporary adjustment factor has been proposed to address this problem, there is an urgent need to collate data from healthy infants studied in different laboratories but using the same protocols, equipment, and quality control, so that reliable, up to date reference equations can be developed. Given the impact of ethnicity on spirometric lung function in older subjects [91], such an initiative should not be restricted to infants of white European descent. Reference equations for tidal breathing, passive respiratory mechanics and plethysmographic FRC derived from healthy white infants studied using modern equipment have been published recently [100] but still require validation using data collected in other departments.

Can We Normalize by Body Size?

Lack of appropriate reference equations has led many centers to try to adjust for the rapid growth that occurs in infancy simply by dividing results such as tidal volume, lung volumes, or compliance by body weight at time of test and expressing results as ml/kg. There is increasing evidence that this practice is misguided and misleading, especially when applied to infants with lung disease in whom growth may be disproportionate [23, 26, 100]. Generally, as in older subjects, height (or in infants, length) is a better determinant of lung function than weight, although age and sex often have to be accounted for as well. Attempts to "normalize" lung function as a ratio in relation to length (i.e., per cm) should never be undertaken as the relationship between outcomes such as tidal or lung volumes and length is not linear, nor does the regression pass close to the origin, such that no consistent ratio occurs with growth in healthy subjects, making interpretation amongst those with lung disease impossible [100] (Box 8.2).

Box 8.2. Interpretation of Infant PFTs: Key Messages

- Limited reference data based on current commercially available equipment with which to identify abnormal lung function in individual infants.
- Prediction equations for infant PFTs should be based on appropriate regression equations with 95 % limits of normality derived from large number of infants (>100/sex), evenly distributed over first 2 years of life.
- Infant PFT results should not be expressed as ratio of body size.

Reference Equations for Preschool PFTs

Given the fact that it is much simpler to study healthy, conscious preschool children than sleeping, sedated infants, it is not surprising that more lung function reference data are available for young children than infants [101]. The applicability of many these equations may, however, be limited by differences in technique, equipment, quality control, number and age range of subjects studied and the type of statistical analysis applied [94] (see Chap. 11 for further details). International collaborative initiatives to address these issues has resulted in recent publication of reference equations for preschool children of White European descent with respect to spirometry [92], specific airways resistance (sRaw) [85], Interrupter resistance (Rint) [90] and multiple breath washout assessments of LCI and FRC using mass spectrometry [89]. All-age multi-ethnic spirometry equations which encompass the preschool age range and which have been endorsed by all the international respiratory societies have now been developed [91] and are currently being implemented into commercial devices (www.lungfunction.org).

Can PFTs Be Used in the Clinical Management of Individual Infants?

Although there is little doubt about the potential value of infant lung function tests as a means of providing objective outcome measures in clinical or epidemiologic research studies [1, 2, 7, 8, 14, 15, 18, 21, 23, 24, 26, 28, 29, 31, 33, 37, 50, 63, 81, 102–106], their potential usefulness with respect to influencing clinical management within an individual infant remains highly debatable. The clinical usefulness of any technique depends not only on its ability to measure parameters that are relevant to the underlying pathophysiology and to discriminate between health and disease, but also on within-subject repeatability both within and between test occasions. As discussed earlier, although highly reproducible measurements of lung function can be made in infants during the same test occasion, little is known about within-subject, between-test repeatability, which severely limits their use in the clinical management of individual infants, except in departments with a high level of expertise and contemporaneous control data collected using identical equipment and software.

Can PFTs Be Used in the Clinical Management of Individual Preschool Children?

The major clinical role of preschool PFTs would be to monitor disease severity over time, evaluate response to treatments, and serve as objective outcome measures in clinical research studies. The results should always be interpreted in the context of other clinical signs and symptoms and, as with any diagnostic test, preschool PFT results should be just one additional piece of evidence utilized by clinicians in their assessment and clinical decision making. A recent report from an official ATS workshop which reviewed five preschool lung function tests (namely spirometry, specific airway resistance, the interrupter technique, forced oscillation, and multiple breath washout), concluded that while such tests were safe and feasible in 3–6 year old children if undertaken by suitably qualified individuals, insufficient evidence currently exists to recommend incorporation of these tests into the routine clinical monitoring of infants and young children with CF, BPD or recurrent wheeze although such tests were considered to be valuable tools with which to address specific concerns [13]. Spirometry can be successfully applied to the preschool population in the clinical setting to identify disease states and track lung function over time. Assessment of sRaw is also extremely feasible in this age group, but further work is required to standardize this technique, especially with regard to the breathing pattern adopted during measurements [85].

Conclusions

Thanks to the development of commercially available devices, it is becoming increasingly feasible to perform infant PFTs, but these assessments require special expertise, are expensive to perform and are very time consuming (both for staff and families). Clinical interpretation of results in individual infants is often limited by lack of appropriate normative data and knowledge of within-subject variability, the need for sedation, and inability to repeat measurements at frequent intervals.

The reason for undertaking such measurements and confidence that meaningful results are likely to be obtained should therefore be clearly established before requesting such tests in infants, particularly those who are clinically unstable. While PFTs are safe and feasible in 3–6-year-old children if undertaken by suitably qualified individuals, insufficient evidence currently exists regarding within and between occasion variability to recommend incorporation of these tests into the routine clinical monitoring of young children with lung disease. Nevertheless, such tests can be valuable tools with which to address specific concerns such as ongoing symptoms or monitoring response to treatment and as outcome measures in clinical research studies.

References

1. Prendergast M, Rafferty GF, Milner AD, Broughton S, Davenport M, Jani J, et al. Lung function at follow-up of infants with surgically correctable anomalies. Pediatr Pulmonol. 2012; 47(10):973–8.
2. Schmalisch G, Wilitzki S, Roehr CC, Proquitte H, Buhrer C. Development of lung function in very low birth weight infants with or without bronchopulmonary dysplasia: longitudinal assessment during the first 15 months of corrected age. BMC Pediatr. 2012;12:37.
3. Lum S, Bush A, Stocks J. Clinical pulmonary function testing for children with bronchopulmonary dysplasia. Pediatr Allergy Immunol Pulmonol. 2011;24(2):77–88.
4. May C, Kennedy C, Milner AD, Rafferty GF, Peacock JL, Greenough A. Lung function abnormalities in infants developing bronchopulmonary dysplasia. Arch Dis Child. 2011; 96(11):1014–9.
5. Prendergast M, May C, Broughton S, Pollina E, Milner AD, Rafferty GF, et al. Chorioamnionitis, lung function and bronchopulmonary dysplasia in prematurely born infants. Arch Dis Child Fetal Neonatal Ed. 2011;96:F270–4.
6. Roehr CC, Wilitzki S, Opgen-Rhein B, Kalache K, Proquitte H, Buhrer C, et al. Early lung function testing in infants with aortic arch anomalies identifies patients at risk for airway obstruction. PLoS One. 2011;6(9):e24903.
7. Balinotti JE, Chakr VC, Tiller C, Kimmel R, Coates C, Kisling J, et al. Growth of lung parenchyma in infants and toddlers with chronic lung disease of infancy. Am J Respir Crit Care Med. 2010;181(10):1093–7.
8. Hoo AF, Gupta A, Lum S, Costeloe KL, Huertas-Ceballos A, Marlow N, et al. Impact of ethnicity and extreme prematurity on infant pulmonary function. Pediatr Pulmonol. 2013; 49(7):679–87.
9. Aurora P, Bush A, Gustafsson P, Oliver C, Wallis C, Price J, et al. Multiple-breath washout as a marker of lung disease in preschool children with cystic fibrosis. Am J Respir Crit Care Med. 2005;171(3):249–56.
10. Aurora P, Stanojevic S, Wade A, Oliver C, Kozlowska W, Lum S, et al. Lung clearance index at 4 years predicts subsequent lung function in children with cystic fibrosis. Am J Respir Crit Care Med. 2011;183:752–8.
11. Gustafsson PM. Inert gas washout in preschool children. Paediatr Respir Rev. 2005;6(4):239–45.
12. Robinson PD, Latzin P, Verbanck S, Hall GL, Horsley A, Gappa M, et al. Consensus statement for inert gas washout measurement using multiple- and single-breath tests. Eur Respir J. 2013;41(3):507–22.
13. Rosenfeld M, Allen J, Arets B, Aurora P, Beydon N, Calogero C, et al. An Official American Thoracic Society Workshop Report: optimal lung function tests for monitoring cystic

fibrosis, bronchopulmonary dysplasia and recurrent wheezing in children <6 years of age. Ann Am Thorac Soc. 2013;10:S1–11.

14. Stocks J, Lum S. Pulmonary function tests in infants and preschool children. In: Wilmott RW, Boat TF, Bush A, Chernick V, Deterding R, Ratjen F, editors. Kendig's disorders of the respiratory tract in children. 8th ed. Philadelphia, PA: Elsevier; 2012. p. 169–210.

15. Latzin P, Roth S, Thamrin C, Hutten GJ, Pramana I, Kuehni CE, et al. Lung volume, breathing pattern and ventilation inhomogeneity in preterm and term infants. PLoS One. 2009;4(2):e4635.

16. Baldwin DN, Pillow JJ, Stocks J, Frey U. Lung-function tests in neonates and infants with chronic lung disease: tidal breathing and respiratory control. Pediatr Pulmonol. 2006;41(5):391–419.

17. Hutten GJ, van Eykern LA, Latzin P, Kyburz M, van Aalderen WM, Frey U. Relative impact of respiratory muscle activity on tidal flow and end expiratory volume in healthy neonates. Pediatr Pulmonol. 2008;43(9):882–91.

18. McEvoy C, Schilling D, Peters D, Tillotson C, Spitale P, Wallen L, et al. Respiratory compliance in preterm infants after a single rescue course of antenatal steroids: a randomized controlled trial. Am J Obstet Gynecol. 2010;202(6):544–9.

19. Gappa M, Pillow JJ, Allen J, Mayer O, Stocks J. Lung function tests in neonates and infants with chronic lung disease: lung and chest-wall mechanics. Pediatr Pulmonol. 2006;41(4):291–317.

20. Malmberg LP, von WL, Kotaniemi-Syrjanen A, Malmstrom K, Pelkonen AS, Makela MJ. Methacholine-induced lung function changes measured with infant body plethysmography. Pediatr Pulmonol. 2011;46(4):362–8.

21. Davis SD, Rosenfeld M, Kerby GS, Brumback L, Kloster MH, Acton JD, et al. Multicenter evaluation of infant lung function tests as cystic fibrosis clinical trial endpoints. Am J Respir Crit Care Med. 2010;182:1387–97.

22. Hulskamp G, Pillow JJ, Dinger J, Stocks J. Lung function tests in neonates and infants with chronic lung disease of infancy: functional residual capacity. Pediatr Pulmonol. 2006;41(1):1–22.

23. Hoo A-F, Thia L, Nguyen TD, Bush A, Chudleigh J, Lum S, et al. Lung function is abnormal in 3 month old infants with cystic fibrosis diagnosed by newborn screening. Thorax. 2012;67:874–81.

24. Nguyen TT, Thia LP, Hoo AF, Bush A, Aurora P, Wade A, et al. Evolution of lung function during the first year of life in newborn screened cystic fibrosis infants. Thorax 2013. doi:10.1136/thoraxjnl-2013-204023.

25. Belessis Y, Dixon B, Hawkins G, Pereira J, Peat J, MacDonald R, et al. Early cystic fibrosis lung disease detected by bronchoalveolar lavage and lung clearance index. Am J Respir Crit Care Med. 2012;185(8):862–73.

26. Hulskamp G, Lum S, Stocks J, Wade A, Hoo AF, Costeloe K, et al. Association of prematurity, lung disease and body size with lung volume and ventilation inhomogeneity in unsedated neonates: a multicentre study. Thorax. 2009;64(3):240–5.

27. Pillow JJ, Frerichs I, Stocks J. Lung function tests in neonates and infants with chronic lung disease: global and regional ventilation inhomogeneity. Pediatr Pulmonol. 2006;41(2):105–21.

28. Bisgaard H, Loland L, Holst KK, Pipper CB. Prenatal determinants of neonatal lung function in high-risk newborns. J Allergy Clin Immunol. 2009;123(3):651. 7.

29. Borrego LM, Stocks J, Leiria-Pinto P, Peralta I, Romeira AM, Neuparth N, et al. Lung function and clinical risk factors for asthma in infants and young children with recurrent wheeze. Thorax. 2009;64(3):203–9.

30. Friedrich L, Pitrez PM, Stein RT, Goldani M, Tepper R, Jones MH. Growth rate of lung function in healthy preterm infants. Am J Respir Crit Care Med. 2007;176(12):1269–73.

31. Jones M. Effect of preterm birth on airway function and lung growth. Paediatr Respir Rev. 2009;10 Suppl 1:9–11.

32. Kozlowska WJ, Bush A, Wade A, Aurora P, Carr SB, Castle RA, et al. Lung function from infancy to the preschool years after clinical diagnosis of cystic fibrosis. Am J Respir Crit Care Med. 2008;178(1):42–9.

33. Linnane BM, Hall GL, Nolan G, Brennan S, Stick SM, Sly PD, et al. Lung function in infants with cystic fibrosis diagnosed by newborn screening. Am J Respir Crit Care Med. 2008;178(12):1238–44.

34. Lum S, Stocks J, Castile R, Davies S, Henschen M, Jones M, et al. ATS/ERS statement: raised volume forced expirations in infants: guidelines for current practice. Am J Respir Crit Care Med. 2005;172(11):1463–71.

35. Lum S, Hulskamp G, Merkus P, Baraldi E, Hofhuis W, Stocks J. Lung function tests in neonates and infants with chronic lung disease: forced expiratory maneuvers. Pediatr Pulmonol. 2006;41(3):199–214.

36. Pillarisetti N, Williamson E, Linnane B, Skoric B, Robertson CF, Robinson P, et al. Infection, inflammation, and lung function decline in infants with cystic fibrosis. Am J Respir Crit Care Med. 2011;184(1):75–81.

37. Rosenfeld M, Ratjen F, Brumback L, Daniel S, Rowbotham R, McNamara S, et al. Inhaled hypertonic saline in infants and children younger than 6 years with cystic fibrosis: the ISIS randomized controlled trial. JAMA. 2012;307(21):2269–77.

38. Stocks J, Sly PD, Tepper RS, Morgan WJ. Infant respiratory function testing. 1st ed. New York: Wiley; 1996.

39. Bates J, Schmalisch G, Filbrun D, Stocks J. Tidal breath analysis for infant pulmonary function testing. Eur Respir J. 2000;16:1180–92.

40. Frey U, Stocks J, Coates A, Sly P, Bates J. Standards for infant respiratory function testing: specifications for equipment used for infant pulmonary function testing. Eur Respir J. 2000;16:731–40.

41. Sly P, Tepper R, Henschen M, Gappa M, Stocks J. Standards for infant respiratory function testing: tidal forced expirations. Eur Respir J. 2000;16:741–8.

42. Stocks J, Sly P, Morris MG, Frey U. Standards for infant respiratory function testing: what(ever) next? Eur Respir J. 2000;16:581–4.

43. Gappa M, Colin AA, Goetz I, Stocks J. Passive respiratory mechanics: the occlusion techniques. Eur Respir J. 2001;17:141–8.

44. Morris MG, Gustafsson P, Tepper R, Gappa M, Stocks J. Standards for infant respiratory function testing: the bias flow nitrogen washout technique for measuring the functional residual capacity. Eur Respir J. 2001;17:529–36.

45. Stocks J, Godfrey S, Beardsmore C, Bar-Yishay E, Castile R. Standards for infant respiratory function testing: plethysmographic measurements of lung volume and airway resistance. Eur Respir J. 2001;17:302–12.

46. Subbarao P, Hulskamp G, Stocks J. Limitations of electronic compensation for measuring plethysmographic airway resistance in infants. Pediatr Pulmonol. 2005;40(1):45–52.

47. Broughton S, Rafferty GF, Milner AD, Greenough A. Effect of electronic compensation on plethysmographic airway resistance measurements. Pediatr Pulmonol. 2008;43(1):104.

48. Vilozni D, Efrati O, Hakim F, Adler A, Livnat G, Bentur L. FRC measurements using body plethysmography in young children. Pediatr Pulmonol. 2009;44(9):885–91.

49. Thamrin C, Gangell CL, Udomittipong K, Kusel MM, Patterson H, Fukushima T, et al. Assessment of bronchodilator responsiveness in preschool children using forced oscillations. Thorax. 2007;62(9):814–9.

50. Stocks J, Thia L, Sonnappa S. Evaluation and use of childhood lung function tests in cystic fibrosis. Curr Opin Pulm Med. 2012;18:602–8.

51. Sonnappa S, Bastardo C, Wade A, Seglani S, McKenzie SA, Bush A, et al. Symptom-pattern phenotype and pulmonary function in preschool wheezers. J Allergy Clin Immunol. 2010;126:519–26.

52. Sonnappa S, Bastardo C, Wade A, Bush A, Stocks J, Aurora P. Repeatability and bronchodilator reversibility of lung function in preschool children. Eur Respir J. 2013;42:116–24.

53. Ren CL, Rosenfeld M, Mayer OH, Davis SD, Kloster M, Castile RG, et al. Analysis of the associations between lung function and clinical features in preschool children with cystic fibrosis. Pediatr Pulmonol. 2012;47(6):574–81.

54. Oostveen E, Dom S, Desager K, Hagendorens M, De BW, Weyler J. Lung function and bronchodilator response in 4-year-old children with different wheezing phenotypes. Eur Respir J. 2010;35(4):865–72.

55. Nielsen KG. Lung function and bronchial responsiveness in young children. Clinical and research applications. Dan Med Bull. 2006;53(1):46–75.

56. Mele L, Sly PD, Calogero C, Bernardini R, Novembre E, Azzari C, et al. Assessment and validation of bronchodilation using the interrupter technique in preschool children. Pediatr Pulmonol. 2010;45(7):633–8.

57. Marchal F, Schweitzer C, Thuy LV. Forced oscillations, interrupter technique and body plethysmography in the preschool child. Paediatr Respir Rev. 2005;6(4):278–84.

58. Kerby GS, Rosenfeld M, Ren CL, Mayer OH, Brumback L, Castile R, et al. Lung function distinguishes preschool children with CF from healthy controls in a multi-center setting. Pediatr Pulmonol. 2012;47(6):597–605.

59. Jeng MJ, Chang HL, Tsai MC, Tsao PC, Yang CF, Lee YS, et al. Spirometric pulmonary function parameters of healthy Chinese children aged 3–6 years in Taiwan. Pediatr Pulmonol. 2009;44(7):676–82.

60. Gangell CL, Horak Jr F, Patterson HJ, Sly PD, Stick SM, Hall GL. Respiratory impedance in children with cystic fibrosis using forced oscillations in clinic. Eur Respir J. 2007;30(5):892–7.

61. Gangell CL, Hall GL, Stick SM, Sly PD. Lung function testing in preschool-aged children with cystic fibrosis in the clinical setting. Pediatr Pulmonol. 2010;45(5):419–33.

62. Galant SP, Nickerson B. Lung function measurement in the assessment of childhood asthma: recent important developments. Curr Opin Allergy Clin Immunol. 2010;10(2):149–54.

63. Brumback LC, Davis SD, Kerby GS, Kloster M, Johnson R, Castile R, et al. Lung function from infancy to preschool in a cohort of children with cystic fibrosis. Eur Respir J. 2013;41(1):60–6.

64. Borrego LM, Stocks J, Almeida I, Stanojevic S, Antunes J, Leiria-Pinto P, et al. Bronchodilator responsiveness using spirometry in healthy and asthmatic preschool children. Arch Dis Child. 2013;98(2):112–7.

65. Beydon N. Assessment of bronchial responsiveness in preschool children. Paediatr Respir Rev. 2006;7 Suppl 1:S23–5.

66. Beydon N, M'buila C, Bados A, Peiffer C, Bernard A, Zaccaria I, et al. Interrupter resistance short-term repeatability and bronchodilator response in preschool children. Respir Med. 2007;101(12):2482–7.

67. Beydon N, Davis SD, Lombardi E, Allen JL, Arets HG, Aurora P, et al. An official American Thoracic Society/European Respiratory Society statement: pulmonary function testing in preschool children. Am J Respir Crit Care Med. 2007;175(12):1304–45.

68. Aurora P, Stocks J, Oliver C, Saunders C, Castle R, Chaziparasidis G, et al. Quality control for spirometry in preschool children with and without lung disease. Am J Respir Crit Care Med. 2004;169(10):1152–9.

69. Mayer OH, Jawad AF, McDonough J, Allen J. Lung function in 3–5-year-old children with cystic fibrosis. Pediatr Pulmonol. 2008;43(12):1214–23.

70. Vilozni D, Livnat G, Dabbah H, Elias N, Hakim F, Bentur L. The potential use of spirometry during methacholine challenge test in young children with respiratory symptoms. Pediatr Pulmonol. 2009;44(7):720–7.

71. Vilozni D, Berkun Y, Levi Y, Weiss B, Jacobson JM, Efrati O. The feasibility and validity of forced spirometry in ataxia telangiectasia. Pediatr Pulmonol. 2010;45(10):1030–6.

72. Bisgaard H, Nielsen KG. Plethysmographic measurements of specific airway resistance in young children. Chest. 2005;128(1):355–62.

73. Beydon N, M'buila C, Peiffer C, Bernard A, Zaccaria I, Denjean A. Can bronchodilator response predict bronchial response to methacholine in preschool coughers? Pediatr Pulmonol. 2008;43(8):815–21.

74. Chan EY, Bridge PD, Dundas I, Pao CS, Healy MJ, McKenzie SA. Repeatability of airway resistance measurements made using the interrupter technique. Thorax. 2003;58(4):344–7.

75. Gochicoa LG, Thome-Ortiz LP, Furuya ME, Canto R, Ruiz-Garcia ME, Zuniga-Vazquez G, et al. Reference values for airway resistance in newborns, infants and preschoolers from a Latin American population. Respirology. 2012;17(4):667–73.

76. Nielsen KG, Bisgaard H. Discriminative capacity of bronchodilator response measured with three different lung function techniques in asthmatic and healthy children aged 2 to 5 years. Am J Respir Crit Care Med. 2001;164(4):554–9.

77. Song TW, Kim KW, Kim ES, Park JW, Sohn MH, Kim KE. Utility of impulse oscillometry in young children with asthma. Pediatr Allergy Immunol. 2008;19(8):763–8.

78. Thamrin C, Albu G, Sly PD, Hantos Z. Negative impact of the noseclip on high-frequency respiratory impedance measurements. Respir Physiol Neurobiol. 2009;165(1):115–8.

79. Thamrin C, Gangell CL, Kusel MM, Schultz A, Hall GL, Stick SM, et al. Expression of bronchodilator response using forced oscillation technique measurements: absolute versus relative. Eur Respir J. 2010;36(1):212.

80. Lum S, Stocks J. Forced expiratory manoeuvres. In: Merkus P, Frey U, editors. Paediatric lung function. Sheffield, UK: ERS Journals Ltd; 2010. p. 46–65.

81. Stocks J, Coates A, Bush A. Lung function in infants and young children with chronic lung disease of infancy: The next steps? Pediatr Pulmonol. 2007;42(1):3–9.

82. Bisgaard H, Jensen SM, Bonnelykke K. Interaction between asthma and lung function growth in early life. Am J Respir Crit Care Med. 2012;185(11):1183–9.

83. Sonnappa S, Bastardo CM, Saglani S, Bush A, Aurora P. Relationship between past airway pathology and current lung function in preschool wheezers. Eur Respir J. 2011;38(6):1431–6.

84. Vilozni D, Hakim F, Adler A, Livnat G, Bar-Yishay E, Bentur L. Reduced vital capacity after methacholine challenge in early childhood–is it due to trapped air or loss of motivation. Respir Med. 2009;103(1):109–16.

85. Kirkby J, Stanojevic S, Welsh L, Lum S, Badier M, Beardsmore C, et al. Reference equations for specific airway resistance in children: the asthma UK initiative. Eur Respir J. 2010;36(3):622–9.

86. Nielsen KG, Pressler T, Klug B, Koch C, Bisgaard H. Serial lung function and responsiveness in cystic fibrosis during early childhood. Am J Respir Crit Care Med. 2004;169(11):1209–16.

87. Kairamkonda VR, Richardson J, Subhedar N, Bridge PD, Shaw NJ. Lung function measurement in prematurely born preschool children with and without chronic lung disease. J Perinatol. 2008;28(3):199–204.

88. Lesnick BL, Davis SD. Infant pulmonary function testing: overview of technology and practical considerations—new current procedural terminology codes effective 2010. Chest. 2011;139(5):1197–202.

89. Lum S, Stocks J, Stanojevic S, Wade A, Robinson P, Gustafsson P, et al. Age and height dependence of lung clearance index and functional residual capacity. Eur Respir J. 2013;41:1371–7.

90. Merkus PJ, Stocks J, Beydon N, Lombardi E, Jones M, McKenzie SA, et al. Reference ranges for interrupter resistance technique: the Asthma UK Initiative. Eur Respir J. 2010;36(1):157–63.

91. Quanjer PH, Stanojevic S, Cole TJ, Baur X, Hall GL, Culver B, et al. Multi-ethnic reference values for spirometry for the 3–95 year age range: the global lung function 2012 equations. Eur Respir J. 2012;40:1324–43.

92. Stanojevic S, Wade A, Cole TJ, Lum S, Custovic A, Silverman M, et al. Spirometry centile charts for young Caucasian children: the Asthma UK Collaborative Initiative. Am J Respir Crit Care Med. 2009;180(6):547–52.

93. Stocks J, Kirkby J, Lum S. How to avoid misinterpreting lung function tests in children: a few practical tips. Pediatr Respir Rev. 2014;14(2):170–80.

94. Stanojevic S, Wade A, Stocks J. Reference values for lung function: past, present and future. Eur Respir J. 2010;36(1):12–9.

95. Stanojevic S, Stocks J, Bountziouka V, Aurora P, Kirkby J, Bourke S, et al. The impact of switching to the new global lung function initiative equations on spirometry results in the UK CF Registry. J Cyst Fibros. 2013;13(3):319–27.

96. Keklikian E, Sanchez-Solis M, Bonina AJ, Meneguzzi A, Pastor-Vivero MD, Mondejar-Lopez P, et al. Do risk factors for persistent asthma modify lung function in infants and young children with recurrent wheeze? Pediatr Pulmonol. 2010;45(9):914–8.
97. Pelkonen AS, Kotaniemi-Syrjanen A, Malmstrom K, Malmberg LP, Makela MJ. Clinical findings associated with abnormal lung function in children aged 3–26 months with recurrent respiratory symptoms. Acta Paediatr. 2010;99(8):1175–9.
98. Stocks J, Modi N, Tepper R. Need for healthy controls when assessing lung function in infants with respiratory disease. Am J Respir Crit Care Med. 2010;182:1340–2.
99. Lum S, Hoo AF, Hulskamp G, Wade A, Stocks J. Potential misinterpretation of infant lung function unless prospective healthy controls are studied. Pediatr Pulmonol. 2010;45: 906–13.
100. Nguyen TTD, Hoo A-F, Lum S, Wade A, Thia LP, Stocks J. New reference equations to improve interpretation of infant lung function. Pediatr Pulmonol. 2013;48(4):370–80.
101. Stanojevic S, Wade A, Lum S, Stocks J. Reference equations for pulmonary function tests in preschool children: a review. Pediatr Pulmonol. 2007;42(10):962–72.
102. Pike KC, Rose-Zerilli MJ, Osvald EC, Inskip HM, Godfrey KM, Crozier SR, et al. The relationship between infant lung function and the risk of wheeze in the preschool years. Pediatr Pulmonol. 2011;46(1):75–82.
103. van der Zalm MM, Uiterwaal CS, Wilbrink B, Koopman M, Verheij TJ, van der Ent CK. The influence of neonatal lung function on rhinovirus-associated wheeze. Am J Respir Crit Care Med. 2011;183(2):262–7.
104. Llapur CJ, Martinez TM, Coates C, Tiller C, Wiebke JL, Li X, et al. Lung structure and function of infants with recurrent wheeze when asymptomatic. Eur Respir J. 2009;33(1): 107–12.
105. Mallol J, Aguirre V, Barrueto L, Wandalsen G, Tepper R. Effect of inhaled fluticasone on lung function in infants with recurrent wheezing: a randomised controlled trial. Allergol Immunopathol (Madr). 2009;37(2):57–62.
106. Sly PD, Brennan S, Gangell C, de Klerk N, Murray C, Mott L, et al. Lung disease at diagnosis in infants with cystic fibrosis detected by newborn screening. Am J Respir Crit Care Med. 2009;180(2):146–52.

Chapter 9
Newer Pulmonary Function Tests

Graham L. Hall and Paul D. Robinson

Abstract The measurement of lung function is an integral component of respiratory medicine. In the past 10–15 years there has been significant progress in the development of newer lung function tests such that there are now standardized guidelines and commercially available equipment for some of these techniques. This chapter focuses on the forced oscillation technique, the interrupter technique and the multiple breath washout test and their application in preschool and school aged children and the potential role of these tests in the diagnosis and management of children with respiratory disease. A primary advantage of these tests is the relatively minimal level of cooperation that is required to obtained acceptable measurements thus making them ideally suited for use in children as young as 2–3 years of age. This creates opportunities to introduce objective measurements of respiratory function at a significantly younger age than previously possible. The aim of this chapter is to provide the reader with an overview of each of these tests and to summarize the evidence that these tests can be used to monitor changes in clinical status.

Keywords Multiple breath washout • Lung clearance index • Forced oscillation technique • Interrupter technique • Respiratory physiology • Lung function testing • Children

G.L. Hall, Ph.D., F.R.A.N.Z.S.R.S. (✉)
Telethon Kids Institute, University of Western Australia,
PO Box 855, West Perth, WA 6872, Australia

Respiratory Medicine, Princess Margaret Hospital for Children, Perth, WA, Australia
e-mail: graham.hall@telethonkids.org.au

P.D. Robinson, M.B.Ch.B., F.R.A.C.P., Ph.D.
Respiratory Medicine, The Children's Hospital at Westmead,
Locked Bag 4001, Sydney, NSW 2145, Australia

Discipline of Paediatrics and Child Health, Faculty of Medicine, The Children's Hospital at Westmead Clinical School, University of Sydney, Sydney, NSW, Australia

The Woolcock Institute of Medical Research, Sydney, NSW, Australia
e-mail: paul.robinson1@health.nsw.gov.au

© Springer Science+Business Media New York 2015
S.D. Davis et al. (eds.), *Diagnostic Tests in Pediatric Pulmonology*,
Respiratory Medicine, DOI 10.1007/978-1-4939-1801-0_9

Introduction

The objective measurement of respiratory function has been an integral component of respiratory medicine for decades. The most commonly used lung function tests in the pediatric respiratory function laboratory will include spirometry, static lung volumes (usually by plethysmography), and the gas transfer of carbon monoxide. As highlighted elsewhere in this book a disadvantage of these lung function tests is the difficulty in using them in infants and young children primarily due to the active cooperation required to achieve acceptable and repeatable outcomes with these tests. In the past 10–15 years there has been significant progress in the development of newer lung function tests from techniques employed in a limited number of specialized research centers with research prototypes to tests able to be performed in a standard pediatric respiratory function laboratory with commercially available equipment. These tests include the raised volume rapid thoracic compression technique and body plethysmography for use in infants; the forced oscillation technique (FOT), the interrupter technique, specific airway resistance and the multiple breath washout (MBW) technique suitable for use in both infants and young children. This chapter will review FOT, the MBW test and the interrupter technique and their application in preschool and school aged children and the potential role of these tests in the diagnosis and management of children with respiratory disease. Readers interested in infant lung function tests are directed to Chap. 9.

These newer lung function tests offer new ways to understand, diagnose, and manage respiratory disease in children. A primary advantage of these tests is the relatively minimal level of cooperation that is required to obtain acceptable measurements thus making them ideally suited for use in children as young as 2–3 years of age. This creates opportunities to introduce objective measurements of respiratory function at a significantly younger age than previously possible. However, there are limitations with each of these tests and their role in the clinical management of individual patients is not clear.

The aim of this chapter is to provide the reader with an overview of each lung function test, including a summary of test protocols; definitions of acceptable and repeatable test outcomes; currently available reference data; the current knowledge of a clinically meaningful difference for each of the tests; and the evidence that these tests can be used to monitor changes in clinical status.

Forced Oscillation Technique

The forced oscillation technique (FOT) was first described by Dubois and colleagues in 1956 [1]. Since that initial description the technique has been applied extensively in preclinical animal models (as reviewed by Sly et al. [2]), infants (for example [3–7]), and preschool and school aged children as well as adults of all ages (as reviewed in [8, 9]). Oscillatory equipment has advanced from discrete single center research prototypes to being commercially available for both animal based research and human research and clinical testing.

The FOT uses the application of a forcing signal to the respiratory system, most commonly at the mouth, to quantify respiratory system mechanics. At the most basic level FOT is similar to that of a ventilator applied sine wave to an intubated patient and the use of the resultant pressures, flows and volumes to derive respiratory system resistance (Rrs) and compliance (being the inverse of respiratory system elastance (Ers)). In practice the majority of research and commercial oscillatory equipment apply a forcing signal that covers a range of frequencies with the response to this signal being the respiratory system impedance (Zrs). The respiratory system impedance is comprised of the Rrs and the respiratory reactance (Xrs) across the range of frequencies being measured. The Rrs represents the resistive elements of the respiratory system, including the airways, lung, and chest wall; however, the airway resistance represents the largest component of Rrs. The respiratory reactance includes both the elastic properties of the lung at lower frequencies and the inertive properties of the airways at higher frequencies. These components are opposite in sign and the frequency at which the elastic and inertive properties are equal (but opposite) is the resonant frequency (Fres) which occurs at the point that Xrs equals zero [10]. Readers seeking detailed information on technical aspects of the technique are directed to comprehensive reviews [9, 10].

The Forced Oscillation Technique Methodology

There are commercially available FOT systems and the most commonly reported are the CareFusion Impulse oscillation system (IOS) and the Cosmed Quark I2M. For the purposes of this chapter the generic term FOT is used to mean all forced oscillation systems and individual commercial systems are only identified if there are equipment specific issues.

The FOT is usually applied in awake individuals but has also been reported in anesthetized children [11] and has been combined with continuous positive airway pressure ventilation [12]. As the focus of this review is the application of the FOT in the pediatric setting we have limited the methodological description below to that used in preschool and school aged children. There are no current international standards for the measurement of forced oscillatory mechanics similar to those used for other lung function tests [13–15]. However, guidelines for the use of FOT in clinical practice [9] and in preschool children [8] are available and readers are encouraged to consult these for full details.

Generally, FOT measurements are performed in a sitting upright position with the subject's head in the midline. Children maintain normal tidal breathing through a mouthpiece (usually incorporating a bacterial filter) while wearing a nose clip. To minimize the impact of shunting in the highly compliant extra-thoracic airways, the cheeks and floor of the mouth need to be firmly supported [16, 17]. In young children this is preferably performed by a staff member to maximize test quality (as seen in Fig. 9.1), but can be performed by a parent. In older children this can be performed by the children themselves.

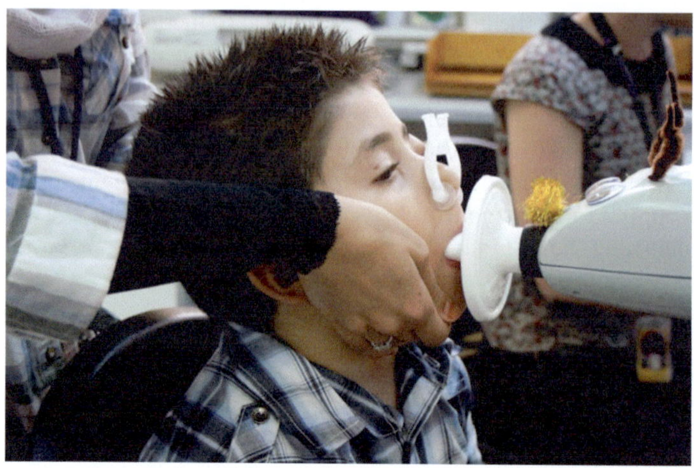

Fig. 9.1 Forced oscillation measurement in a 5-year-old child. Children should be seated upright with their head in the midline and neutral position. The child breathes through a mouthpiece incorporating a bacterial filter with a nose clip in place. Firm support of the cheeks and roof of the mouth is important to minimize the pressure loss of the oscillatory signal

Acceptability and Repeatability of FOT Measurements

Acceptable measurements should be free of artifact including leak, swallowing, mouth movements, talking and other noises and obstruction of the mouthpiece with the child's tongue. These criteria can be assessed through visual inspection of the Zrs spectra and the individual pressure and flow recordings. In young children additional feedback from the staff member supporting the cheeks and the floor of the mouth can be very helpful. A minimum of three to five acceptable measurements should be obtained and the average and standard deviation (SD) of all acceptable measurements are reported [8, 9]. The most commonly reported FOT outcomes are the Rrs and Xrs at individual specific frequencies and reported as Rrsf and Xrsf (for example Rrs and Xrs at 8 Hz are denoted as Rrs8 and Xrs8), the resonant frequency (Fres) and the area under the reactance curve (AX; defined as the area under the Xrs curve from a defined frequency to the resonant frequency) [18]. Figure 9.2 illustrates these commonly reported outcomes in a healthy child and a child with cystic fibrosis (CF).

To date there is insufficient evidence to allow the definition of intra-test repeatability that can be used to state that a test session is repeatable. The mean within-test coefficient of variability (CV: defined as the standard deviation (SD)/mean and expressed as a percentage) has been reported as ranging between 5 and 10 % for Rrs and up to 20 % for Xrs [19–22]. Until such time as definitive criteria for repeatability are available users should retain all acceptable measurements and exercise caution when deciding to exclude apparently acceptable data based on repeatability criteria alone.

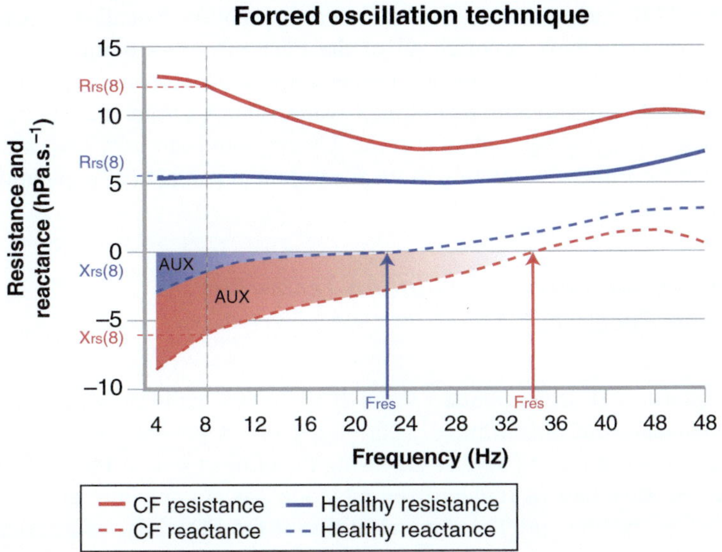

Fig. 9.2 Respiratory impedance spectra from a healthy child (shown in *blue*) and a child with cystic fibrosis (shown in *red*) of similar age and heights. The respiratory resistance (Rrs: *solid line*) tends to be increased and show negative frequency dependence at lower frequencies while respiratory reactance (Xrs: *dashed lines*) is decreased (more negative) in children with lung disease. Commonly reported FOT outcomes include the Rrs and Xrs at a specific frequency (shown here as Rrs and Xrs at 8 Hz: Rrs8 and Xrs8, respectively). The resonant frequency (Fres) is the frequency at which Xrs is equal to zero and represents the point at which the respiratory system recoil (or compliance) and inertance (reflecting the properties of the central airways) are balance. The area under the reactance curve (AUX) is the sum of the Xrs curve from the lowest frequency measured to the resonant frequency

The between test (inter-test) coefficient of repeatability (twice the SD of the difference between two measurements) in healthy children ranges between 1.1 and 2.6 hPa s/L for Rrs and equates to a relative change of 12–30 % [23–25] with similar short- and long term repeatability reported in children with lung disease [19, 20, 26]. The repeatability of Xrs is reported as absolute value due to the proximity of Xrs values to zero and ranges from 1.2 to 2.0 hPa s/L [19, 20, 23–26].

Reference Ranges in Preschool and School Aged Children Using Forced Oscillations

There is a range of reference equations available for use in preschool and school aged children and to date the majority of these studies are in Caucasian children [24, 27–29] although reference data in children from Mexico [30], Iran [31], Korea [32], and Vietnam [33] are now available. It is not clear what impact ethnicity will have on reported FOT outcomes and this area deserves attention. Not all studies reporting reference equations have reported all of the FOT outcomes outlined above. It is important to note that the frequency range of the FOT outcomes reported by the CareFusion IOS is different to that of the Cosmed Quark I2M and as such reference equations are currently equipment specific. Users should carefully review the available studies for suitability relating to local equipment and patient populations.

The Role of the Forced Oscillation Technique in Clinical Practice

The use of the FOT in the management of individual children with lung disease remains unclear with only limited information on its potential use. The primary reasons for this shortage of studies assessing the clinical role of the FOT are likely to be the historical lack of standardized methodological guidelines and availability of commercial equipment. The clinical utility of the FOT in young children with recurrent wheeze and/or asthma, CF and in those children born preterm with or without bronchopulmonary dysplasia (BPD) has recently been comprehensively reviewed as part of an ATS workshop report on optimal lung function tests in young children [34], while the role of the FOT in older children with lung disease remains to be formally assessed.

The change in FOT outcomes following bronchodilator inhalation considered to be clinically relevant is reasonably consistent across multiple studies. A clinically relevant bronchodilator response is defined using the 5th/95th centiles of the response to bronchodilators in healthy populations. These have been reported to be between −33 and −42 % for Rrs, 61 and 70 % for Xrs and approximately 80 % for AX, irrespective of the dose of the salbutamol [25, 27, 33, 35–37]. The ability of the FOT to assist in the diagnosis and/or management of asthmatic and/or wheezy children either before or after bronchodilator inhalation remains unclear. Some studies demonstrated no differences in the baseline lung function or bronchodilator responsiveness between healthy and asthmatic children [22, 35–37]. In contrast, other studies have reported that FOT may provide some benefit in the identification of children with asthma [38–41]. One study from Shi et al. [42] suggest that FOT outcomes may predict loss of asthma control and therefore may have a role in the management of children with asthma and further work in this area is needed.

The FOT has been used to assess lung function in children with CF; however, the majority of these studies have been cross-sectional with only limited assessment of pulmonary infection or inflammation and therefore the ability of FOT to assist in the clinical management of younger children with CF is unclear. Brennan et al. assessed the relationship of respiratory mechanics derived from the low-frequency FOT [43] in a group of infants and young children with CF at the time of an annual bronchoalveolar lavage and reported increased pulmonary inflammation, but not infection, was associated with increased respiratory resistance. However, this variation of FOT is not easily transferred to a clinical setting. Most studies using commercially available FOT equipment suggest that the FOT is not sensitive to the early CF lung disease either cross-sectionally or longitudinally [26, 44–48]. In contrast, increased Rrs and decreased Xrs have been reported in young children with CF in the presence of respiratory symptoms [19].

The primary impact of preterm birth and BPD on the respiratory system is likely to be the peripheral lung with altered alveolar structure [49]. As such the FOT should be a particularly suitable test for use in infants and children following preterm birth, particularly those born very preterm (<32 weeks gestational age). Despite this the FOT has not been used widely in infants and children born preterm. Using the low-frequency FOT Pillow et al. demonstrated that oscillatory mechanics can be measured in preterm infants around term [3]. Studies using commercially available equipment have demonstrated that FOT outcomes are abnormal in both preschool and school aged preterm children, both with and without BPD and that these differences are more pronounced in measures of respiratory reactance than resistance suggesting that the FOT is sensitive to the altered peripheral lung pathophysiology evident in these children [20, 50, 51]. There are limited reports of the FOT being applied in children with upper airway dysfunction and further research in this patient group is required [52–54].

Future Work and Conclusions

The measurement of respiratory system impedance has the potential to provide a great deal of information on a variety of conditions during the early years of life; however, further work is required if the FOT is yet to reach its full clinical potential. In the short term it is important to identify which FOT outcomes are most sensitive to each specific pediatric lung disease with the knowledge that the pathophysiological mechanisms of many respiratory diseases exhibit strong peripheral lung involvement during early life. In the longer term it is important to gain an understanding of how respiratory mechanics alters longitudinally during development and what kind of deviation from this path requires intervention.

The Multiple Breath Washout Technique

Inert gas washout was first described over 60 years ago following the advent of fast responding gas analysers [55, 56], but it was not until the development of personal computers that breath-by-breath analysis became feasible and enabled MBW analysis techniques as we know them today. The choice of a suitable inert gas for MBW testing should consider if the inert tracer gas is safe for patients to inhale and does not participate in gas exchange or dissolve significantly in the blood or other tissues. Inert gases may either be resident within the lung (i.e., present within room air, e.g., Nitrogen (N_2) or Argon) or non-resident (e.g., Sulfur hexafluoride, SF_6, or Helium).

Inert gas washout tests allow the distribution of ventilation to be assessed. Ventilation within the lung is determined by the structure of the respiratory airway tree and the gas exchange unit or alveoli. Gas transport and mixing by convection (i.e., bulk flow) predominates in the conducting airways. In the lung periphery, bulk flow is minimal and gas transport by molecular diffusion dominates. In the region of the entry of the acinus, the relative contributions of convection and diffusion to gas mixing are equal, generating a "diffusion-convection front" in the healthy adult lung [57]. Pathological processes affecting the dimensions of these peripheral airways in a *heterogeneous*, or patchy, manner, affect the distribution of ventilation. It is this *unevenness* of ventilation that is detected by tests such as the MBW technique. A typical MBW test is performed over a series of tidal breaths, requiring minimal cooperation or coordination, offering feasibility across the *entire* pediatric age range. Improved sensitivity to detect lung disease, in comparison to conventional spirometry, across a number of important pediatric lung diseases [58–61].

The Technique Methodology

The MBW examines the pattern by which an inert gas is washed out of the lungs during tidal breathing. Standardization guidelines for equipment validation, MBW test performance and subsequent analysis have recently been developed for use in all age groups and are covered in more detail elsewhere [62]. Inert gas washout is based on accurate measurement of respiratory flow and inert gas concentration signals, which need to be correctly aligned in time prior to subsequent analyses. The majority of equipment in publications prior to the early to mid-2000s has been custom-made and based on a variety of flow measurement devices and inert gas analysers. In recent years commercial systems have been developed, based on SF_6 measurement for the infant age range (Exhalyzer D, ECO Medics AG, Switzerland) or on N_2 measurement suitable for preschoolers and above (Exhalyzer D, ECO Medics AG, Switzerland; Easyone Pro, ndd Medical Technologies, Switzerland). Recent advances in equipment validation [63] appear to have provided robust clinical devices suitable for widespread use.

For the patient, minimal cooperation and coordination are required: an adequate mouthpiece/facemask seal must be maintained to prevent leaks, and a regular breathing pattern needs to be maintained. A facemask is used in infants and may be used for preschool children due to difficulty maintaining an adequate mouthpiece seal. A regular breathing pattern is achieved in infants by performing the test during natural sleep or under sedation (in the supine position), or in older children, sitting upright and using distraction with an interesting video [62].

In N_2-based MBW the nitrogen is washed out of the lung by switching the patient into breathing 100 % O_2. Non-resident inert gases require an additional wash-in phase during which the inhaled inert gas concentration (typically 4 % SF_6 or 4 % He with 21 % O_2 and the balance N_2) equilibrates within the lung, before being washed out by breathing room air. Initial MBW studies demonstrated feasibility using N_2 as the inert gas [64–66], but inhalation of pure O_2 in infants was subsequently shown to alter normal tidal breathing patterns [67], with potential effects on subsequent calculated indices. As a result interest in non-resident inert marker gases increased, with strong feasibility subsequently demonstrated for SF_6-based MBW [58, 68–70]. The clinical utility of the MBW may be hampered by the test duration which may be up to an hour in some children. Recent efforts to shorten the MBW protocol suggest the test duration can be shortened [71, 72]. Feasibility within the busy clinical environment and in more remote settings has also recently been demonstrated [73, 74].

Available MBW Indices

Each MBW test is conventionally performed until the end-tidal inert gas concentration reaches 1/40 of its starting concentration (i.e., approximately 2 % for N_2 MBW and 0.1 % for SF_6/He MBW at the concentrations mentioned prior) (Fig. 9.3). Three technically acceptable tests should be the target of each testing session. In addition to providing information about ventilation distribution, lung volume data (functional residual capacity, FRC), trapped gas and measures of the volume of the conducting airways (Fowler [75] and Langley [76] airways dead space) can also be determined. These ventilation inhomogeneity parameters can be grouped into those reflecting the presence of overall global abnormalities, such as the Lung Clearance Index (LCI) [77] and moment ratios [78], and those based on more sophisticated phase III slope analysis providing additional information about the location of any abnormality [79].

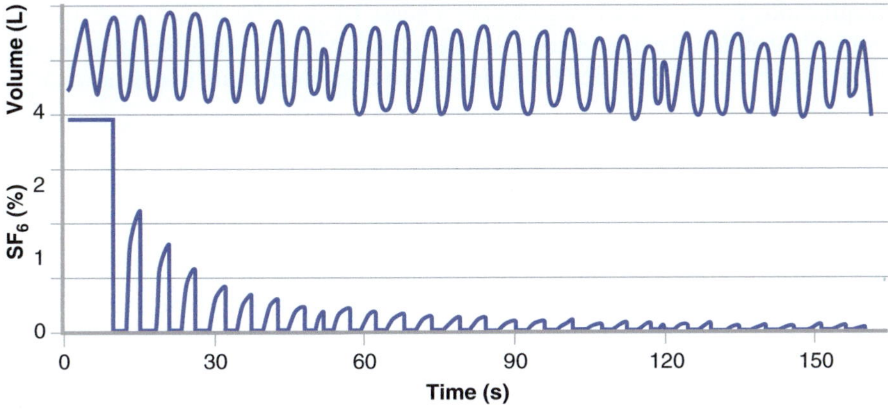

Fig. 9.3 Real time tracings from a MBW test. Tidal volume (*upper panel*) and inert gas SF_6 concentration (*lower panel*) are displayed. The washout phase of the MBW test commences after equilibration of SF_6 concentration within the lungs to approximately 4 % and continues until SF_6 concentration has decreased to below 1/40th or 0.1 %

LCI is the simplest parameter to calculate, the easiest for physicians and patients/parents to understand conceptually, and the most popular index reported in the recent pediatric literature. It represents the number of lung volume turnovers (TO, or FRCs) required to clear the lungs of the inert marker gas to 1/40 of the starting concentration. Moment ratios (calculated using an approach termed "moment analysis") are more complicated and describe the degree of skewing of the washout curve, with increased skewing representing increased release of inert gas at a later stage of the washout [78]. Calculation of moment ratios are described in more detail elsewhere [80]. The proposed advantage of moment analysis is that it may compensate for the impact of variation in respiratory rate and tidal volume during the washout [65, 81].

Phase III slope analysis from MBW is the main index reported in the adult literature, and has been developed from theoretical [79], experimental [82, 83], and adult lung modelling data [83–85], to separate ventilation inhomogeneity arising from conductive airway zones (termed convection-dependent inhomogeneity or CDI) and within more distal acinar zones (where diffusion and convection interact to generate inhomogeneity, termed diffusion-convection-dependent inhomogeneity or DCDI). The CDI and DCDI can be expressed as the clinical indices, S_{cond} and S_{acin}, respectively [86]. The original method for calculation proposed in adults required a strict breathing protocol (tidal volumes 1.0–1.3 L and breathing rate of 10–12 breaths/min), to try to avoid variation in pre-inspiratory lung volume, inspired and expired volumes and flow [57, 87–94] affecting the magnitude of the phase III slope. Adaptation of this method for pediatric testing, where a structured breathing protocol is not feasible ≤16 years, has required the incorporation of a tidal volume compensation for phase III slope values [62]. The use of the strict adult breathing protocol in children has been shown to significantly affect MBW outcomes [45]. Phase III slope parameters do not appear as robust as LCI to variations in breathing pattern, which compromises feasibility to a degree in the preschool age range, whilst the low parenchymal-to-airway volume ratio encountered in infants makes identification and accurate assessment of a phase III slope from tidal breath expirograms challenging. These indices remain exploratory in the pediatric range at present and have not demonstrated the same degree of clinical utility to date as LCI.

Acceptability and Repeatability of MBW Measurements

The majority of the data presented in this section is based on SF_6-based MBW, whereas the recent availability of commercial N_2-based equipment is starting to generate equivalent data. Strong feasibility exists across all age ranges: in infants 76–90 % during natural sleep (aged <6 weeks) [95, 96] and 87 % in sedated infants [70], compared to 80 % in preschoolers (ranging from 50 % of 2–3-year-olds to 87 % of 5–6-year-olds) [58]. Within-session variability ranges from 3 to 8 % across studies in preschoolers and above, with between-session variability approximately 5 % [97], equating to a statistically significant change of ±1 TO for LCI. A collaborative multiple center approach has led to publication of recent SF_6 mass spectrometer based normative data for the entire pediatric age range [98]. Recently preliminary data describing normative N_2-based LCI data has also been published from 7 to 70 years of age [99]. Both these sets of normative data illustrate the higher LCI values encountered at the extremes of age (e.g., infancy) but show largely stable values in between, making LCI an attractive longitudinal tool.

The Role of LCI in Clinical Practice

LCI is now strongly supported as a research tool in clinical studies in CF, due to a large body of evidence supporting potential clinical utility in this disease group [51]. The heterogeneous distribution of CF lung disease has been nicely illustrated by recent imaging studies [100], and includes the peripheral airways [101].

Abnormal LCI values are frequently present in CF subjects, from infancy onwards, and disparity between health and disease appears to increase over time, based on this cross-sectional data. Improved sensitivity of LCI to detect lung disease despite normal spirometry exists across a number of studies from the preschool age range onwards [58, 60, 69, 102]. Strong correlation between LCI and high resolution computed tomography (HRCT) measured structural lung damage has also been described in several studies, from infancy [103–106]. Prognostic value is also starting to emerge, with preschool LCI values predicting those subjects with abnormal spirometry at school age [107]. LCI improves with treatment intervention [108–110], and its potential to detect significant changes despite small cohort sizes is exciting for future intervention studies. However, heterogeneity of response encountered in established disease [80] may limit utility in more severe subjects.

As in CF, the heterogeneous distribution of the disease process in asthma, involving the *entire* airway tree, not just the central airways, has been demonstrated in imaging and pathology studies [111–113], predicting potential utility for MBW. Pediatric asthmatics have increased global ventilation inhomogeneity (LCI and moment ratio values), compared to controls [65, 114]. Phase III analysis describes a predominant conducting airways pattern of abnormality (elevated S_{cond}) [115]. Improved sensitivity to detect disease involvement, in comparison to spirometry, is suggested by both pathological gas trapping in childhood and adolescent asthmatics [116], and elevated LCI values in well controlled childhood asthmatics [61], despite normal baseline spirometry in both groups. Whether this represents established airway remodelling is unclear. Increased ventilation inhomogeneity has also been suggested as an important mechanism for airway hyperresponsiveness in adult asthmatics [113, 117].

In younger preschool recurrent wheeze phenotypes, MBW also appears to differentiate between multi-trigger wheeze and viral-induced wheeze phenotypes (increased LCI and S_{cond} values) [118]. Establishing a predictive value to detect those who subsequently develop classical asthma will require longitudinal studies. Utility in challenge testing is suggested by the ability to detect a marked peripheral airways response, missed by spirometry, on challenge testing [119], but the time-consuming nature of the test compromises routine clinical utility in this setting. The same applies for assessment of bronchodilator response. Response to treatment with therapy targeting the peripheral airways (e.g., fine particle inhaled corticosteroid) has been demonstrated in adults [120], but corresponding pediatric data is lacking.

Discussion of clinical utility of MBW in infants with BPD illustrates the importance of disease distribution when assessing potential utility. "Old" BPD cross-sectional studies describe elevated gas trapping (as assessed by FRC_{pleth} and FRC_{N2}) and LCI (or moment ratios) in BPD infants during the newborn period, in comparison to healthy controls [81, 121]. However, recent larger multicenter studies, of "new" BPD, show little difference between groups [95, 96]. This probably reflects both improved study design, adequately correcting for important confounders such as prematurity and intrauterine growth, and the more diffuse nature of "new" BPD, generating less marked ventilation unevenness.

Future Work and Conclusions

The availability of robust commercial equipment and improved standardization of the MBW technique represent essential steps if exciting potential utility suggested by research studies to date is to translate into feasibility in the busy clinical laboratory. Strongest utility is currently suggested for CF, but may also exist for asthma and other disease groups. Efforts in the future to shorten test duration are important and evaluation of current commercial equipment is ongoing. Longitudinal studies will provide a clearer idea of true utility.

The Interrupter Technique

The interrupter technique allows the measurement of the resistance of the respiratory system, including the airway tree, lung tissue and chest wall. The primary advantage of the technique is that it requires minimal cooperation from the individual being tested and hence is of particular interest in infants and young children. There have been a number of studies conducted in sedated and unsedated sleeping infants [122–128] and spontaneously breathing children as young as 2 years [24, 129–133]. Historically, there was little standardization of the technique. The availability of commercial equipment and the release of guidelines for its use in preschool children [8] should lead to an improved understanding of its role in the clinical management of young children [34].

The classical description of the interrupter technique involves the rapid occlusion of the airway opening and the measurement of the flow immediately preceding the interruption and the changes in airway opening pressure (Pao) following the interruption. The interrupter resistance (Rint) is derived from the change in Pao by the flow. An alternative approach derives the Rint using the change in Pao and the flow immediately after the interruption [134]. The outcomes derived from these two approaches differ and cannot be used interchangeably [135]. The classical approach is the most commonly used and unless specified otherwise is the technique for which details are provided in this chapter.

The Interrupter Technique Methodology

Commercial equipment for both the classical and the alternative methods of measuring the Rint are available. The interrupter technique assumes that following the interruption to airflow the alveolar pressure rapidly equilibrates with the airway opening and that the change in Pao reflects the pressure drop across the whole airway tree and therefore equates to the alveolar pressure [128, 136, 137]. Following occlusion two distinct phases are seen in the Pao trace (Fig. 9.4). There is an initial rapid rise in Pao that reflects the resistive drop across the airway tree and a component of the resistive properties of the lung and chest wall. This is followed by a slower rise to a plateau and reflects the stress relaxation of the respiratory tissues.

The Rint is influenced by the closure time of the occlusion valve [128], the compliance of the upper airways [128], the type of patient interface (face mask or mouthpiece) used [126, 138, 139] and the method of determining the change in Pao following the interruption [126, 140, 141]. The most commonly used approach for the derivation of the Pao is to use the linear back extrapolation of Pao between 30 and 70 ms following the interruption [8].

In infants Rint is measured with the infant in a supine position during quiet sleep. The facemask is placed over the nose and mouth of the infant and supported firmly to minimize pressure loss across the cheeks and floor of the mouth [126]. The use of equipment designed for older children and not adapted for infants is not recommended, with low success rates and poor repeatability of Rint reported [122, 123].

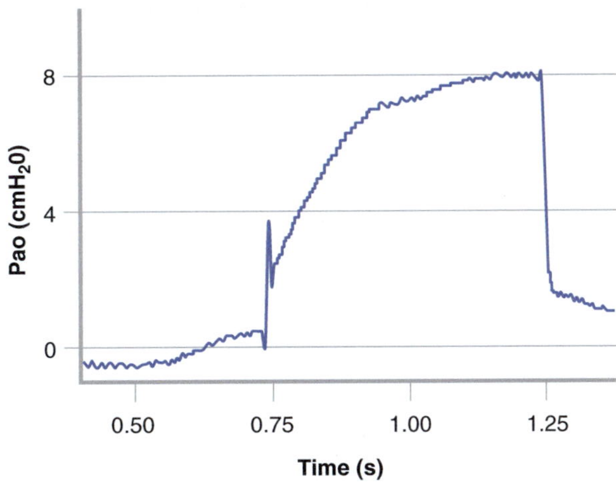

Fig. 9.4 Interrupter resistance (Rint) measurement in an infant. The airway opening pressure (Pao) has an initial rapid, followed by a slower, secondary rise. The pre-occlusion flow and post occlusion Pao are used to derive Rint

Recommendations for the measurement of Rint in young children are available and in the absence of detailed guidelines in older children should be used for all measurements of interrupter resistance in cooperative children [8]. In preschool and school aged children measurements are made with the child seated and looking directly ahead while breathing through a mouthpiece and with a nose clip in place and the cheeks firmly supported during measurements. The airway is occluded during expiration with the interrupter valve for a period of 100 ms at a flow equating to the peak tidal expiratory flow. A minimum of ten interruptions should be obtained with at least five acceptable measurements retained.

Acceptability and Repeatability of Interrupter Technique Measurements

Measurements should show a smooth increase in airway opening pressure to a peak and be free of leak or unusual changes in pressure and/or flow at the time of the interruption. The median of all acceptable measurements is reported. The within-test repeatability of Rint in healthy infants is dependent on the analysis technique [126] and the mean (or median) coefficient of variation has been reported to range 16.6–19.3 % [124–126] The data available for the between test repeatability of Rint in infants is scarce with Fuchs et al. reporting the mean between test difference in 22 unsedated 6 week old infants to be 1.4 hPa s/L with the limits of agreement being −21.2 and 23.9 hPa s/L [124].

In contrast there are many studies that have assessed the within- and between-test repeatability of Rint in preschool and school aged children and these are extensively reviewed elsewhere [8, 34]. The coefficient of variability of a single testing session ranges between 10 and 12 % of the median Rint value [133, 142–145]. The short term (15–30 min) and longer term (2 weeks to up to 3 months) repeatability of the Rint has been assessed in healthy children and in children with lung disease. The coefficient of repeatability (equating to two times the standard deviation of the measurement) ranges from 1.7 to 4.4 hPa s/L [132, 146, 147].

Reference Ranges for Interrupter Resistance in Infants, Preschool and School Aged Children

Fuchs et al. [124] reported upper limits of normal for Rint in unsedated infants aged 5–7 weeks of age. To date only one study reported reference ranges for the Rint in sedated infants over a broader age range [125]. Measurements of Rint in healthy preschool and school aged children have been reported in Caucasian children [24, 132, 133, 143, 148] as well as children of differing ethnic backgrounds [125, 148–150]. Collated reference values for the classical technique in children aged 3–13 years have been developed and offer the most robust references ranges currently available [151].

The Role of the Interrupter Technique in Clinical Practice

The potential role for measurements of Rint in infants has not been assessed. The lack of appropriate commercially available equipment and standardized methodology guidelines in this age group limit the ability of health professionals and researchers to assess the ability of Rint to assist in the diagnosis and/or management of infants with lung disease.

The clinical role of Rint in preschool children has been extensively reviewed by the ATS workshop report on optimal lung function tests in young children [34]. While studies reporting measurements of Rint in older, school aged children show responsible agreement with other clinically available lung function tests [144] its primary role is likely to be in younger children unable to perform these tests accurately.

The limits of agreement for the determination of a clinically relevant bronchodilator response in Rint obtained with the classical technique are similar and are reported as a decrease in Rint of >2.5 hPa s/L or >32–35 % of baseline [143, 152, 153].

The majority of studies using the interrupter technique have been in children with a history of recurrent wheeze or cough and asthma. The majority of studies have reported that children with asthma have increased Rint compared to healthy controls; however, the proportion of asthmatic children with Rint outside of the normal range varies significantly and these differences are likely to relate to subject selection (community versus hospital/clinic asthmatics) and current asthma treatments [36, 131, 133, 144, 145, 152]. Children with asthma or recurrent wheeze tend to have larger decreases in Rint following bronchodilator inhalation when compared to healthy children, and studies have reported sensitivity and specificity ranges from 24 to 76 % and 70 to 92 %, respectively to distinguish between asthmatic and healthy children [36, 148, 152]. However, each of these studies expressed the bronchodilator responses differently making direct comparisons difficult. A number of investigators have assessed the Rint in placebo controlled clinical trials of asthma medications [131, 154–156] with significant improvements in Rint seen in some [131, 155] but not all trials [154, 156], and provide early evidence that Rint may be a useful clinical trial outcome measure in young children with asthma.

Studies measuring Rint in children with CF are primarily cross-sectional [26, 142, 157–160] with only two studies tracking Rint longitudinally [26, 160]. While children with CF tend to have increased Rint when compared to healthy children, there is a large overlap and in the longitudinal studies Rint was not altered with changing clinical status. The sensitivity of Rint to predict pulmonary infection and/or exacerbations or to track the effectiveness of treatments in children with CF has not been assessed.

There are only limited data using the interrupter technique in children born preterm. Vrijlandt et al. reported increased Rint in preterm children with and without BPD when compared to healthy controls. However, there were no significant differences in the baseline Rint or response to bronchodilators between the preterm groups [50]. In a group of preterm children attending tertiary respiratory clinics Kairamkonda and coworkers reported preterm children with a history of BPD had significantly increased Rint compared to preterm children without BPD [161]. As described previously the likely anatomical site of altered physiology in children born preterm will be in the peripheral lung and the emerging evidence that respiratory reactance from the FOT (a measure of peripheral lung function) has increased sensitivity compared to respiratory resistance suggests that the clinical utility of the interrupter technique in preterm children may be limited.

Future Work and Conclusions

Further development of the interrupter technique in infants is required including the most appropriate triggering flow, interruption duration and airway opening pressure analysis method. In preschool children the data available to date suggest the interrupter technique is going to be most informative in children with a history of recurrent wheeze and in the assessment of airway responsiveness including both bronchodilator responsiveness and inhaled bronchial challenge tests. Future studies should focus on longitudinal measurement of Rint and prospectively collected clinical information to provide a better understanding of the sensitivity of Rint to changing clinical status.

Summary

The advent of newer pulmonary function tests and in particular the availability of commercial equipment and standardized guidelines has provided renewed interest in the objective measurement of lung function in pediatric lung disease. The ability of these tests to allow the quantification of lung function from as young as 2 years of age provides a window of opportunity for pediatric health professionals and researchers alike to accurately characterize the natural history of pediatric lung disease and in the diagnosis and management of children with a range of respiratory disorders.

The current status for each of these tests is similar as is the way forward. Robust reference ranges across a range of ethnicities are required. Longitudinal studies incorporating some or all of these techniques are required to allow appropriate conclusions to be drawn on the relative merits of each test within the context of the disease pathophysiology and the determination of the minimal meaningful clinical difference to assist in the management of our patients with lung disease.

References

1. Dubois AB, et al. Oscillation mechanics of lungs and chest in man. J Appl Physiol. 1956;8:587–94.
2. Sly PD, et al. Measuring lung function in murine models of pulmonary disease. Drug Discov Today Dis Models. 2004;1:337–43.

 3. Pillow JJ, et al. Partitioning of airway and parenchymal mechanics in unsedated newborn infants. Pediatr Res. 2005;58:1210–5.
 4. Wohl ME, et al. Resistance of the total respiratory system in healthy infants and infants with bronchiolitis. Pediatrics. 1969;43:495–509.
 5. Frey U, et al. High-frequency respiratory impedance measured by forced-oscillation technique in infants. Am J Respir Crit Care Med. 1998;158:363–70.
 6. Hall GL, et al. Altered respiratory tissue mechanics in asymptomatic wheezy infants. Am J Respir Crit Care Med. 2001;164:1387–91.
 7. Sly PD, et al. Measurement of low-frequency respiratory impedance in infants. Am J Respir Crit Care Med. 1996;154:161–6.
 8. Beydon N, et al. An official American Thoracic Society/European Respiratory Society statement: pulmonary function testing in preschool children. Am J Respir Crit Care Med. 2007;175:1304–45.
 9. Oostveen E, et al. The forced oscillation technique in clinical practice: methodology, recommendations and future developments. Eur Respir J. 2003;22:1026–41.
10. Bates JHT, et al. Oscillation mechanics of the respiratory system. Compr Physiol. 2011;1:1233–72.
11. Petak F, et al. Airway and tissue mechanics in anesthetized paralyzed children. Pediatr Pulmonol. 2003;35:169–76.
12. Farre R, et al. A system to generate simultaneous forced oscillation and continuous positive airway pressure. Eur Respir J. 1997;10:1349–53.
13. Macintyre N, et al. Standardisation of the single-breath determination of carbon monoxide uptake in the lung. Eur Respir J. 2005;26:720–35.
14. Miller MR, et al. Standardisation of spirometry. Eur Respir J. 2005;26:319–38.
15. Wanger J, et al. Standardisation of the measurement of lung volumes. Eur Respir J. 2005;26:511–22.
16. Cauberghs M, Van de Woestijne KP. Effect of upper airway shunt and series properties on respiratory impedance measurements. J Appl Physiol. 1989;66:2274–9.
17. Peslin R, et al. Respiratory impedance measured with head generator to minimize upper airway shunt. J Appl Physiol. 1985;59:1790–5.
18. Goldman MD, et al. Clinical applications of forced oscillation to assess peripheral airway function. Respir Physiol Neurobiol. 2005;148:179–94.
19. Gangell CL, et al. Respiratory impedance in children with cystic fibrosis using forced oscillations in clinic. Eur Respir J. 2007;30:892–7.
20. Udomittipong K, et al. Forced oscillations in the clinical setting in young children with neonatal lung disease. Eur Respir J. 2008;31:1292–9.
21. Lall CA, et al. Airway resistance variability and response to bronchodilator in children with asthma. Eur Respir J. 2007;30:260–8.
22. Harrison J, et al. Lung function in preschool children with a history of wheezing measured by forced oscillation and plethysmographic specific airway resistance. Pediatr Pulmonol. 2010;45:1049–56.
23. Hall GL, et al. Respiratory function in healthy young children using forced oscillations. Thorax. 2007;62:521–6.
24. Klug B, Bisgaard H. Specific airway resistance, interrupter resistance, and respiratory impedance in healthy children aged 2–7 years. Pediatr Pulmonol. 1998;25:322–31.
25. Malmberg LP, et al. Determinants of respiratory system input impedance and bronchodilator response in healthy Finnish preschool children. Clin Physiol Funct Imaging. 2002;22:64–71.
26. Nielsen KG, et al. Serial lung function and responsiveness in cystic fibrosis during early childhood. Am J Respir Crit Care Med. 2004;169:1209–16.
27. Calogero C, et al. Respiratory impedance and bronchodilator responsiveness in healthy children aged 2–13 years. Pediatr Pulmonol. 2013;48(7):707–15.
28. Dencker M, et al. Reference values for respiratory system impedance by using impulse oscillometry in children aged 2–11 years. Clin Physiol Funct Imaging. 2006;26:247–50.

29. Frei J, et al. Impulse oscillometry: reference values in children 100 to 150 cm in height and 3 to 10 years of age. Chest. 2005;128:1266–73.
30. Shackleton C, et al. Reference ranges for Mexican preschool-aged children using the forced oscillation technique. Arch Bronconeumol. 2013;49:326–9.
31. Amra B, et al. Respiratory resistance by impulse oscillometry in healthy Iranian children aged 5–19 years. Iran J Allergy Asthma Immunol. 2008;7:25–9.
32. Lee JY, et al. Reference values of impulse oscillometry and its utility in the diagnosis of asthma in young Korean children. J Asthma. 2012;49:811–6.
33. Vu LT, et al. Respiratory impedance and response to salbutamol in healthy Vietnamese children. Pediatr Pulmonol. 2008;43:1013–9.
34. Rosenfeld M, et al. An Official American Thoracic Society Workshop report: optimal lung function tests for monitoring cystic fibrosis, bronchopulmonary dysplasia and recurrent wheezing in children <6 years of age. Ann Am Thorac Soc. 2013;10:S1–11.
35. Hellinckx J, et al. Bronchodilator response in 3–6.5 years old healthy and stable asthmatic children. Eur Respir J. 1998;12:438–43.
36. Nielsen KG, Bisgaard H. Discriminative capacity of bronchodilator response measured with three different lung function techniques in asthmatic and healthy children aged 2 to 5 years. Am J Respir Crit Care Med. 2001;164:554–9.
37. Thamrin C, et al. Assessment of bronchodilator responsiveness in preschool children using forced oscillations. Thorax. 2007;62:814–9.
38. Komarow HD, et al. A study of the use of impulse oscillometry in the evaluation of children with asthma: analysis of lung parameters, order effect, and utility compared with spirometry. Pediatr Pulmonol. 2012;47:18–26.
39. Oostveen E, et al. Lung function and bronchodilator response in 4-year-old children with different wheezing phenotypes. Eur Respir J. 2010;35:865–72.
40. Shin YH, et al. Oscillometric and spirometric bronchodilator response in preschool children with and without asthma. Can Respir J. 2012;19:273–7.
41. Vu LT, et al. Respiratory impedance and response to salbutamol in asthmatic Vietnamese children. Pediatr Pulmonol. 2010;45:380–6.
42. Shi Y, et al. Peripheral airway impairment measured by oscillometry predicts loss of asthma control in children. J Allergy Clin Immunol. 2013;131:718–23.
43. Brennan S, et al. Correlation of forced oscillation technique in preschool children with cystic fibrosis with pulmonary inflammation. Thorax. 2005;60:159–63.
44. Ren CL, et al. Analysis of the associations between lung function and clinical features in preschool children with cystic fibrosis. Pediatr Pulmonol. 2012;47:574–81.
45. Yammine S, et al. Impact of different breathing protocols on multiple-breath washout outcomes in children. J Cyst Fibros. 2014;13:190–7.
46. Mazurek HK, et al. Specificity and sensitivity of respiratory impedance in assessing reversibility of airway obstruction in children. Chest. 1995;107:996–1002.
47. Lebecque P, Stanescu D. Respiratory resistance by the forced oscillation technique in asthmatic children and cystic fibrosis patients. Eur Respir J. 1997;10:891–5.
48. Kerby GS, et al. Lung function distinguishes preschool children with CF from healthy controls in a multi-center setting. Pediatr Pulmonol. 2012;47:597–605.
49. Jobe AH, Bancalari E. Bronchopulmonary dysplasia. Am J Respir Crit Care Med. 2001;163:1723–9.
50. Vrijlandt EJ, et al. Respiratory health in prematurely born preschool children with and without bronchopulmonary dysplasia. J Pediatr. 2007;150:256–61.
51. Kent L, et al. Lung clearance index: evidence for use in clinical trials in cystic fibrosis. J Cyst Fibros. 2014;13:123–38.
52. Harrison J, et al. Lung function in children with repaired tracheo-oesophageal fistula using the forced oscillation technique. Pediatr Pulmonol. 2010;45:1057–63.
53. Hoijer U, et al. The ability of noninvasive methods to detect and quantify laryngeal obstruction. Eur Respir J. 1991;4:109–14.
54. Rigau J, et al. Oscillometric assessment of airway obstruction in a mechanical model of vocal cord dysfunction. J Biomech. 2004;37:37–43.

55. Siri WE. A mass spectroscope for analysis in the low mass range. Rev Sci Instrum. 1947;18:540.
56. Lilly JC. Mixing of gases within respiratory system with a new type nitrogen meter. Am J Physiol. 1950;161:342–51.
57. Paiva M. Gas transport in the human lung. J Appl Physiol. 1973;35:401–10.
58. Aurora P, et al. Multiple-breath washout as a marker of lung disease in preschool children with cystic fibrosis. Am J Respir Crit Care Med. 2005;171:249–56.
59. Fuchs SI, et al. A novel sidestream ultrasonic flow sensor for multiple breath washout in children. Pediatr Pulmonol. 2008;43:731–8.
60. Gustafsson PM, et al. Evaluation of ventilation maldistribution as an early indicator of lung disease in children with cystic fibrosis. Eur Respir J. 2003;22:972–9.
61. Macleod KA, et al. Ventilation heterogeneity in children with well controlled asthma with normal spirometry indicates residual airways disease. Thorax. 2009;64:33–7.
62. Robinson PD, et al. Consensus statement for inert gas washout measurement using multiple- and single-breath tests. Eur Respir J. 2013;41:507–22.
63. Singer F, et al. A realistic validation study of a new nitrogen multiple-breath washout system. PLoS One. 2012;7:e36083.
64. Wall MA. Moment analysis of multibreath nitrogen washout in young children. J Appl Physiol. 1985;59:274–9.
65. Kraemer R, Meister B. Fast real-time moment-ratio analysis of multibreath nitrogen washout in children. J Appl Physiol. 1985;59:1137–44.
66. Hjalmarson O, Sandberg K. Abnormal lung function in healthy preterm infants. Am J Respir Crit Care Med. 2002;165:83–7.
67. Schibler A, et al. Moment ratio analysis of multiple breath nitrogen washout in infants with lung disease. Eur Respir J. 2000;15:1094–101.
68. Schibler A, et al. Measurement of lung volume and ventilation distribution with an ultrasonic flow meter in healthy infants. Eur Respir J. 2002;20:912–8.
69. Aurora P, et al. Multiple breath inert gas washout as a measure of ventilation distribution in children with cystic fibrosis. Thorax. 2004;59:1068–73.
70. Lum S, et al. Early detection of cystic fibrosis lung disease: multiple-breath washout versus raised volume tests. Thorax. 2007;62:341–7.
71. Robinson PD, et al. Abbreviated multi-breath washout for calculation of lung clearance index. Pediatr Pulmonol. 2013;48:336–43.
72. Yammine S, et al. Multiple-breath washout measurements can be significantly shortened in children. Thorax. 2013;68:586–7.
73. Gray DM, Willemse L, Alberts A, Simpson S, Sly PD, Hall GL, Zar HJ. Lung function in African infants: a pilot study. Pediatr Pulmonol. DOI 10.1002/ppul.22965. 2013.
74. Singer F, et al. Practicability of nitrogen multiple-breath washout measurements in a pediatric cystic fibrosis outpatient setting. Pediatr Pulmonol. 2013;48:739–46.
75. Fowler WS. Lung function studies; the respiratory dead space. Am J Physiol. 1948;154:405–16.
76. Langley F, et al. Ventilatory consequences of unilateral pulmonary artery occlusion. Les Colloques des l'Institut National de la Sante' et de la Recherche Me'dicale. 1975;51:209–12.
77. Bouhuys A. Pulmonary nitrogen clearance in relation to age in healthy males. J Appl Physiol. 1963;18:297–300.
78. Saidel GM, et al. Moment analysis of multibreath lung washout. J Appl Physiol. 1975;38:328–34.
79. Paiva M. Two new pulmonary functional indexes suggested by a simple mathematical model. Respiration. 1975;32:389–403.
80. Robinson PD, et al. Inert gas washout: theoretical background and clinical utility in respiratory disease. Respiration. 2009;78:339–55.
81. Shao H, et al. Impaired gas mixing and low lung volume in preterm infants with mild chronic lung disease. Pediatr Res. 1998;43:536–41.

82. Paiva M, et al. Slope of phase III in multibreath nitrogen washout and washin. Bull Eur Physiopathol Respir. 1982;18:273–80.
83. Verbanck S, Paiva M. Model simulations of gas mixing and ventilation distribution in the human lung. J Appl Physiol. 1990;69:2269–79.
84. Dutrieue B, et al. A human acinar structure for simulation of realistic alveolar plateau slopes. J Appl Physiol. 2000;89:1859–67.
85. Paiva M, Engel LA. Model analysis of gas distribution within human lung acinus. J Appl Physiol Respir Environ Exerc Physiol. 1984;56:418–25.
86. Verbanck S, et al. Ventilation distribution during histamine provocation. J Appl Physiol. 1997;83:1907–16.
87. Cumming G, et al. The influence of gaseous diffusion on the alveolar plateau at different lung volumes. Respir Physiol. 1967;2:386–98.
88. Fowler WS. Lung function studies; uneven pulmonary ventilation in normal subjects and in patients with pulmonary disease. J Appl Physiol. 1949;2:283–99.
89. Jones JG. The effect of preinspiratory lung volume on the result of the single breath O_2 test. Respir Physiol. 1967;2:375–85.
90. Crawford AB, et al. Effect of airway closure on ventilation distribution. J Appl Physiol. 1989;66:2511–5.
91. Crawford AB, et al. Effect of lung volume on ventilation distribution. J Appl Physiol. 1989;66:2502–10.
92. Lacquet LM, van Muylem A. He and SF6 single-breath expiration curves. Comparison with the paiva-engel model. Bull Eur Physiopathol Respir. 1982;18:239–46.
93. Crawford AB, et al. Effect of tidal volume on ventilation maldistribution. Respir Physiol. 1986;66:11–25.
94. Gronkvist M, et al. Effects of body posture and tidal volume on inter- and intraregional ventilation distribution in healthy men. J Appl Physiol. 2002;92:634–42.
95. Hulskamp G, et al. Association of prematurity, lung disease and body size with lung volume and ventilation inhomogeneity in unsedated neonates: a multicentre study. Thorax. 2009;64:240–5.
96. Latzin P, et al. Lung volume, breathing pattern and ventilation inhomogeneity in preterm and term infants. PLoS One. 2009;4:e4635.
97. Fuchs SI, et al. Lung clearance index: normal values, repeatability, and reproducibility in healthy children and adolescents. Pediatr Pulmonol. 2009;44:1180–5.
98. Lum S, et al. Age and height dependence of lung clearance index and functional residual capacity. Eur Respir J. 2013;41(6):1371–7.
99. Houltz B, et al. Tidal N_2 washout ventilation inhomogeneity indices in a reference population aged 7–70 years. Eur Respir J. 2012;40:694s.
100. van Beek EJ, et al. Assessment of lung disease in children with cystic fibrosis using hyperpolarized 3-Helium MRI: comparison with Shwachman score, Chrispin-Norman score and spirometry. Eur Radiol. 2007;17:1018–24.
101. Hamutcu R, et al. Clinical findings and lung pathology in children with cystic fibrosis. Am J Respir Crit Care Med. 2002;165:1172–5.
102. Horsley AR, et al. Lung clearance index is a sensitive, repeatable and practical measure of airways disease in adults with cystic fibrosis. Thorax. 2008;63:135–40.
103. Gustafsson PM, et al. Multiple-breath inert gas washout and spirometry versus structural lung disease in cystic fibrosis. Thorax. 2008;63:129–34.
104. Owens CM, et al. Lung clearance index and HRCT are complementary markers of lung abnormalities in young children with CF. Thorax. 2011;66:481–8.
105. Ellemunter H, et al. Sensitivity of lung clearance index and chest computed tomography in early CF lung disease. Respir Med. 2010;104:1834–42.
106. Hall GL, et al. Air trapping on chest CT is associated with worse ventilation distribution in infants with cystic fibrosis diagnosed following newborn screening. PLoS One. 2011;6:e23932.
107. Aurora P, et al. Lung clearance index at 4 years predicts subsequent lung function in children with cystic fibrosis. Am J Respir Crit Care Med. 2011;183:752–8.

108. Robinson PD, et al. Using index of ventilation to assess response to treatment for acute pulmonary exacerbation in children with cystic fibrosis. Pediatr Pulmonol. 2009;44:733–42.
109. Amin R, et al. Hypertonic saline improves the LCI in paediatric CF patients with normal lung function. Thorax. 2010;65:379–83.
110. Amin R, et al. The effect of dornase alfa on ventilation inhomogeneity in patients with cystic fibrosis. Eur Respir J. 2011;37:806–12.
111. Hamid Q, et al. Inflammation of small airways in asthma. J Allergy Clin Immunol. 1997;100:44–51.
112. Carroll N, et al. The structure of large and small airways in nonfatal and fatal asthma. Am Rev Respir Dis. 1993;147:405–10.
113. Venegas JG, et al. Self-organized patchiness in asthma as a prelude to catastrophic shifts. Nature. 2005;434:777–82.
114. Saniie J, et al. Real-time moment analysis of pulmonary nitrogen washout. J Appl Physiol. 1979;46:1184–90.
115. Gustafsson PM, et al. Peripheral airway involvement in asthma assessed by single-breath SF6 and He washout. Eur Respir J. 2003;21:1033–9.
116. Gustafsson PM, et al. Pneumotachographic nitrogen washout method for measurement of the volume of trapped gas in the lungs. Pediatr Pulmonol. 1994;17:258–68.
117. Downie SR, et al. Ventilation heterogeneity is a major determinant of airway hyperresponsiveness in asthma, independent of airway inflammation. Thorax. 2007;62:684–9.
118. Sonnappa S, et al. Symptom-pattern phenotype and pulmonary function in preschool wheezers. J Allergy Clin Immunol. 2010;126:519–26.
119. Aljassim F, et al. A whisper from the silent lung zone. Pediatr Pulmonol. 2009;44:829–32.
120. Verbanck S, et al. The functional benefit of anti-inflammatory aerosols in the lung periphery. J Allergy Clin Immunol. 2006;118:340–6.
121. Wauer RR, et al. Assessment of functional residual capacity using nitrogen washout and plethysmographic techniques in infants with and without bronchopulmonary dysplasia. Intensive Care Med. 1998;24:469–75.
122. Adams AM, et al. Measurement and repeatability of interrupter resistance in unsedated newborn infants. Pediatr Pulmonol. 2009;44:1168–73.
123. Chavasse RJ, et al. Comparison of resistance measured by the interrupter technique and by passive mechanics in sedated infants. Eur Respir J. 2001;18:330–4.
124. Fuchs O, et al. Normative data for lung function and exhaled nitric oxide in unsedated healthy infants. Eur Respir J. 2011;37:1208–16.
125. Gochicoa LG, et al. Reference values for airway resistance in newborns, infants and preschoolers from a Latin American population. Respirology. 2012;17:667–73.
126. Hall GL, et al. Evaluation of the interrupter technique in healthy, unsedated infants. Eur Respir J. 2001;18:982–8.
127. Lanteri CJ, Sly PD. Changes in respiratory mechanics with age. J Appl Physiol. 1993;74:369–78.
128. Sly PD, Bates JH. Computer analysis of physical factors affecting the use of the interrupter technique in infants. Pediatr Pulmonol. 1988;4:219–24.
129. Bridge PD, et al. Measurement of airway resistance using the interrupter technique in preschool children in the ambulatory setting. Eur Respir J. 1999;13:792–6.
130. McKenzie SA, et al. Airway resistance and atopy in preschool children with wheeze and cough. Eur Respir J. 2000;15:833–8.
131. Nielsen KG, Bisgaard H. The effect of inhaled budesonide on symptoms, lung function, and cold air and methacholine responsiveness in 2- to 5-year-old asthmatic children. Am J Respir Crit Care Med. 2000;162:1500–6.
132. Lombardi E, et al. Reference values of interrupter respiratory resistance in healthy preschool white children. Thorax. 2001;56:691–5.
133. Merkus PJ, et al. Interrupter resistance in preschool children: measurement characteristics and reference values. Am J Respir Crit Care Med. 2001;163:1350–5.
134. Bisgaard H, Klug B. Lung function measurement in awake young children. Eur Respir J. 1995;8:2067–75.

135. Oswald-Mammosser M, et al. The opening interrupter technique for respiratory resistance measurements in children. Respirology. 2010;15:1104–10.
136. Bates JH, et al. A theoretical analysis of interrupter technique for measuring respiratory mechanics. J Appl Physiol. 1988;64:2204–14.
137. Bates JH, et al. Interrupter resistance elucidated by alveolar pressure measurement in open-chest normal dogs. J Appl Physiol. 1988;65:408–14.
138. Oswald-Mammosser M, et al. Measurements of respiratory system resistance by the interrupter technique in healthy and asthmatic children. Pediatr Pulmonol. 1997;24:78–85.
139. Thamrin C, Frey U. Effect of bacterial filter on measurement of interrupter resistance in preschool and school-aged children. Pediatr Pulmonol. 2008;43:781–7.
140. Phagoo SB, et al. Accuracy and sensitivity of the interrupter technique for measuring the response to bronchial challenge in normal subjects. Eur Respir J. 1993;6:996–1003.
141. Phagoo SB, et al. Evaluation of the interrupter technique for measuring change in airway resistance in 5-year-old asthmatic children. Pediatr Pulmonol. 1995;20:387–95.
142. Beydon N, et al. Pulmonary function tests in preschool children with cystic fibrosis. Am J Respir Crit Care Med. 2002;166:1099–104.
143. Beydon N, et al. Pre/postbronchodilator interrupter resistance values in healthy young children. Am J Respir Crit Care Med. 2002;165:1388–94.
144. Beydon N, et al. Baseline and post-bronchodilator interrupter resistance and spirometry in asthmatic children. Pediatr Pulmonol. 2012;47:987–93.
145. Beydon N, et al. Interrupter resistance short-term repeatability and bronchodilator response in preschool children. Respir Med. 2007;101:2482–7.
146. Beelen RM, et al. Short and long term variability of the interrupter technique under field and standardised conditions in 3–6 year old children. Thorax. 2003;58:761–4.
147. Chan EY, et al. Repeatability of airway resistance measurements made using the interrupter technique. Thorax. 2003;58:344–7.
148. McKenzie SA, et al. Airway resistance measured by the interrupter technique: normative data for 2–10 year olds of three ethnicities. Arch Dis Child. 2002;87:248–51.
149. Li AM, et al. Interrupter respiratory resistance in healthy Chinese preschool children. Chest. 2009;136:554–60.
150. Rech VV, et al. Airway resistance in children measured using the interrupter technique: reference values. J Bras Pneumol. 2008;34:796–803.
151. Merkus PJ, et al. Reference ranges for interrupter resistance technique: the Asthma UK Initiative. Eur Respir J. 2010;36:157–63.
152. Beydon N, et al. Pulmonary function tests in preschool children with asthma. Am J Respir Crit Care Med. 2003;168:640–4.
153. Mele L, et al. Assessment and validation of bronchodilation using the interrupter technique in preschool children. Pediatr Pulmonol. 2010;45:633–8.
154. Kooi EM, et al. Fluticasone or Montelukast for preschool children with asthma-like symptoms: randomized controlled trial. Pulm Pharmacol Ther. 2008;21:798–804.
155. Pao CS, McKenzie SA. Randomized controlled trial of fluticasone in preschool children with intermittent wheeze. Am J Respir Crit Care Med. 2002;166:945–9.
156. Schokker S, et al. Inhaled corticosteroids for recurrent respiratory symptoms in preschool children in general practice: randomized controlled trial. Pulm Pharmacol Ther. 2008;21:88–97.
157. Carter ER, et al. Evaluation of the interrupter technique for the use of assessing airway obstruction in children. Pediatr Pulmonol. 1994;17:211–7.
158. Davies PL, et al. The interrupter technique to assess airway responsiveness in children with cystic fibrosis. Pediatr Pulmonol. 2007;42:23–8.
159. Oswald-Mammosser M, et al. Interrupter technique versus plethysmography for measurement of respiratory resistance in children with asthma or cystic fibrosis. Pediatr Pulmonol. 2000;29:213–20.
160. Terheggen-Lagro SW, et al. Radiological and functional changes over 3 years in young children with cystic fibrosis. Eur Respir J. 2007;30:279–85.
161. Kairamkonda VR, et al. Lung function measurement in prematurely born preschool children with and without chronic lung disease. J Perinatol. 2008;28:199–204.

Chapter 10
Selection and Appropriate Use of Spirometric Reference Equations for the Pediatric Population

Sanja Stanojevic and Margaret Rosenfeld

Abstract Spirometry is an important tool for the diagnosis and monitoring of pediatric pulmonary diseases. Interpretation of spirometry results is facilitated by reference equations, which compare an individual's lung function to that of a healthy reference population of the same body shape, sex, and age. A plethora of reference equations exist, and since interpretation of results can differ based on the chosen equation, it is difficult to select one equation that is most appropriate for an individual laboratory or patient. In this chapter we explain why reference equations are fundamental to the interpretation of pulmonary function test results, how they are created, and how to select an appropriate reference equation.

Keywords Reference ranges • Spirometry • Normative data • Children

Spirometry is an important tool for the diagnosis and monitoring of pediatric pulmonary diseases. Interpretation of spirometry results is facilitated by reference equations, which compare an individual's lung function to that of a healthy reference population of the same body shape, sex, and age. A plethora of reference equations exist, and since interpretation of results can differ based on the chosen equation [1–4], it is difficult to select one equation that is most appropriate for an individual laboratory or patient. In this chapter we explain why reference equations are fundamental to the interpretation of pulmonary function test results, how they are created, and how to select an appropriate reference equation.

S. Stanojevic, Ph.D. (✉)
Division of Respiratory Medicine, The Hospital for Sick Children,
555 University Avenue, Toronto, ON, Canada M5G 1X8
e-mail: sanja.stanojevic@sickkids.ca

M. Rosenfeld, M.D., M.P.H.
Division of Pulmonary Medicine, Seattle Children's Hospital, 4800 Sand Point Way NE,
Seattle, WA 98105, USA

© Springer Science+Business Media New York 2015 181
S.D. Davis et al. (eds.), *Diagnostic Tests in Pediatric Pulmonology*,
Respiratory Medicine, DOI 10.1007/978-1-4939-1801-0_10

What Is a Reference Equation?

The interpretation of many medical observations relies on the availability of normative reference data with which to distinguish the effects of disease from normal variability in the population. The use of reference equations may also help to monitor test results over time. The principles behind reference data rely on the idea that a summary measure of values obtained from "normal" individuals will represent the range of values expected in a healthy population. For many biological outcomes the range of normal values changes with age and/or height. Lung growth in particular is related to increasing body size, dimensions of the thoracic cavity, sex, and age (i.e., maturity). During childhood and adolescence, growth is particularly rapid with lung function increasing 20-fold during the first 10 years of life [5]. Furthermore, during adolescence the forced vital capacity (FVC) increases proportionately more than the forced expiratory volume in 1 s (FEV_1) until the start of the adolescent growth spurt [6]. Once peak lung function has been attained during early adulthood, this peak being some 5 years later in males than females, there is a steady age-related decline in most lung function outcomes (Fig. 10.1). Therefore the correct description of the range of normal values requires that these physiological factors are taken into account.

Interpretation of Reference Data

Interpretation of reference ranges is often based on the assumption that the values observed in the sample population are normally distributed, such that 95 % of the values will fall within approximately two standard deviations (SD) of the mean.

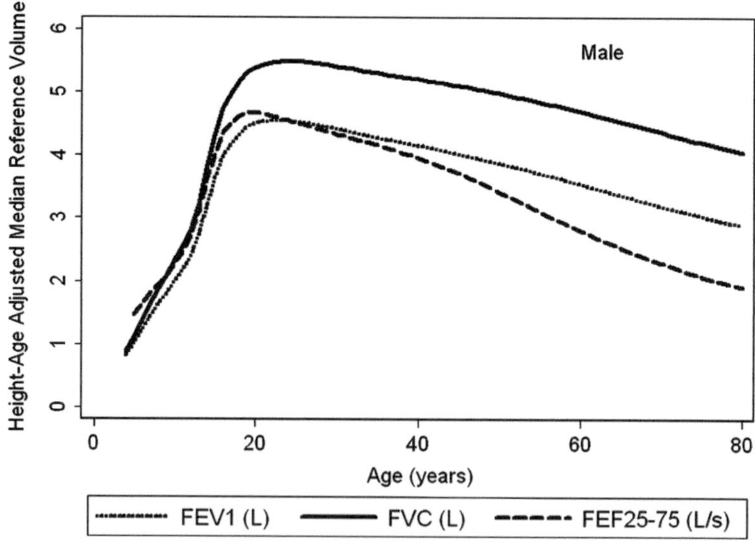

Fig. 10.1 Height- and age-adjusted spirometry outcomes across the life-span among healthy males. Figure re-drawn from tables published in Stanojevic et al. [7]

Values outside the reference interval (mean ± 2 SD) do not necessarily indicate abnormality or pathology, but rather they imply that the result is unusual in that it lies outside the range within which approximately 95 % of the reference population lies. Test results outside the reference ranges should be investigated further, with repeat assessments or additional investigations. Reference ranges also facilitate the standardization of results, such that individuals can be monitored over time to identify significant declines in lung function. Accurate identification and interpretation of changes in lung function as a result of disease or treatment require knowledge of normal variability over time within healthy subjects [8]. Since interpretation of longitudinal data may be biased when cross-sectional equations are used to interpret repeated measurements [3], longitudinal reference equations are preferable to understand how an individual lung function should change with growth. However, in the absence of longitudinal growth charts, repeated measurements should be interpreted in the context of the patient's somatic growth and clinical symptoms.

How Is a Reference Equation Constructed?

Most spirometry reference equations have been developed using linear regression techniques expressing each outcome (e.g., FEV_1, FVC) measurement as a function of both height and age, with separate equations for males and females. The relationship between lung function and age is complex, particularly during adolescents, when somatic growth and lung growth are not synchronized (Fig. 10.2).

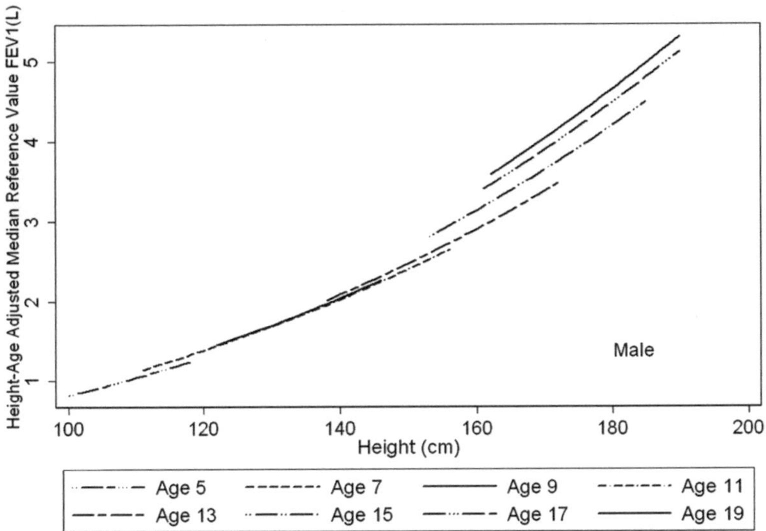

Fig. 10.2 Height trends in FEV_1 at eight specific ages. The age trend demonstrates that, for any given height, age is as important to consider in determining the reference range, especially during puberty. In contrast to adulthood where there is a decline with age, throughout childhood, at any given height an older subject can be expected to have higher values of lung function. This effect is most marked during puberty. Figure adapted with permission of the American Thoracic Society (from Stanojevic et al., AJRCCM 2008 [9]). Copyright 2013 American Thoracic Society

As a result various strategies have been used to address this asymmetric growth, for example, logarithmic transformations, age-specific equations, and more recently the LMS (Lambda, Mu, Sigma) method.

Physicians and parents will be familiar with growth charts for height and weight. The LMS method is a statistical technique designed specifically to construct growth charts (birth weight, height, weight, BMI, blood pressure), and has been used widely for this purpose. The method is an extension of regression analysis that depends on fewer assumptions. When applied to lung function data, the growth charts become three dimensional since lung function measures depend on both height and age.

Obtaining Good-Quality Pulmonary Function Data

Appropriate interpretation of PFT results relies on the assumption that spirometry has been performed according to standard guidelines and that flow-volume curves are inspected for acceptability and reproducibility [10–12]. Poorly performed maneuvers may give the appearance of disease where none is present.

Obtaining a good-quality result in young children (ages 3–6 years) is challenging but not impossible. Indeed, children of preschool age generally have short attention spans and are easily distracted, and at one time they were also thought to lack the coordination to perform tests which required active participation [13]. Young children, typically those under 6 years, are unable to meet the quality standards set for adults [14, 15]. This is partly due to the fact that spirometry measures the volume and speed (flow) with which air can be forcefully expired from the lungs after a maximal inspiration and therefore depends on both the coordination and strength of the chest wall muscles to maintain pressure. Many preschool children have not developed the chest wall strength necessary to maintain prolonged exhalation. Furthermore, the natural development of the lungs means that young children have relatively large airways compared to their lung volumes, increasing the likelihood that they will expire to residual volume in less than 1 s [16]. This means that attempts to maintain a forced expiration for 6 s, as specified by adult quality control criteria [11], are not feasible, and in some cases nor is the assessment of FEV_1. Consequently, measures of the forced expiratory volume in 0.75 s ($FEV_{0.75}$) may be more relevant in young children with small lung volumes [17, 18]; it has been shown that $FEV_{0.75}$ provides similar information to FEV_1 [15, 19].

Manufacturers of PFT equipment have also developed age-appropriate breath-activated software animations that help to maintain the child's interest during measurements. The animations help to break down the technique into components, so that the child learns in a way that is appropriate to its development. Furthermore, the level of difficulty is adjusted for lung volume and experience, to encourage an appropriate effort for each individual child [20]. There are now published and accepted standards for preschool children, which will facilitate future studies [10]. Since these adaptations have been implemented, there has been an increasing volume of literature demonstrating the feasibility of performing spirometry in preschool children and the clinical utility of these techniques.

Interpretation of Pulmonary Function Data

Clinicians in respiratory medicine have become familiar with the concept of expressing lung function as percent predicted ([observed/predicted] $\times$ 100), where the predicted value is derived from reference equations. The limitation of using percent predicted is that it does not take into account the natural variability of the measurement in healthy individuals, which is different depending on the lung function parameter, age, height, and sex. For example, as shown in Fig. 10.3, for FEV_1 in 20–30-year-old adults, the between-subject coefficient of variation (CV) is 10 %, so the normal range (encompassing 95 % of the population at that age) corresponds to 80–120 % predicted. However, for older individuals and younger children the coefficient of variation is higher, leading to a wider range of normal (60–140 % predicted) (Fig. 10.4).

A better approach to reporting lung function measures is to express results as z scores (or standard deviation (SDS) scores). The z score is a mathematical combination of the percent predicted and the between-subject variability to give a single number that accounts for age- and height-related lung function variability expected within comparable healthy individuals. For clinical interpretation of spirometric results a one-sided approach is used, where the 5th centile or -1.645 z score defines the lower limit of normal (LLN). Unlike percent predicted the same cutoff of -1.64 for z scores applies across all ages, genders, ethnic groups, and spirometric pulmonary function indices. z Scores also facilitate more appropriate interpretation of repeated measurements in the same individual.

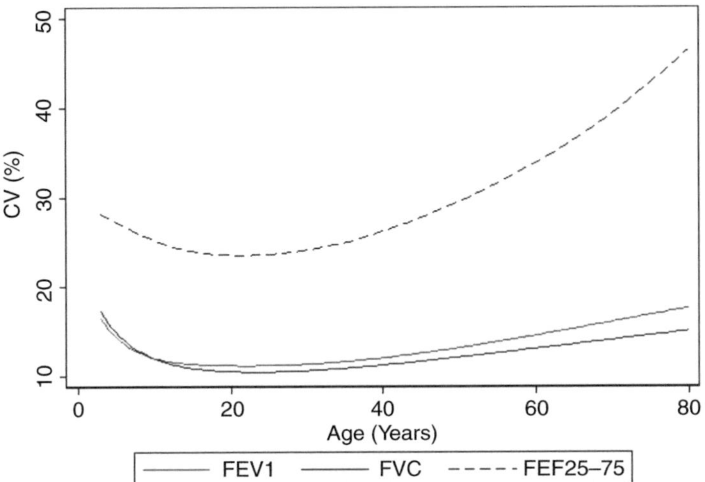

Fig. 10.3 Between-subject variability, expressed as the coefficient of variation (CV) for each of the three spirometric outcomes (FEV_1, FVC, and FEF_{25-75}). A CV of 10 % corresponds to the 95 % limits of normal (80–120 % predicted). As can be seen, the CV for FVC and FEV_1 is near 10 % only over the age range of 15–35 years. The variability at other ages and for FEF_{25-75} at all ages is considerably greater. Figure adapted with permission of the American Thoracic Society (Stanojevic et al., AJRCCM 2009 [7]). Copyright 2014 American Thoracic Society

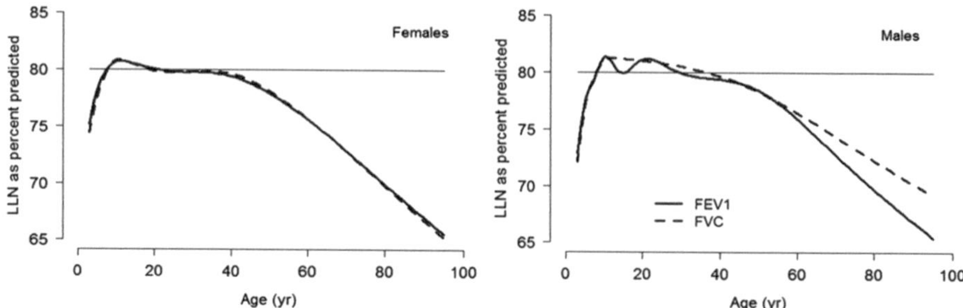

Fig. 10.4 Age-dependent lower limit of normal, in contrast to a fixed cutoff of 80 % predicted. Despite considerable debate on the limitations of percent predicted to express PFT results [21–23], its usage remains commonplace in clinical settings. Overdependence on fixed cutoffs to define abnormality, irrespective of well-recognized age-related changes, further magnifies these problems [11, 24–27]. Figure adapted with permission of the European Respiratory Society (Quanjer et al. [28])

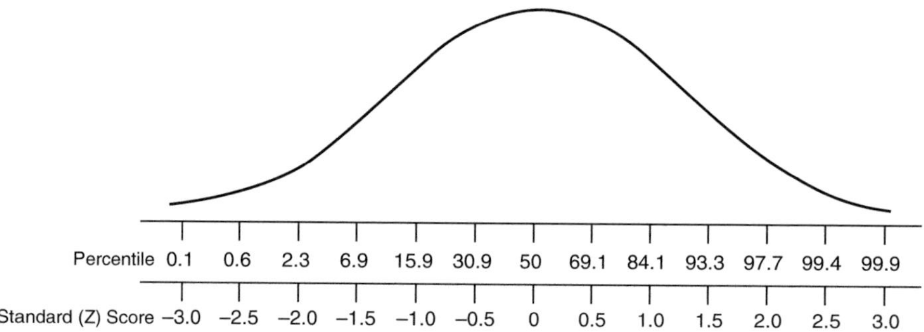

Fig. 10.5 Comparison of percentiles and z scores (SDS scores)

z Scores or SD scores quantify how far from the population mean an individual observation is reported. z Scores provide the direction and magnitude of an individual observation, in the context of the natural variability of measurements within the population. Alternatively, z scores can be converted into centiles, such as are employed in pediatric growth charts, which are more intuitive and easier to explain to patients, such that a z score of 0 equates to the 50th centile. Centiles and z scores are equivalent (Fig. 10.5); however at the extremes of the distribution, z scores are more informative.

Both the American Thoracic Society and European Respiratory Society recommend the use of the lower limit of normal (LLN), or upper limit where appropriate (i.e., plethysmographic lung volumes), to delineate between health and suspected disease. Since by convention the LLN is set at the 5th centile, whereby 90 % of the healthy population falls within the normal range, it must be appreciated that using this cutoff results in a 5 % false-positive rate.

Regardless of whether z scores, centiles, or percent predicted are used to express results, the age-specific normal range should always be included in the lung function report. In addition, the cutoffs for abnormal results do not necessarily need to be

±1.645 z scores, but any clinically or physiologically appropriate threshold. When interpreting results, it is important to remember that there will always be a degree of within-person variability, so that by chance a measurement may be just outside the "normal range" on one occasion, but just within it on the next. It is also essential to take other clinical information into account, and to weigh the consequences of an erroneous decision against that of a correct diagnosis. Particular caution is required when interpreting results which lie close to the somewhat arbitrary "cutoffs" between health and suspected disease, especially when results are limited to a single test occasion.

How to Choose a Reference Equation

The overwhelming number of published reference equations often complicates the selection of an appropriate reference. The use of inappropriate reference equations and misinterpretation even when potentially appropriate equations are used can lead to serious errors in both under- and overdiagnosis, with its associated burden in terms of financial and human costs [1, 4]. Observed differences between reference equations may be explained by differences in population characteristics; in addition equipment, software, and measurement technique used may also explain some of the variations [29, 30]. Secular trends in the population may also explain changes in body size and lung function; therefore outdated equations should be used with caution, particularly in developing countries where there have been rapid improvements in growth and nutrition. Importantly, the sample of subjects should be unbiased, and large enough to ensure that the extreme limits of "normal" can be estimated with reasonable precision and are representative of the population being tested. Criteria for choosing an appropriate reference equation are summarized in Table 10.1.

Table 10.1 Recommendation for selecting a reference equation [12, 32, 33]

Selection	Predicted values should be obtained from a reference population with the same anthropometric characteristics (height, age, sex, race, ethnicity) as the patient being tested
Equipment	Instruments and lung function testing protocols should be similar to the lab where the reference population was derived
Reference equations	Reference values should take into account height, age, and sex
	All parameters (FEV1, FVC, etc.) should, if possible, be taken from the same reference source
	Race/ethnic-specific equations should be used whenever possible
	Consideration should be given to updating reference equations on a regular basis, e.g., every 10 years
Use	Extrapolation beyond the height and age of the reference population should be avoided
	Height and weight should be measured for each patient at the time of testing to the nearest decimal
	For each lung function parameter, values below the 5th percentile (−1.64 SD) of the reference population are considered to be below the expected "normal range"

Despite the important influence that choice of reference equation may have on interpretation of results, many users of lung function equipment, and indeed clinicians who request such tests, are often not aware of which equations are used to interpret results, simply relying on default values set by manufacturers at the time of installation. Ideally, the reference range applied to interpret results should be derived from the same population from which the test subjects come, using the same equipment and methodologies as those applied [24]. Logistically, center-specific reference data are difficult to obtain, since the recruitment of a reference population is both time consuming and costly. Furthermore, a large sample is required to ensure that interpretation is not influenced by sampling bias [31]. This applies to both validation of existing reference equations and deriving new ones.

Which Reference Equations Should I Use?

Many studies have demonstrated that applying different reference equations to the same lung function data yields discrepant results in terms of z score [1–4] (Fig. 10.6). An example of how different equations can lead to different interpretations is

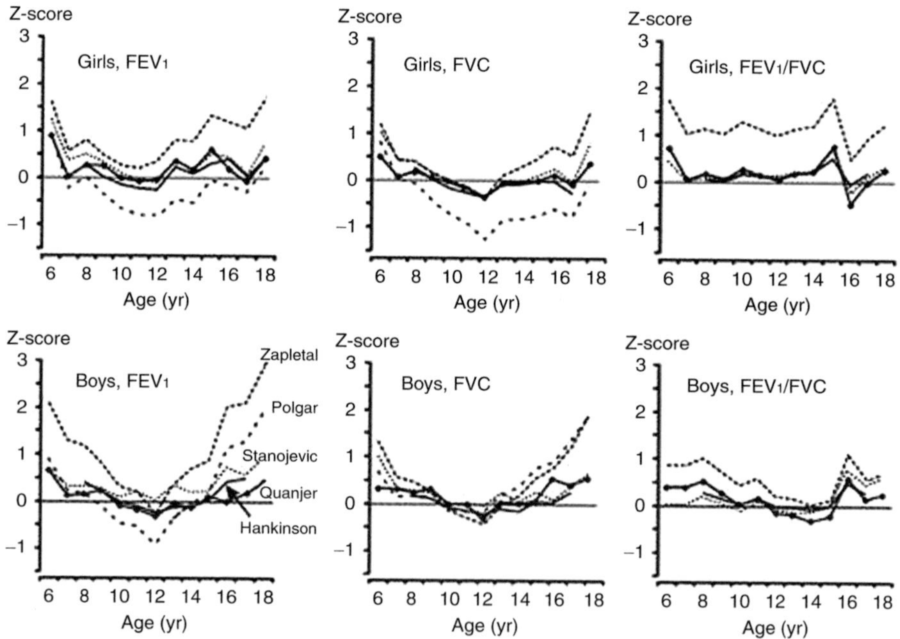

Fig. 10.6 Median values of z scores for FEV1, FVC, and FEV1/FVC for a cross section of healthy Dutch children aged 8–18 years, by five different reference equations. Figure adapted with permission of the American Thoracic Society (from Quanjer et al. [3]). Copyright 2013 American Thoracic Society

Table 10.2 Comparison of FEV_1 results for two subjects using six available pediatric equations

| | Mean FEV_1 z score (95 % confidence intervals) | | | |
| | 110 cm Boy ($FEV_1 = 0.87$ L) | | 130 cm Boy ($FEV_1 = 1.35$ L) | |
	% Predicted	z Score	% Predicted	z Score
Quanjer—GLI [28]	78	−1.7	81	−1.6
Rosenthal [33]	88	−0.9	81	−1.5
Eigen [13]	79	−2.2	79	−2.2
Nystad [34]	77	−1.5	78	−2.1
Zheng [35]	87	−0.3	100	0.0
Zapletal [36]	80	−2.9	81	−2.8

It is possible to interpret results quite differently depending on which equation is chosen, and whether percent predicted (% predicted) or z scores are used

displayed numerically in Table 10.2; for a group of healthy children the average z scores can vary by more than 1 z score when different equations are used. The differences between equations also introduce problems when children switch from one pulmonary function laboratory to another, during the transition to adult care, and in some cases within a laboratory when there is a switch in reference equations. The switching of reference equations from different populations and different age ranges introduces biases ranging from −14 to 38 % at the transition from adolescence to adulthood [3].

The American Thoracic Society (ATS) previously recommended the use of the ethnic-specific NHANES III reference equations for the interpretation of pulmonary function test results [2]. These equations however were limited to children older than 8 years of age. Therefore in many laboratories, pediatric equations from Wang et al. [37] in children <8 years were combined with the NHANES III (National Health and Nutrition Examination Survey) equation [38] during adolescence. The "stitching of equations" however introduced potential errors at the transition point [Rosenfeld M, Personal Communication]. The NHANES III and Wang equations are also limited by the fact that they do not include reference equations for $FEF_{25–75}$, which is particularly important when interpreting tests in young children.

Discontinuities in reference equations between different age groups have long been a limitation to interpretation of PFT results in children. In 2008 the "all-age spirometry" study [9] described the relationship between lung function, height, and age while also being applicable to adults and the critical transition between the two. By collating the raw data for healthy individuals collected in different studies, these equations provided smoothly changing reference curves during periods of rapid growth and transition to produce a single reference across a wide age range (3–80 years) in Caucasians. Furthermore, they describe a multiplicative and allometric relationship, where $FEV_{0.75}$, FEV_1, FVC, and $FEF_{25–75}$ are proportional to height raised to the power 2.5. For example a 1 % increase in height corresponds to a 2.5 % increase in FEV_1.

The "all-age reference" also demonstrates that the between-subject variability in lung function is highly age dependent. The practical implication of these findings is that the "normal range" for FVC or FEV_1 is considerably wider than the frequently quoted "80–120 % predicted" both for young children and for subjects older than 30 years.

Ignoring this age-dependent variability means many patients will be flagged incorrectly as "abnormal." Subsequent studies have shown that this approach of collating data to produce reference equations is robust [31]. The potential and minimal inflation of the limits of normality when using a collated dataset are balanced against a greater bias in predicted values when smaller datasets are used. In practice it is advisable for laboratories to adopt reference equations derived from large studies. The major limitation of the all-age equation is the lack of appropriate equations for ethnic groups other than those of white European descent, especially among younger children.

Ethnicity

The differences in lung function between different racial/ethnic groups are well recognized in adults and some studies have observed differences in children [35, 38–41]. African-American/Afro-Caribbean children tend to have reduced lung function (spirometry and plethysmographic lung volumes) compared with Caucasian children of the same height [39, 42]. Since the timing and tempo of somatic growth and puberty are likely under genetic control, there must be an ethnic/racial component [43]. The observed differences in somatic growth will affect the dimensions of the chest wall and the strength of the chest wall muscles [41, 42, 44, 45]. Furthermore, several studies have demonstrated the importance of trunk:leg ratio to explain racial/ethnic differences in African-Americans [39, 41, 44]. Sitting height is a good proxy for the trunk:leg ratio and has been shown to explain as much as 53 % of the observed racial differences between Caucasian and African-American subjects [41]. In addition to anthropometric differences between ethnic/racial groups, socioeconomic status has been shown to at least partially explain the ethnic/racial differences observed within the same population, as a number of factors may be involved in the interrelationship between socioeconomic status and respiratory disease [45, 46].

The observed differences and strong evidence from physiological studies suggest that ethnic-specific reference equations are necessary. However, ethnic-specific reference equations are not necessarily a satisfactory alternative since this approach requires large and representative samples, which are not readily available. The ATS recommends an adjustment factor for African-American between 12 and 15 % lower than that predicted for Caucasians; however the ethnic differences observed within this thesis highlight the fact that ethnic adjustments are complex and inconsistent [39]. In addition, ethnicity itself is difficult to define, especially given the growing number of multiethnic/multiracial children.

The Global Lungs Initiative (GLI)

To address the limitations of the all-age equations, the Global Lungs Initiative presents spirometry prediction equations that span ages 3–95 years for ethnic and geographic groups from 26 countries [28]. These all-age ethnic reference equations use the same methodology (LMS method) as the all-age equations and are generalizable across many populations. They are available for the following four ethnic groups: *Caucasians*, which includes Europe, Israel, Australia, the USA, Canada, Mexican Americans, Brazil, Chile, Mexico, Uruguay, Venezuela, Algeria, and Tunisia; *African Americans*; *South East Asians*, which includes Thailand, Taiwan, and China (including Hong Kong) south of the Huaihe River and Qinling Mountains; and *North East Asians* which includes Korea and China north of the Huaihe River and Qinling Mountains. For individuals not represented by these four groups, or of mixed ethnic origins, a composite equation taken as the average of the above equations is provided to facilitate interpretation until a more appropriate solution is developed. The spirometric equations are now endorsed by six international societies. The GLI study confirms the existence of proportional differences in pulmonary function between ethnic groups, signifying proportionate scaling of lung size due to differences in body build, so that the FEV_1/FVC ratio is generally independent of ethnic group. This has clinical advantages in that it allows a uniform definition of airway obstruction (i.e., pathological airflow limitation) based on the LLN for FEV_1/FVC across ethnic groups. Indeed, there is very little difference between the two equations except that the GLI provides a more detailed description of the desynapsis between FEV_1 and FVC during puberty in males. The GLI results also confirm a recent study reexamining the NHANES III data, which showed no statistical justification to produce separate reference equations for Hispanic Caucasians and non-Hispanic Caucasians [47]. Despite new ethnic-specific equations it is important to bear in mind that ethnicity itself is extremely difficult to define, especially given the growing multiethnic population, and may be politically sensitive; some nations now forbid recording of such details. Further research is required into the causal mechanisms behind ethnic differences in lung function.

Interpretation of Other Pulmonary Function Tests

The principles and recommendations described for spirometric reference equations apply to reference equations for other pulmonary function tests as well, particularly ones that change with growth. Selection of appropriate equations should be based on the criteria described in Table 10.1. At this time we are unable to recommend specific equations for other lung function measures since they generally lack robust equations derived from large cohorts using sophisticated statistical methods. It is important to be aware of which equations are used, as interpretation can be influenced by the choice of reference equations.

Summary

Reference equations are vital for the appropriate interpretation of pulmonary function test results. Recent advances in how we define the normal range have facilitated the use of a single reference equation across all ages, and multiple ethnic groups.

Clinicians should be aware of the reference equations used in their pulmonary function test equipment, and recognize the strengths and limitations of the reference equations selected when interpreting individual results. When possible, a single equation should be used to follow patients over time, both within and between care centers. Reference equations are necessary for the interpretation of spirometry results, but results should always be interpreted in the context of the clinical history and current symptoms of the patient.

References

1. Rosenfeld M, et al. Effect of choice of reference equation on analysis of pulmonary function in cystic fibrosis patients. Pediatr Pulmonol. 2001;31(3):227–37.
2. Pellegrino R, et al. Interpretative strategies for lung function tests. Eur Respir J. 2005;26(5): 948–68.
3. Quanjer PH, et al. Cross-sectional and longitudinal spirometry in children and adolescents: interpretative strategies. Am J Respir Crit Care Med. 2008;178(12):1262–70.
4. Subbarao P, et al. Comparison of spirometric reference values. Pediatr Pulmonol. 2004;37(6):515–22.
5. Quanjer PH, et al. Compilation of reference values for lung function measurements in children. Eur Respir J Suppl. 1989;4:184S–261.
6. Quanjer PH, et al. Changes in the FEV(1)/FVC ratio during childhood and adolescence: an intercontinental study. Eur Respir J. 2010;36(6):1391–9.
7. Stanojevic S, et al. Spirometry centile charts for young Caucasian children: the asthma UK collaborative initiative. Am J Respir Crit Care Med. 2009;180(6):547–52.
8. van Pelt W, et al. Discrepancies between longitudinal and cross-sectional change in ventilatory function in 12 years of follow-up. Am J Respir Crit Care Med. 1994;149(5):1218–26.
9. Stanojevic S, et al. Reference ranges for spirometry across all ages: a new approach. Am J Respir Crit Care Med. 2008;177(3):253–60.
10. Beydon N, et al. An official American Thoracic Society/European Respiratory Society statement: pulmonary function testing in preschool children. Am J Respir Crit Care Med. 2007;175(12):1304–45.
11. Miller MR, et al. Standardisation of spirometry. Eur Respir J. 2005;26(2):319–38.
12. Pellegrino R, et al. Quality control of spirometry: a lesson from the BRONCUS trial 1. Eur Respir J. 2005;26(6):1104–9.
13. Eigen H, et al. Spirometric pulmonary function in healthy preschool children. Am J Respir Crit Care Med. 2001;163(3):619–23.
14. Arets HG, Brackel HJ, van der Ent CK. Forced expiratory manoeuvres in children: do they meet ATS and ERS criteria for spirometry? Eur Respir J. 2001;18(4):655–60.
15. Crenesse D, et al. Spirometry in children aged 3 to 5 years: reliability of forced expiratory maneuvers. Pediatr Pulmonol. 2001;32(1):56–61.
16. Aurora P, et al. Quality control for spirometry in preschool children with and without lung disease. Am J Respir Crit Care Med. 2004;169(10):1152–9.
17. Cogswell JJ, et al. Lung function in childhood. I. The forced expiratory volumes in healthy children using a spirometer and reverse plethysmograph. Br J Dis Chest. 1975;69(1):40–50.
18. Polgar G, Promadhat V. Pulmonary function tests in children: techniques and standards. Philadelphia, London: Saunders; 1971.
19. Piccioni P, et al. Reference values of forced expiratory volumes and pulmonary flows in 3–6 year children: a cross-sectional study. Respir Res. 2007;8:14.
20. Kozlowska WJ, Aurora P. Spirometry in the pre-school age group 1. Paediatr Respir Rev. 2005;6(4):267–72.

21. Sobol BJ, Sobol PG. Per cent of predicted as the limit of normal in pulmonary function testing: a statistically valid approach. Thorax. 1979;34(1):1–3.
22. Quanjer PH. Predicted values: how should we use them? Thorax. 1988;43(8):663–4.
23. Harber P, Tockman M. Defining "disease" in epidemiologic studies of pulmonary function: percent of predicted or difference from predicted? Bull Eur Physiopathol Respir. 1982;18(6):819–28.
24. Crapo RO. The role of reference values in interpreting lung function tests. Eur Respir J. 2004;24(3):341–2.
25. Swanney MP, et al. Using the lower limit of normal for the FEV1/FVC ratio reduces the misclassification of airway obstruction. Thorax. 2008;63(12):1046–51.
26. Miller MR, et al. Defining the lower limit of normal for FEV1/FVC. Am J Respir Crit Care Med. 2007;176(1):101. author reply 101–2.
27. Quanjer PH, et al. Avoiding bias in the annualized rate of change of FEV1. Am J Respir Crit Care Med. 2007;175(3):291–2. author reply 292.
28. Quanjer PH, et al. Multi-ethnic reference values for spirometry for the 3–95-yr age range: the global lung function 2012 equations. Eur Respir J. 2012;40(6):1324–43.
29. Orfei L, et al. Early influences on adult lung function in two national British cohorts. Arch Dis Child. 2008;93(7):570–4.
30. Chinn S, et al. Sources of variation in forced expiratory volume in one second and forced vital capacity. Eur Respir J. 2006;27(4):767–73.
31. Quanjer PH, et al. Influence of secular trends and sample size on reference equations for lung function tests. Eur Respir J. 2011;37(3):658–64.
32. Pittman JE, Rosenfeld M. Appropriate pediatric spirometry reference equations and interpretation. Pediatr Allergy Immunol Pulmonol. 2011;24(2):63–8.
33. Rosenthal M, et al. Lung function in white children aged 4 to 19 years: II – single breath analysis and plethysmography. Thorax. 1993;48(8):803–8.
34. Nystad W, et al. Feasibility of measuring lung function in preschool children. Thorax. 2002;57(12):1021–7.
35. Zhang QL, et al. Feasibility and predicted equations of spirometry in Shenzhen preschool children. Zhonghua Er Ke Za Zhi. 2005;43(11):843–8.
36. Zapletal A, et al. Maximum expiratory flow-volume curves and airway conductance in children and adolescents. J Appl Physiol. 1969;26(3):308–16.
37. Wang X, et al. Pulmonary function between 6 and 18 years of age. Pediatr Pulmonol. 1993;15(2):75–88.
38. Hankinson JL, Odencrantz JR, Fedan KB. Spirometric reference values from a sample of the general U.S. population. Am J Respir Crit Care Med. 1999;159(1):179–87.
39. Whitrow MJ, Harding S. Ethnic differences in adolescent lung function: anthropometric, socioeconomic, and psychosocial factors. Am J Respir Crit Care Med. 2008;177(11):1262–7.
40. Ip MS, et al. Lung function reference values in Chinese children and adolescents in Hong Kong. I. Spirometric values and comparison with other populations. Am J Respir Crit Care Med. 2000;162(2 Pt 1):424–9.
41. Harik-Khan RI, Muller DC, Wise RA. Racial difference in lung function in African-American and White children: effect of anthropometric, socioeconomic, nutritional, and environmental factors. Am J Epidemiol. 2004;160(9):893–900.
42. Greenough A, et al. Importance of using lung function regression equations appropriate for ethnic origin. Pediatr Pulmonol. 1991;11(3):207–11.
43. Butte NE, Garza C, de Onis M. Evaluation of the feasibility of international growth standards for school-aged children and adolescents. Food Nutr Bull. 2006;27(4 Suppl Growth Standard):S169–74.
44. Donnelly PM, et al. What factors explain racial differences in lung volumes? Eur Respir J. 1991;4(7):829–38.
45. Yang TS, et al. A review of the racial differences in the lung function of normal Caucasian, Chinese and Indian subjects. Eur Respir J. 1991;4(7):872–80.
46. Harik-Khan RI, et al. The effect of anthropometric and socioeconomic factors on the racial difference in lung function. Am J Respir Crit Care Med. 2001;164(9):1647–54.
47. Kiefer EM, Hankinson JL, Barr RG. Similar relation of age and height to lung function among Whites, African Americans, and Hispanics. Am J Epidemiol. 2011;173(4):376–87.

Chapter 11
Polysomnography for the Pediatric Pulmonologist

Iman R. Sami and Judith A. Owens

Abstract Sleep affects control of breathing and ventilation both in children and adolescents who are healthy as well as those who have underlying respiratory, cardiovascular, or neurologic disorders. This chapter discusses the utility of nocturnal in-lab polysomnography in assessing children for sleep-related breathing disorders. The diagnostic and treatment indications for pediatric polysomnography are reviewed based on recently published guidelines. The respiratory and nonrespiratory components of a polysomnogram are reviewed, so are the reported parameters from such a study. Challenges involved in conducting and interpreting pediatric polysomnograms are discussed, including diagnostic and treatment (positive airway pressure titration) studies.

Keywords Sleep • Polysomnography • Pediatric pulmonologist • Sleep-related breathing disorders • Evaluation and treatment

Introduction

Sleep is a physiologic function of the body with profound effects on virtually all the major organ systems. In the respiratory system, sleep affects both the control of breathing and the mechanics of ventilation. Even healthy normal individuals develop different breathing patterns during sleep (usually slower and regular during slow-wave sleep, and irregular during rapid eye movement {REM} sleep). Airway resistance in the upper airways increases and the cough reflex is diminished during sleep. The gas exchange is impaired due to relative hypoventilation that results both in elevation of the levels of carbon dioxide and/or in oxygen desaturation. The response to hypoxia also diminishes during sleep especially among newborns and prematurely born infants.

I.R. Sami, M.D., M.R.C.P. (✉) • J.A. Owens, M.D., D,A.B.S.M.
Division of Pulmonary and Sleep Medicine, Children's National Health System,
111 Michigan Avenue NW, Washington, DC 20010, USA
e-mail: ISami@childrensnational.org

© Springer Science+Business Media New York 2015
S.D. Davis et al. (eds.), *Diagnostic Tests in Pediatric Pulmonology*,
Respiratory Medicine, DOI 10.1007/978-1-4939-1801-0_11

The presence, duration, and severity of these abnormalities differ between the different stages of sleep but in a healthy individual these alterations have little clinical importance. However, any underlying respiratory, cardiovascular, or neurologic disorder may exacerbate the physiologic effects of sleep leading to clinically significant changes and in turn they may be adversely affected by the effects of sleep, thus creating a vicious cycle. For example patients with muscle weakness are going to develop more profound hypoventilation than a healthy individual. The cough reflex diminishes during sleep in all individuals but it will have much more profound effect in patients who are prone to develop aspiration.

Nocturnal in-lab polysomnography (NPSG) is an important tool in the diagnostic evaluation of sleep-related breathing disorders (SRBD) in children. It can be used to identify events such as apneas (obstructive and/or central) and hypopneas, hypoventilation, as well as alterations in gas exchange (i.e., hypoxemia and/or hypercapnia) during sleep. The following conditions can often be differentiated and the degree of severity assessed:

- Primary snoring (snoring without associated ventilatory abnormalities)
- Obstructive sleep apnea syndrome (OSAS)
- Central sleep apnea
- Central hypoventilation
- Hypoventilation due to neuromuscular weakness or pulmonary disease

NPSG is also indicated for the institution and evaluation of treatment of SRBD in children, for example titration of positive airway pressure and/or degree of mechanical ventilator support required during sleep.

While the focus of this chapter is on NPSG in respiratory disorders, it should be pointed out that NPSG can be useful in the assessment of non-respiratory sleep disorders.

A polysomnogram is a tool that measures and records the presence or absence of airflow as well as the pattern of breathing, in relation to the respiratory effort, and the stage of sleep. It also relates these events to gas exchange reflected by oxygenation plus/minus end-tidal carbon dioxide measurements.

Components of Diagnostic NPSG

In assessing the need for and utility of NPSG in diagnosing SRBD, it is important to recognize the specific information that is recorded during a typical sleep study.

NPSG monitors simultaneously a number of physiologic functions:

(a) Movement of the rib cage and abdomen monitored by respiratory inductance plethysmography via leads on the chest and abdomen.
(b) Airflow in the nose and in the mouth, via a dual probe ("nasal-oral thermistor").
(c) Airflow via a nasal pressure transducer.
(d) Gas exchange, via pulse oximetry for oxygen saturation and end-tidal CO_2 monitoring via capnometry.

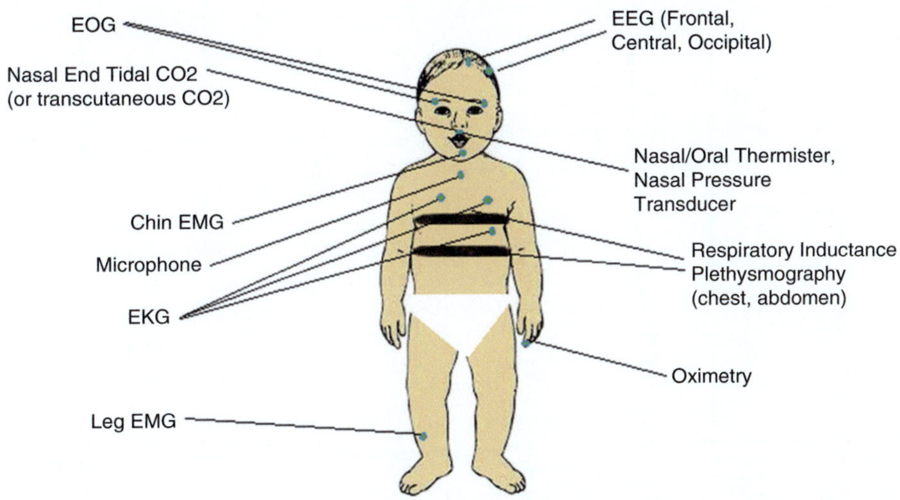

Fig. 11.1 Placement of sensors and variables collected during PSG

(e) Cardiac function, via continuous electrocardiogram (ECG).
(f) Sleep staging via continuous electroencephalogram (EEG) and electromyogram (EMG) in order to document the exact sleep stage in which abnormalities in any or all of the above occur. The leads are placed in the following locations (Fig. 11.1):

- Frontal, central, and occipital EEG
- R. outer canthus and L. outer canthus EOG
- Chin EMG
- R. and L. anterior tibia EMG

(g) Body position, and presence or absence of snoring via a video camera and microphone.

Optional recordings available in some labs and/or by special request include transesophageal balloon manometry (records intrathoracic pressure swings and may be useful in the diagnosis of suspected SRBD with negative PSG findings, such as upper airway resistance syndrome (UARS)), extended EEG montage for nocturnal seizure assessment, and pH probe recording for evaluation of gastroesophageal reflux.

The PSG is divided into 30-s segments ("epochs") (Fig. 11.2). The study is then divided into different stages according to the patient's sleep stage. The latter is being determined on the basis of the EEG (brain activity), EOG (eye movement), and EMG (skeletal muscle tone). The *sleep/wake stages are the following*:

1. Wake or W
2. Stage 1 or N1 (transitional sleep)
3. Stage 2 or N2 (sleep characterized by specific EEG features—K complexes and sleep spindles)

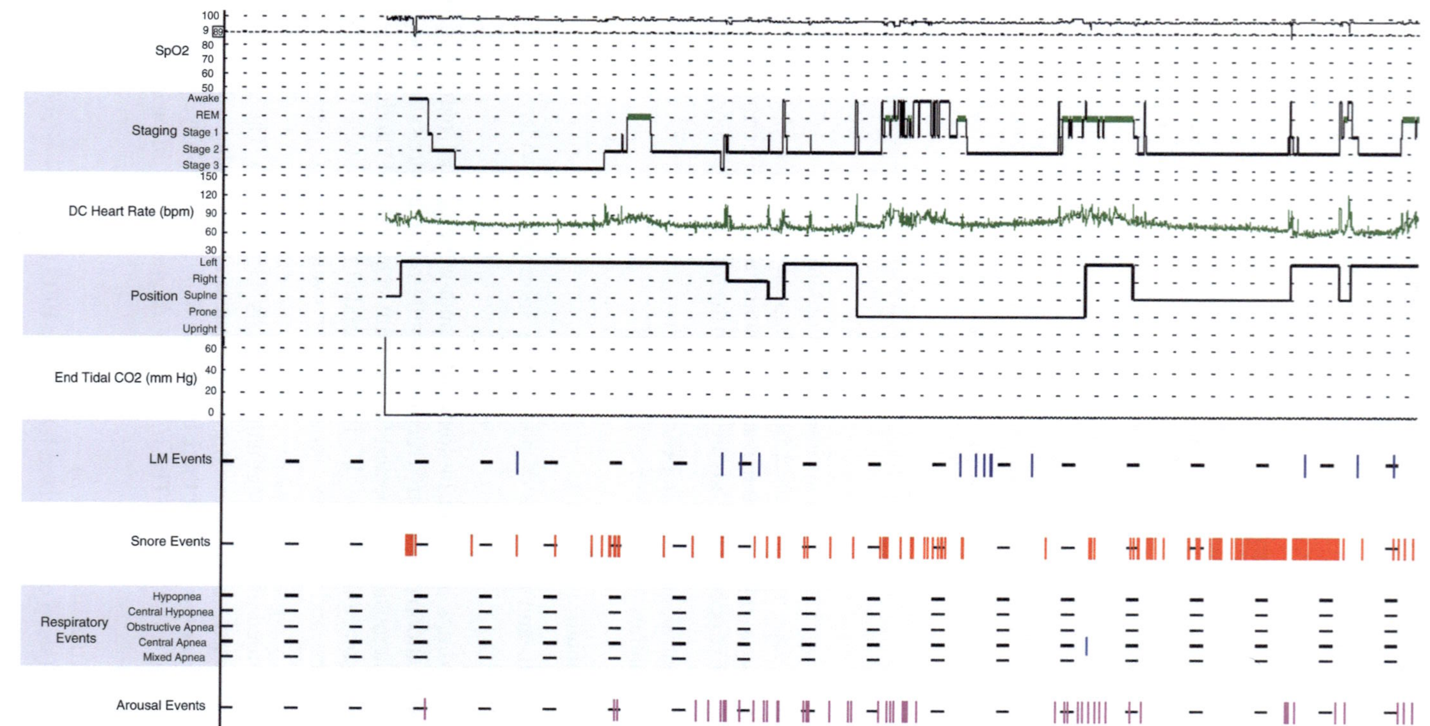

Fig. 11.2 Hypnogram shows mild sleep disruption, snoring, and increased arousals. REM sleep latency is prolonged. Leg movements are noted in stage II sleep. Oxygen saturation is normal. Only one central apnea event is noted during the latter portion of the night

4. Stage 3 or N3 (combines prior stages 3 and 4; slow-wave, deep, or delta sleep)
5. REM or stage R (rapid eye movement sleep)

The determination of the sleep stages allows the generation of several *sleep-specific parameters* which are reported as follows:

1. Lights out/on
2. Total recording time (TRT—lights out to lights on)
3. Total sleep time (TST)
4. Sleep latency (SL)—time to first epoch of sleep
5. Stage R latency (sleep onset to first epoch of stage R)
6. Wake after sleep onset (WASO)
7. Sleep efficiency (SE) = TST/TRT × 100
8. Time in each stage
9. Percent of TST in each stage
10. Arousals:

    (a) Total number
    (b) Arousal index (no. of arousals per hour of sleep time)

Respiratory parameters are determined by airflow (nasal/oral thermistor and nasal pressure transducer) and respiratory effort (RIP), as well as EEG arousals to assess sleep fragmentation associated with respiratory events:

1. Number of apneas (obstructive, mixed, central), hypopneas, apneas + hypopneas
2. Indices (index = number of events per hour of sleep): Apnea index (usually reported separately as central AI and obstructive AI), hypopnea index (HI), apnea + hypopnea index (AHI): This last parameter is the one most frequently used to determine the presence and severity of SRBD and is often subdivided into total (includes central events) and obstructive AHI.
3. Optional:

    (a) Number of respiratory efforts related to arousals (RERAs) and RERA index (number of events/hour)
    (b) Paradoxical breathing (asynchronous chest and abdominal wall muscle movement indicating increased respiratory effort)

Oxygenation (pulse oximeter) and *ventilatory status* (end-tidal CO_2 or transcutaneous CO_2) parameters reported are the following:

1. Number of oxygen desaturations >3 or 4 % from prior reading
2. Oxygen desaturation index (number of desaturation episodes >3 %/h)
3. Mean oxygen saturation
4. Minimum oxygen saturation (and whether or not there is an association with any respiratory events)
5. End-tidal carbon dioxide (optional in adult studies, but essential in pediatric studies)
6. Occurrence of hypoventilation, periodic breathing, or Cheyne-Stokes pattern (see Definitions)

Cardiac events as assessed by EKG:

1. Average heart rate (HR)
2. Maximum HR during recording, and during sleep
3. Bradycardia, tachycardia, asystole, and other arrhythmias.

Movement events as assessed by bilateral EMG anterior tibialis monitors and EEG arousals:

1. These can be limb movements or periodic limb movements (PLMS). Periodic limb movements are scored when there are four or more limb movements in succession with an interval that ranges from 5 to 90 s. The total numbers are reported for each one as well as the index (no. of events per hour of sleep).
2. Number of PLMS with arousals as well as PLM arousal index (no. of events per hour of sleep).

The hypnogram (Fig. 11.2) is a visual display that gives an overview picture of the study night and sleep architecture, cardiorespiratory, and movement-related parameters.

Respiratory Indications for NPSG in Children

The indications for performing a PSG have been addressed in several recent publications by the American Academy of Sleep Medicine (AASM) in March 2011 and the American Academy of Pediatrics (AAP) in October 2012. A synopsis of the AASM diagnostic and treatment practice parameters is as follows (descending strength of evidence level is indicated by standard (S), guideline (G), and option (O)):

Diagnostic Indications (Children and Adolescents)

1. Nocturnal in-lab PSG is a reliable and valid measure of the presence of OSAS.

    (a) Nap (abbreviated) PSG is not recommended for the evaluation of OSAS in children as it is likely to underestimate the presence and severity of SRBD (low sensitivity) (O).
    (b) There is currently insufficient data to support the use of unattended in-home portable PSG testing in the clinical diagnosis of SRBD in children. While there is an increasing trend towards the use of portable monitoring in adults with suspected SRBD, the feasibility and diagnostic accuracy of these devices in the pediatric population have yet to be determined.

2. NPSG is indicated when the clinical assessment suggests the diagnosis of OSAS in children (S).

    (a) OSAS in children should be diagnosed based on clinical and PSG data.

(b) The clinical evaluation (history and physical exam, audio/visual recordings, screening questionnaires, etc.) alone does not have sufficient sensitivity/specificity to establish the diagnosis.

3. NPSG should be strongly considered if there is the slightest clinical suspicion of SRBD in the following high-risk conditions:

   (a) Craniofacial anomalies (Pierre Robin sequence, achondroplasia)
   (b) Congenital CNS malformations (Arnold-Chiari, meningomyelocele, spina bifida)
   (c) Cerebral palsy
   (d) Neuromuscular diseases (Duchenne muscular dystrophy)
   (e) Obesity
   (f) Prader-Willi syndrome
   (g) Down syndrome

   Intermediate risk conditions, in which the clinician should have a low threshold for ordering NPSG in the presence of signs/symptoms of SRBD, include the following:

   (a) Prematurity
   (b) African American race
   (c) Family history of SRBD
   (d) Sickle cell disease

   However, there is insufficient evidence to support routine PSG in the following respiratory disorders unless there is a clinical suspicion for an accompanying sleep-related breathing disorder (O):

   (a) Chronic asthma
   (b) Cystic fibrosis
   (c) Bronchopulmonary dysplasia
   (d) Pulmonary hypertension

4. PSG is indicated when the clinical assessment suggests the diagnosis of sleep-related hypoventilation due to neuromuscular or chest wall deformities (G).
5. PSG is indicated when the clinical assessment suggests the diagnosis of congenital central alveolar hypoventilation syndrome (G).

Diagnostic Indications (Infants)

1. PSG is indicated only in selected cases of primary sleep apnea of infancy (G). There is insufficient evidence to support the utility of routine PSG in establishing primary sleep apnea of infancy diagnosis and most infants are diagnosed by clinical history and direct observation.
2. PSG is indicated in selected populations of infants who have experienced an acute life-threatening event (ALTE) when there is clinical evidence of a sleep-related breathing disorder (G). While subtle PSG abnormalities have been identi-

fied in some infants with ALTEs, PSG findings have not been found to be predictive of recurrence and most infants have normal PSGs. Infants with ALTEs who subsequently develop SRBD generally have other risk factors (craniofacial dysmorphology, etc.).

3. PSG is not routinely indicated to assess sudden infant death (SIDS) risk in infants, as PSG abnormalities in SIDS are neither sufficiently distinctive nor predictive.
4. PSG may have clinical utility in evaluating the presence and severity of SRBD before and after surgical intervention in infants with laryngomalacia.

Treatment Indications

1. PSG is indicated in children being considered for T&A to treat OSAS (G). As noted above, clinical assessment alone is insufficient to reliably identify the presence of OSAS. In addition, PSG is required to establish the severity of SRBD, which is important from the standpoint not only of increased risk of postoperative complications including respiratory compromise in severe OSAS and requirements for inpatient postoperative monitoring, but also determines the need for a repeat PSG after surgery.
2. PSG is indicated following T&A to assess for residual OSAS in children with preoperative evidence of high-risk conditions (S):

    (a) Moderate-to-severe OSAS
    (b) Obesity
    (c) Craniofacial anomalies
    (d) High-risk congenital conditions (Down's syndrome, Prader-Willi syndrome, etc.)

3. Children with mild OSAS preoperatively should have clinical evaluation following T&A to assess for residual symptoms of OSAS. If residual symptoms are present, PSG should be performed (S).
4. PSG is indicated after treatment of children with OSAS with rapid maxillary expansion or an oral appliance (O), as there is currently insufficient evidence to support clinical assessment of efficacy.
5. PSG is indicated for positive airway pressure titration in children with OSA syndrome (S).
6. Follow-up PSG in children on chronic PAP support is indicated to determine whether pressure requirements have changed (G). While there are no specific guidelines as to how frequently repeat PAP titrations should be performed, a reasonable approach, especially in younger children, would be to conduct these on an annual basis. More frequent titration may be indicated if growth parameters change significantly, SRBD symptoms recur, or additional treatments have been instituted.
7. PSG is indicated for noninvasive positive pressure ventilation (NIPPV) titration in children with other sleep-related breathing disorders in NMD (O). Children treated with mechanical ventilation may also benefit from periodic evaluation with PSG to adjust ventilator settings (O).

8. Children treated with tracheostomy for sleep-related breathing disorders benefit from PSG as part of the evaluation prior to decannulation (O).
9. Children considered for treatment with supplemental oxygen do *not* routinely require PSG for management of oxygen therapy (O), as home oximetry is generally sufficient to establish O_2 requirements.

It should be noted that there is no universal agreement with the above AASM practice parameters, particularly in regard to the recommendations that NPSG is required to establish the diagnosis of OSAS and that it is necessary to conduct a sleep study prior to adenotonsillectomy. While recent otolaryngology guidelines (2011) acknowledge that NPSG is the most reliable and objective test to assess for the presence and severity of OSAS, they also state that PSG is not necessary to perform routinely, and the diagnosis of SDB in children may be based on other clinical parameters such as history and physical exam, nocturnal oximetry, or limited PSG. Similarly, the revised AAP Clinical Practice Guidelines (2012) for the Diagnosis and Management of OSAS (in otherwise healthy typically developing children and excluding infants), while upholding NPSG as the "gold standard" for diagnosis of OSAS, also specify that if in-lab NPSG is not available, then "referral to a specialist (ENT, sleep) for more extensive evaluation or alternative diagnostic tests [nocturnal video recording, nocturnal oximetry, daytime nap or ambulatory PSG] may be considered." The recommendations state that in the event that these tests fail to demonstrate OSAS in a patient with a high pretest probability, full PSG should be conducted.

NPSG can also be useful in the assessment of non-respiratory sleep disorders. Briefly, these include the following:

– Periodic limb movement disorder (a PLM index of 5 or more per hour is considered abnormal in children).
– Nocturnal seizures (generally requires extended EEG montage).
– Narcolepsy (generally requires additional daytime nap study—Multiple Sleep Latency Test (MSLT)): The MSLT consists of five nap opportunities conducted at 2-h intervals, following an overnight PSG. Each nap opportunity lasts for 20–39 min depending on whether sleep occurs and when. The mean sleep latency is calculated; a SOL of <8 min is considered abnormal in adults. The presence of REM during naps is also documented and the appearance of REM in two or more of the naps is consistent with a diagnosis of narcolepsy.

A sleep study may also be helpful in the evaluation of unexplained daytime sleepiness despite adequate nocturnal sleep and unexplained failure to thrive or polycythemia which could be related to an undiagnosed sleep-related breathing disorder. Occasionally NPSG findings (e.g., frequent arousals and sleep fragmentation, alpha-wave intrusion into slow-wave sleep in pain syndromes, arrhythmias, and nocturnal hypoxia in cardiopulmonary disorders) may provide clinically useful supporting data in other chronic medical conditions, but are rarely indicated for diagnostic assessment. In addition, parasomnias such as sleepwalking, sleep terrors, and sleep-related rhythmic movement disorders (i.e., head banging, bruxism) can also be documented during a polysomnogram, but NPSG is not typically required for the diagnosis of these disorders, especially those which are episodic in nature.

Finally, polysomnography is seldom indicated in the assessment of primarily behaviorally based or circadian rhythm sleep disorders such as insomnia or delayed sleep-phase disorder, unless a comorbid sleep-related breathing disorder is suspected on the basis of the clinical history.

Conducting and Interpreting Pediatric Diagnostic NPSG

There are many unique challenges to providing at the very least a minimum standard of diagnostic sleep services for children. First, the sleep lab staff (both healthcare providers and technologists) need to possess a knowledge base regarding pediatric respiratory pathophysiology and neurophysiology, normal developmental changes in sleep architecture, and cognitive/motor/language/social developmental milestones. Required technical skills in conducting and scoring pediatric sleep studies necessitate initial specialized training, ongoing education, and exposure to an adequate volume of patients.

Young and/or medically complicated children and developmentally delayed children are particularly difficult, often requiring extended setup and monitoring times and a high technician-to-patient ratio (2:1 or 1:1).

Conducting sleep studies in children also requires specific accommodations to the physical space (sleeping accommodations for parents, cribs), to the emotional and physical needs of children across a range of ages and their caregivers, and the implementation of pediatric specific procedures to insure comfort and safety. Recognizing that caregivers are an integral component of pediatric care, sleep programs should have specific policies which provide family-centered and child-friendly care.

For these reasons, pediatric PSGs should be performed in a lab that has the expertise to deal with the challenges presented by this population. While currently there are no specific standards for primarily adult sleep labs in regard to conducting studies in children, at minimum, it is recommended that the lab be accredited by the American Academy of Sleep Medicine (a list of accredited labs may be found at aasmnet.org) to ensure a high standard of care. Ideally, the diagnostic lab should be part of a comprehensive sleep center which also offers clinical assessment and treatment for pediatric patients.

In order to insure that the study is conducted properly and the appropriate information recorded and documented, it is *absolutely critical* that the referring physician provide certain basic information to the medical director reviewing and approving all referrals and the sleep lab staff conducting the test to ensure the best outcome during the study. This information is also essential in allowing the interpreting physician to make appropriate clinical decisions and recommendations. Information required includes the following:

1. Specific diagnostic test requested (baseline NPSG, PAP titration, NPSG + MSLT, etc.)
2. Specific reason for referral

3. Presenting complaints and clinical symptoms related to referral question, including key SRBD symptoms (snoring, witnessed apnea) and risk factors (obesity, enlarged tonsils, craniofacial abnormalities)
4. Other pertinent medical history, including previous interventions such as adenotonsillectomy, concurrent respiratory therapies, and all medications
5. Current weight and BMI, including BMI percentile for age and gender
6. Dates and findings from previous PSGs (attach reports if available)
7. Additional sleep-related symptoms (insomnia, circadian rhythm disruptions, parasomnias)
8. Presence of daytime sleepiness and/or impairments
9. Pertinent psychiatric/neurodevelopmental history, such as comorbid anxiety disorders or autism spectrum disorders, and all medications
10. Other special concerns (language barriers, behavioral issues, allergies)
11. Usual sleep–wake schedule (a 2-week sleep diary is very helpful and required for interpreting an MSLT)
12. Additional specific testing instructions from the ordering physician
13. Family expectations

During the study, documentation of events by the sleep lab tech such as seizures, parasomnias, and unusual sleeping positions is essential to scoring and interpretation of the study. A "morning after" questionnaire completed by the accompanying parent regarding sleep and breathing on the study night compared to "usual" is also helpful to the interpreting physician.

Once the study has been completed, the raw data is reviewed and sleep staging, arousals, cardiorespiratory events, and body movements are scored for each 30-s epoch by a trained scoring technologist. This process takes up to 3 h for each study. The scored study is then reviewed, epoch by epoch, by sleep-certified physician and interpreted or "read" using pediatric rules and norms. For example, for purposes of sleep staging interpretation it is important to bear in mind the age of the child, and expected values for parameters such as amount of sleep and proportion of time spent in each stage. Interpretation of sleep-onset latency will depend on the age of the child and prior night sleep period. Adolescents and toddlers generally have the hardest time falling asleep in the sleep lab. This may translate into a decreased sleep efficiency which is often attributed to the "first night effect." If the child wakes up and has difficulty settling down the sleep architecture will be fragmented as well.

While there have been relatively few large-scale studies assessing normative PSG parameters in children of different ages, the following table (Table 11.1) provides average values and standard deviations as a reference for the most commonly reported PSG variables across the pediatric age spectrum.

The referring physician must therefore take all of this into account when reviewing a PSG report so that the correct interpretation can be made that supports the clinical history and physical findings, and appropriate management strategies can be instituted.

Table 11.1 Normal PSG values for children aged 3–9

Parameter	3–6 Years old: mean (SD)	6–9 Years old: mean (SD)
Total sleep time	475 (42)	472 (43)
Stage 1 %	6.6 (4.8)	7.1 (5.5)
Stage 2 %	41.6 (7.1)	46.1 (8.5)
Stage 3 %	6.6 (2.6)	5.5 (2.9)
Stage 4 %	21.6 (6.2)	18.5 (6.6)
SWS %	29 (9)	25 (10)
REM %	23.6 (4.8)	22.6 (5.2)
Sleep efficiency	90 (7)	89.3 (7.5)
Sleep-onset latency	24.1 (25.6)	23 (25.3)
Latency to REM	87.8 (41.2)	132 (57.7)
Arousal index	9.0 (3.4)	9.5 (5.3)
Periodic limb movement index	1.4 (1.4)	0.91 (1.2)
Periodic limb movement arousal index	0.04 (0.12)	0.10 (0.24)
Obstructive apnea index	0.03 (0.1)	0.05 (0.11)
Mixed apnea index	0.01 (0.05)	0.01 (0.06)
Central apnea index	0.03 (0.01)	0.45 (0.49)
Apnea index	0.86 (0.75)	0.50 (0.52)
Apnea hypopnea index	0.9 (0.78)	0.68 (0.75)
Obstructive apnea/hypopnea index	0.08 (0.16)	0.14 (0.22)
Nadir SpO_2	92.7 (4.5)	92.6 (3.6)
Desaturation index (>4 %)	0.29 (0.35)	0.47 (0.96)
Mean end-tidal CO_2	40.6 (4.6)	40.7 (4.5)
Heart rate (6–11 years of age) adapted from Archbold 2010 (values averaged across samples)		
Male		76 (8.2)
Female		79.6 (9.2)

Adapted from (Montgomery-Downs et al. 2006)

Diagnostic Criteria for SRBD

While there are no universal standardized criteria for differentiating "primary snoring" from clinically significant sleep-disordered breathing, the following PSG parameter definitions are generally accepted as pathologic, with the caveat that these numerical data must be interpreted in the context of the clinical information in each individual case. Obstructive sleep apnea syndrome (OSAS) is defined as repeated episodes of upper airway obstruction during sleep in the face of continued or increased respiratory effort. This results in complete or partial cessation of airflow at the nose and/or mouth. Intermittent hypoxia, hypercapnia, arousals, and daytime symptoms often accompany OSAS. The PSG diagnostic criteria for OSAS are the following:

- AHI >1.5 or AI >1 event per hour (up to 12 years of age—at age 13 adult criteria can be used although some sleep labs elect to use pediatric criteria until the age of 18 years): In adults an AHI of 5 or greater is required to make the diagnosis.

– OSA is classified as moderate in children if the AHI is >5, and severe if it is >10. For adults it is moderate if >15, and severe if greater than 30.
– Oxygen desaturation nadir <91 %.
– Change in oxygen nadir from baseline >3 %.
– Maximum end-tidal carbon dioxide >54 mmHg.
– End-tidal carbon dioxide >50 mmHg for more than 25 % of TST.
– Increased EEG arousals.

NPSG and Treatment of SRBD

Positive Airway Pressure Titration Studies

Continuous positive airway pressure (CPAP) is the most commonly prescribed treatment for obstructive sleep apnea syndrome. It is indicated in situations where adenotonsillectomy is not indicated, or where it has failed to resolve the symptoms. It is also used preoperatively in children with severe OSAS. A flow generator creates the CPAP, which is delivered through a hose connected to an interface. There are three kinds of interfaces:

– Nasal masks
– Full face masks
– Nasal pillows

Prior to starting PAP, proper mask fitting is crucial to the success of this treatment. The use of warm humidity, a ramp feature, and expiratory pressure relief have also made this treatment modality more comfortable, and improved compliance. After a 2–4-week period of "desensitization" where the child wears the mask initially while awake, and then during sleep to acclimatize to the pressure prior to the study, an overnight PSG is performed to determine the optimal CPAP pressure. Optimal pressures are determined when:

– All obstructive apnea events are eliminated.
– Desaturation events are eliminated or minimized.
– Good sleep efficiency is achieved.

It is essential to achieve this during supine REM sleep. Over-titration of the patient may cause central apnea events.

In children who do not tolerate CPAP, or who hypoventilate, bilevel PAP (BIPAP—where the inspiratory pressure—IPAP is higher than the expiratory pressure—EPAP) may offer an alternative modality of delivering PAP. However studies have shown that in children with uncomplicated OSAS the use of BIPAP does not appear to offer an advantage over conventional CPAP in terms of compliance.

Patients with neuromuscular weakness or pulmonary disease require separate consideration. These children need to use their accessory muscles to assist with ventilation. This is particularly problematic during REM sleep because of muscle atonia resulting in hypoxemia and hypercarbia from hypoventilation. When there is central apnea or hypoventilation, BIPAP with the option of adding a ventilation rate can provide noninvasive positive pressure ventilatory support (NIPPV) during sleep. A large pressure difference between the IPAP and EPAP is particularly important in patients with neuromuscular weakness.

Oxygen titration studies to determine whether the addition of supplemental oxygen at various concentrations will eliminate oxygen desaturation and apnea events. These studies are usually performed in ex-premature infants to facilitate discharge planning.

Children with chronic respiratory failure and requiring chronic ventilatory support can also be assessed with a sleep study to assess whether rate and pressure settings are adequate during sleep.

Tracheostomy studies: Whether or not an NPSG is required prior to decannulation is controversial, and several publications have attempted to address this question. The opinion of many otolaryngologists is that if a child can tolerate a Passy-Muir valve for prolonged periods of time, and has an adequate airway on direct visualization by a rigid bronchoscope, then decannulation can be performed without resorting to an NPSG. On the other hand, in children with chronic tracheostomy (greater than 6 months), who undergo an NPSG prior to decannulation, there is a very high correlation between a "favorable" study and successful decannulation, and vice versa. Specifically in children with tracheostomies and other comorbid conditions such as hypotonia, craniofacial abnormalities, or concomitant lung disease, an NPSG with the tracheostomy occluded can provide valuable information on whether decannulation will be tolerated. It is important to assess the child with an NSPG after decannulation especially if it was placed to enable prolonged mechanical ventilation as there is a very high prevalence of sleep-disordered breathing in this patient population.

Definitions

Obstructive apnea: Cessation of airflow ($\leq$90 % of baseline) >10-s duration or two baseline breaths (in children) with continued or increased respiratory effort. This is scored on the nasal thermistor channel. An oxygen desaturation is not required to score the event.

Central apnea: Cessation of airflow without respiratory effort $\geq$20 s *or* if less than 20 s must be associated with arousal/awakening *or* $\geq$3 % O_2 desaturation.

Mixed apnea: Initial central apnea followed by chest and abdominal movements with a lack of airflow >10 s in duration (or at least two breaths in children).

Hypopnea: $\geq$30 % reduction airflow associated with arousal/awakening *or* $\geq$3 % O_2 desaturation. When scoring obstructive hypopneas the nasal pressure transducer channel is used.

Periodic breathing: At least three central apneas in succession which are a minimum duration of 3 s, and are separated by no more than 20 s of regular respiration: This is a pattern of breathing seen more commonly in infants, especially premature babies.

Normal values for premature infants are <5 % of sleep time, and for term infants <3 % of sleep time. This pattern disappears as the infant matures and its continued presence may reflect underlying central nervous system immaturity or anemia.

Hypoventilation: End-tidal carbon dioxide greater than 50 mmHg for more than 25 % of the total sleep time. Hypoventilation is assessed by measuring end-tidal CO_2.

Cheyne-Stokes respiration: Central apneas and hypopneas alternate with periods of hyperventilation, producing a waxing and waning pattern of tidal volume.

References

1. Wise MS, Nichols CD, Grigg-Damberger MM, Marcus CL, Witmans MB, Kirk VG, D'Andrea LA, Hoban TF. Executive summary of respiratory indications for polysomnography in children: an evidence-based review. Sleep. 2011;34(3):389–98.
2. Aurora RN, Zak RS, Karippot A, Lamm CI, Morgenthaler TI, Auerbach SH, Bista SR, Casey KR, Chowdhuri S, Kristo DA, Ramar K. Practice parameters for the respiratory indications for polysomnography in children. Sleep. 2011;34(3):379–88.
3. Baugh RF, Archer SM, Mitchell RB, Rosenfeld RM, Amin R, Burns JJ, Darrow DH, Giordano T, Litman RS, Li KK, Mannix ME, Schwartz RH, Setzen G, Wald ER, Wall E, Sandberg G, Patel MM. Clinical practice guidelines: tonsillectomy in children. Otolaryngol-Head Neck Surg. 2011;144:S1–30.
4. Beck SE, Marcus CL. Pediatric polysomnography. Sleep Med Clin. 2009;4(3):393–406.
5. Marcus CL, Brooks LJ, Draper KA, Gozal D, Halbower AC, Jones J, Schechter MS, Ward SD, Sheldon SH, Shiffman RN, Lehmann C, Spruyt K, American Academy of Pediatrics. Diagnosis and management of childhood obstructive sleep apnea syndrome. Pediatrics. 2012;130(3): e714–55.
6. Montgomery-Downs HE, O'Brien LM, Gulliver TE, Gozal D. Polysomnographic characteristics in normal preschool and early school-aged children. Pediatrics. 2006 Mar;117(3):741–53.
7. Lorenzi-Filho G, Genta PR, Figueiredo AC, Inoue D. Cheyne-stokes respiration in patients with congestive heart failure: causes and consequences. Clinics (Sao Paulo). 2005;60(4):333–44.

Chapter 12
Cardiopulmonary Exercise Testing Techniques to Evaluate Exercise Intolerance

David Thomas and Daniel P. Credeur

Abstract The use of exercise testing is an important tool for the pediatric pulmonologist. Physical stress often reveals cardiorespiratory abnormalities that are not apparent on conventional static tests. There is little doubt the information acquired from exercise tests have diagnostic and prognostic value, but exercise tests may also be critical to determine success or failure of treatment strategies. The purpose of this chapter is to provide the pediatric specialist with an overview of exercise evaluation that may assist in the diagnosis of and management of disease in pediatric and adolescent patients with physical activity intolerance, especially those with cardio-respiratory diseases. The specific aims of this chapter are to: (1) describe various exercise tests and the biomechanical and physiological principles of those tests necessary to assess patients; (2) discuss methods to assess the physical fitness profile of patients with cardiorespiratory diseases and physical limitations; (3) provide specific strategies for an exercise prescription based on the fitness and clinical profile of the patient and; (4) assist the provider in developing a center for exercise evaluation. Although each aim provides unique information, the overall goal of this chapter is to stimulate the pediatric pulmonologist to develop an understanding of indications for cardiopulmonary exercise testing (CPET) and implement strate-gies to systematically assess each patient's fitness profile; to track patient's disease or training progression or alternatively to monitor responses of medical interventions; and to prescribe a well-rounded exercise prescription to maximize functional ability and wellness of individual patients. This chapter is not intended to be an in depth review for exercise physiologists, but is designed to assist the practicing clinician in the logistics of developing a program and a comfort in interpreting studies.

D. Thomas, M.D., Ph.D. (✉)
Pediatric Center for Respiratory, Exercise and Sleep Medicine,
Athletic Training Facility Football Operations,
Louisiana State University, Baton Rouge, LA, USA

Louisiana Healthcare Connections, 8585 Archive Blvd Suite 301,
Baton Rouge, LA 70809, USA

D.P. Credeur, Ph.D.
Department of Medical Pharmacology and Physiology, University of Missouri,
1 Hospital Dr., Medical Sciences Bldg. M415, Columbia, MO 65212, USA

© Springer Science+Business Media New York 2015
S.D. Davis et al. (eds.), *Diagnostic Tests in Pediatric Pulmonology*,
Respiratory Medicine, DOI 10.1007/978-1-4939-1801-0_12

Keywords Exercise testing • Exercise evaluation • Pediatric pulmonology • Treatment strategies • Cardiorespiratory disease • Physical fitness profile • Cardiovascular exercise testing

Introduction

Exercise testing consists of an analysis of the functional capacity to engage in activities of daily living (ADL) and higher levels of physical activity and or exercise. Humans engage in various forms of physical activity through integrated skeletal muscle movements requiring energy. Any physical activity in which work is performed by skeletal muscle can be regarded as exercise. It is important to differentiate between resistance and endurance exercises. Resistance exercise consists of brief periods of muscle contraction, such as weight lifting, and endurance exercise consists of rhythmic contractions for extended periods of time, such as in walking or running. The energy used for skeletal muscle use is derived from the chemical breakdown of carbohydrates, fats, and protein to energize mitochondria within muscle cells to contract and relax. This energy pathway is composed of a system of enzymes, substrates, and oxygen that eventually result in the production of (adenosine triphosphate) ATP. There are many good textbooks and reviews which describe the processes on bioenergetics of muscular activity and concepts of clinical exercise testing for diagnostic purpose [1–8]. The authors especially recommend the chapter written by Morton in Pediatric Pulmonary Medicine [5]. This chapter (Morton) is an outstanding overview of exercise physiology and applies these principles to pediatrics.

The use of physical stressors often reveal cardiopulmonary abnormalities that are not evident on resting pulmonary function or cardiovascular evaluations like electrocardiograms (ECG), echocardiograms, and spirometry to name a few. This chapter is not intended to be a footprint of previous textbooks and but is to assist clinicians in developing a program to utilize exercise techniques and equipment for the purpose of evaluating exercise intolerance and developing exercise prescription. Understanding the type of evaluation needed allows the clinician to develop organization and logistics to determine which personnel and equipment will be required to perform the tests, execution of the evaluation, and to interpret results to develop an individualized exercise prescription to treat exercise intolerance in the pediatric or adolescent patient.

Understanding the basic concepts of cardiopulmonary exercise testing (CPET) has never been more important than present. Reduced physical activity and a sedentary lifestyle are associated with chronic conditions including coronary artery disease, musculoskeletal and metabolic disorders such as type-II diabetes and obesity [9]. Childhood obesity rates continue to climb and physical inactivity in children and adults present significant challenges to public health [10]. Obesity and physical inactivity usually begin in childhood and often become a lifelong issue with a plethora of health disparities as illustrated in Fig. 12.1. Unfortunately, we deal with many outside influences which confuse the true science and medicine around these problems. Such interferences include the Internet, blogs, social media, sports news,

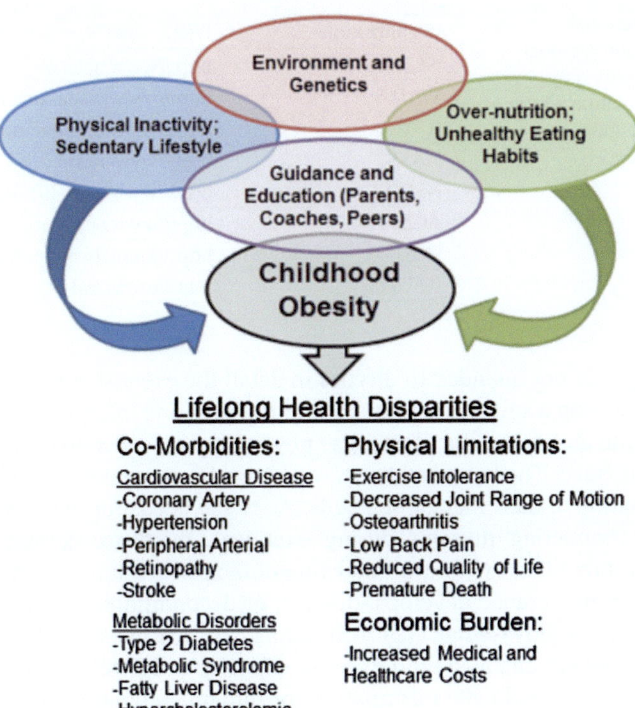

Fig. 12.1 Health disparities. Integration of comorbidities resulting in childhood obesity and lifelong health disparities of impairment and risk

and journalists. There are many practitioners in the field of exercise and training with no significant education in physiology and biomechanics of exercise, who often recommend techniques and diets which are unhealthy and generate revenue [11]. This is especially true in the supplement market which has potential to do more harm than improve performance [12]. The aware clinician interested in providing a comprehensive exercise evaluation and prescription should also be informed of dietary and sleep needs of patients as these may affect physical activity and capacity [13]. This is especially true of those who are dealing with performance athletes [14]. Performance athletes are susceptible to these external stimuli as the level of competition has much higher stakes including scholarships and professional contracts. Performance athlete coaches and trainers and sometimes team physicians have little to no experience in exercise science and may encourage behaviors and prescribe methods that are clearly incorrect and can actually lead to disability of their athlete. Prohibited and dangerous methods of training, dietary supplementation, and drug use are clearly defined by organizations like the National Collegiate Athletic Association (NCAA) and others listed in Table 12.1, but very few high school athletic associations regulate or investigate inappropriate use of supplements and training practices [15]. Organizations such as those listed in Table 12.1 study the effects of exercise in all age groups and provide education, training, and certification in the principles of exercise testing and prescription.

Table 12.1 National, international, and regional organizations providing education, regulation and/or certification of sports and exercise training

Organization	URL
NCAA	http://www.ncaa.org
WADA	http://www.wada-ama.org
IOC	http://www.olympic.org/ioc
NASM	http://www.nasm.org
NSCA	http://www.nsca-lift.org/Home/
ACSM	http://www.acsm.org
PES	http://journals.humankinetics.com/pe
USUHS	http://usuhs.mil

This chapter is not intended to discuss in detail the exercise science beyond that required to develop a suitable laboratory environment and interpret clinical studies. However, some understanding of exercise physiology is needed to evaluate physical activity intolerance. The heart and lungs work together as a unit to supply oxygen to tissues in relation to their metabolic needs. As tissue needs for oxygen increase (as they do in contracting muscles during exercise), there are certain predictable responses in individuals with a normal functioning heart, lungs, and vasculature. When exercise intolerance develops, disease, or deconditioning may be present in either the (1) cardiovascular, (2) respiratory, or (3) musculoskeletal system. Behavioral problems can also limit exercise capacity and a well conducted exercise test can also provide valuable information for initiating cognitive behavior therapy [16]. Adverse responses to exercise and physical activity are predictable deviations from the normal. Exercise tests, with measurements of both cardiovascular and respiratory function, are often called cardiorespiratory or cardiopulmonary exercise (CPET) testing. The CPET can provide valuable noninvasive information about the functioning of both the cardiovascular and respiratory systems. To assist the clinician in understanding the indications and interpretation of exercise intolerance, important concepts in exercise physiology and testing are briefly reviewed in Table 12.2.

Defining Maximal Oxygen Uptake

The relationship between the amounts of oxygen consumed and work performed is predictable, and since the body has limited capacity for storing oxygen, the rate of oxygen uptake at the lung represents rate of cellular oxygen consumption. Oxygen uptake (VO_2) is proportional to the external work of physical activities. Maximal oxygen uptake is defined as the maximal amount of oxygen distributed and used by the body while performing heavy exercise. A high VO_2 requires the respiratory system to exchange oxygen and carbon dioxide within blood; the cardiovascular system to pump and distribute oxygen-laden blood (hemoglobin) to active skeletal muscle; and the ability of the skeletal muscle to convert stored substrates to power muscular

Table 12.2 Exercise testing components and description

Component	Description
1. VO_2 (maximal oxygen uptake)	– Maximal amount of oxygen taken up by the respiratory system, distributed by the cardiovascular system and utilized by metabolically active tissue (i.e., contracting skeletal muscle) during heavy aerobic exercise
2. Importance of oxygen uptake	– Ensures adequate supply, delivery, and utilization of oxygen to sustain metabolic processes and muscular work
3. Measurement of VO_2	– Measuring the volume of oxygen consumed through spirometry, arterial-venous oxygen differences, and or using validated estimation equations based on heart rate and workload (i.e. Bruce Treadmill protocol, YMCA cycle test)

4. Variables obtained during CPET testing	– Volume of oxygen consumed (VO_2)
	– Volume of carbon dioxide produced (VCO_2)
	– Pulmonary ventilation (L/min)
	– Ventilatory threshold (V_T)
	– Lactate threshold (LT)
	– Respiratory exchange ratio (RER)
	– Rating of perceived exertion (RPE)
	    • Borg scale
	    • Dyspnea scale
	    • Angina scale

5. Exercise testing for diagnostic purposes	– ECG recordings
	    • Monitor heart rate and myocardial electrical disturbances
	    • Blood pressure responses

6. Methods for CPET	– Bruce treadmill protocol – YMCA cycle test

7. Methods to determine exercise intolerance in performance athletes	– Sport-specific exercise tests
	    • Shuttle runs
	    • Burpees
	    • Box jumps
	    • Beep tests

8. Age influences on physiological adjustments to exercise with respect to *age appropriate* physiology	– Cardiorespiratory responses
	    • Increased cardiac output (Blunted in elderly, greater in children and adolescents)
	    • Increased arterial–venous O_2 difference(Blunted in elderly, greater in children and adolescents)
	    • Increased skeletal muscle blood (Blunted in elderly, greater in children and adolescents)
	    • Increased ventilation (Blunted in elderly, greater in children and adolescents)
	    • Increased arterial blood pressure (Increased in elderly)

contraction. Maximal oxygen uptake is abbreviated VO_2 max; where V represents the volume of oxygen per minute, O_2 represents oxygen, and max represents maximal amount or conditions. Thus, VO_2 max is the maximal volume of oxygen used by the body per minute [1–8]. This value is usually expressed in absolute terms as liters per minute (L min^{-1}) or in relative terms as milliliters per kilogram of body weight

Table 12.3 VO_2 max prediction equations

Modality of exercise	Equation
1. Treadmill (walking)	$- VO_2 = 0.1$(speed in m/min) $+ 1.8$(speed in m/min) (grade %) $+ 3.5$
2. Treadmill (running)	$- VO_2 = 0.2$(speed in m/min) $+ 0.9$(speed in m/min) (grade %) $+ 3.5$
3. Stepping	$- VO_2 = 0.2$(Step rate in steps/min) $+ 2.4$(Step height) (Step rate in steps/min) $+ 3.5$
4. Leg ergometry	$- VO_2 = 1.8$(Work rate)/bodyweight in kg $+ 7$ • Work rate (kg × m/min) = force setting in kg × pedal distance × pedal rate
5. Arm ergometry	$- VO_2 = 3$(Work rate)/bodyweight in kg $+ 3.5$ • Work rate (kg × m/min) = force setting in kg × pedal distance × pedal rate

6. Recovery HR (BPM)	– *Following stepping:*
	• 15 s count HR × 4 = BPM
	  ° Male, VO_2 max $= 111.33 - (0.42 \times HR)$
	  ° Female, VO_2 max $= 65.81 - (0.1847 \times HR)$
	– *Walk/run tests*
	• 12 min walk/run (male and female)
	  ° VO_2max $= 3.126$ x (meters covered) $- 11.3$
	• 1.5 mile run test (male and female)
	  ° VO_2 max $= 3.5 + 483$/time

per minute (mL/kg min^{-1}). VO_2 max is considered the gold standard measure of maximal aerobic capacity or aerobic power. Because VO_2 max is a measure of energy transfer, it is also considered a measure of aerobic power rather than just volume or capacity [1–8]. The by-product of aerobic power production is carbon dioxide (CO_2), and the volume of CO_2 eliminated per minute from the body is the VCO_2. This variable is important and provides information regarding cardiopulmonary efficiency especially at the onset of nonaerobic or "anaerobic" metabolism (anaerobic glycolysis or lactic acid system) [1–8]. Except for steady state exercise, there is an additional variable of total metabolism from anaerobic processes. Indeed, aerobic metabolism persists in longer duration physical events; however, it is important to recognize that aerobic metabolism is only one component of metabolic rate during maximal exercise. At maximal exercise, metabolism (rate of energy transfer) is the sum of maximal aerobic power (VO_2 max) and maximal anaerobic power. Some commonly used calculations to estimate VO_2 are listed in Table 12.3. However, one should be cautious when using normative calculations in the pediatric population; especially for maximal heart rate calculations [17, 18]. Children are born with a set number of muscle cells, but development of strength which is characterized by increased diameter of muscle fibers (cells) is dependent upon changes into puberty. The emergence into Tanner 4–5 stages can be variable and use of age related calculations can be problematic.

Historically, the measurement of VO_2 max can be a costly and time consuming operation confined to research laboratories. With the development of rapidly responding gas analyzers and volume measuring devices, along with advances in

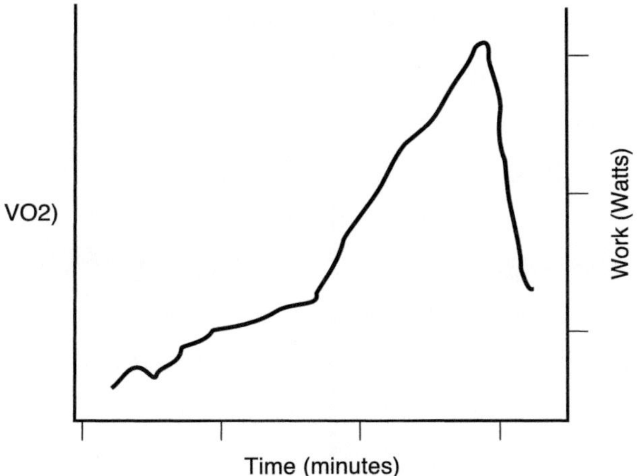

Fig. 12.2 VO$_2$ max (peak). At VO$_2$ max (peak) work rate will usually peak or plateau. After the plateau, work rate may continue to increase with no further increase in VO$_2$ and this represents the physiological limit of aerobic power

computer technology, this measurement is now accessible to scientists, clinicians, and fitness personnel. In fact there are now portable and even hand held VO$_2$ testing devices available on the market [19–22]. When work rate increases on an ergonometric device (e.g., speed and grade on a treadmill or cycle ergometer) or during any physical activity, so does VO$_2$ as long as the subject is not limited or deficient in any of the aforementioned physiological systems (i.e., cardiovascular, respiratory, hematologic, and musculoskeletal system). When approaching VO$_2$ max work rate will usually peak or plateau. After the plateau, work rate may continue to increase with no further increase in VO$_2$ (Fig. 12.2). Therefore, VO$_2$ max represents the physiological limit of aerobic power. Although work rate may continue to increase following a plateau of VO$_2$, this increase may be a product of other energy systems such as anaerobic power or metabolism [1–8]. Nonetheless, sustained work output will soon subside as muscular fatigue sets in. The magnitude increase in work rate beyond plateau does not affect the measurement of VO$_2$ max, but instead can be used as an index anaerobic power as well as psychological motivation and persistence (Fig. 12.3) [1–8]. Table 12.4 lists important variables obtained during a CPET.

Determining VO$_2$ max

In the classic definition, VO$_2$ max was presumed to occur when there was less than a 2.1 mL/kg min^{-1} increase in VO$_2$ with an increase in treadmill grade of 2.5 % at speed of 7 mph. Thus, there would be an increase of less than 0.6 METs (metabolic equivalent of task) or about 25 % of the expected increase of 2.5 METS [1–5]. A metabolic equivalent is a physiological measure of the energy cost of physical

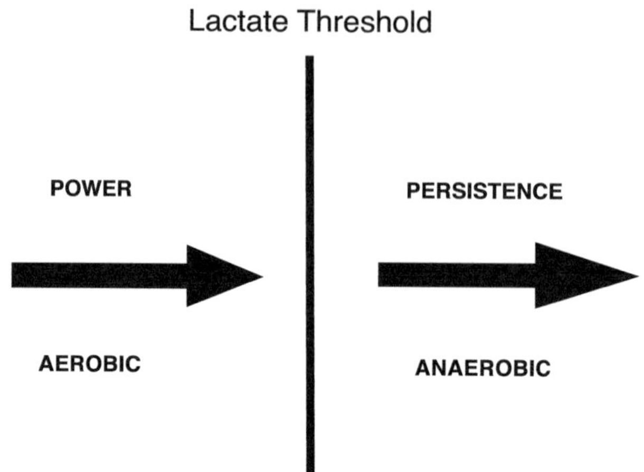

Fig. 12.3 Power and persistence. Once LT is achieved, power (work) is more a measure of anaerobic capacity and theoretical persistence or desire to continue

Table 12.4 Key variables of a CPET assessment

Peak VO_2: (max)	Oxygen utilization ($mLO_2 \cdot kg^{-1} \cdot min^{-1}$): A measure of aerobic capacity; normal values are influenced by age and sex
VT (AT estimate)	VO_2 at the ventilatory threshold ($mLO_2\,kg^{-1} \cdot min^{-1}$): A measure of submaximal exercise tolerance. Anerobic threshold (AT)
Peak RER:	The ratio of exhaled CO_2 to inhaled O_2
VO_2/w (mL/min/w):	Characterizes the ability of exercising muscle to extract oxygen (power) Low VO_2/w relationship suggests cardiac or pulmonary impairment
O_2 pulse (mL O_2/heart beat):	Approximates stroke volume
$PetCO_2$:	End-tidal CO_2 or the level of CO_2 in the air exhaled from the body (measured in mm Hg). Reduced values indicate VQ mismatching, and is consistent with worsening cardiac or pulmonary disease severity, and worse prognosis
VE (L O2/min): Ventilation	(based on tidal volume and respiratory rate) during exercise. Peak VE can be assessed relative it can help determine if exercise intolerance or dyspnea relate to a pulmonary limitation
VE/MVV:	Assessment of the maximum minute ventilation during exercise relative to maximum voluntary ventilation which is determined during PFTs at rest. The VE/MVV ratio is normally 80 % (and consistent with the premise that the pulmonary system is not limiting the exercise capacity
VE/VCO_2 slope:	Measurement of ventilatory efficiency (ie, minute ventilation relative to CO_2 exhalation). Whereas VE/VCO_2 slope is normally <30, efficiency decreases with cardiomyopathy intrinsic lung disease, and/or pulmonary hypertension, VE/VCO_2 slope increases in each instance
VD/VT	Dead space ventilation
Pulse oximetry (% O_2 saturation)	Decline in hemoglobin oxygenation levels, 90 % indicative of diminished ability to adequately increase alveolar-pulmonary capillary oxygen transfer during exercise

Table 12.5 Criteria for achievement of VO_2 max

Criteria	Description
1. Plateau in VO_2	– Oxygen consumption plateaus or decreases despite an increase in workload
2. Blood lactate > 8 mmol	– Indicates increased glycolytic production of lactic acid
3. RER > 1.0	– Respiratory exchange ratio, or respiratory quotient (VCO_2/VO_2) indicative of carbohydrate utilization (i.e. muscle glycogen) for continued energy production
4. Age predicted maximum heart rate	– Traditional, 220—Age (max heart Rate declines with age) – More recently, 206.9—(0.67 × Age)
5. Perceived exertion = 20	– Subjective Perception of maximal exercise
6. Rate pressure product = Systolic BP × heart rate (fivefold)	– RPP is an index of myocardial O_2 demand
7. ST-segment shifts	– Indicative of cardiac ischemia and/or injury

activity defined as the ratio of metabolic rate (rate of energy consumption) during a specific physical activity to a reference metabolic rate, set by convention to 3.5 ml O_2/kg min^{-1}.

Other criteria for achievement of VO_2 max in well-motivated subjects include (1) a respiratory exchange ratio (RER) greater than 1.0 and (2) a blood lactate concentration greater than 8 mmol L^{-1} (Table 12.5, [1–3]). In several studies involving both younger and older subjects, less than 50 % of these individuals could reach a plateau in VO_2 at maximal work rates. Åstrand was the first to document that many children and adolescents complete a progressive exercise test to exhaustion without a plateau in VO_2. Subsequent studies have confirmed only a minority of young people exhibit a classical VO_2 plateau [23].

Lactate or Anaerobic Threshold (LT or AT)

After plateau, work rate may continue to increase with no further increase in VO_2. Therefore, VO_2 max represents the physiological limit of aerobic power. Although work rate may continue to increase following a plateau of VO_2, this increase is a product of anaerobic power or metabolism [1–4]. Nonetheless, sustained work output will soon subside as muscular fatigue develops. As previously mentioned, the magnitude increase in work rate beyond plateau does not affect the measurement of VO_2 max, but instead can be used as an index anaerobic power as well as psychological motivation or persistence as represented by Fig. 12.3 [1–8]. The easiest method to determine the lactate threshold is known as the V-slope method by determining the ventilator anaerobic threshold (Fig. 12.4). The upward inflection in VCO_2 is the VO_2 at which ventilatory anaerobic threshold (VAT) is determined. The increase in $VECO_2$ occurs when ventilatory buffering is needed to compensate for increased lactate driven metabolic acidosis. The magnitude of cardiac and ventilatory

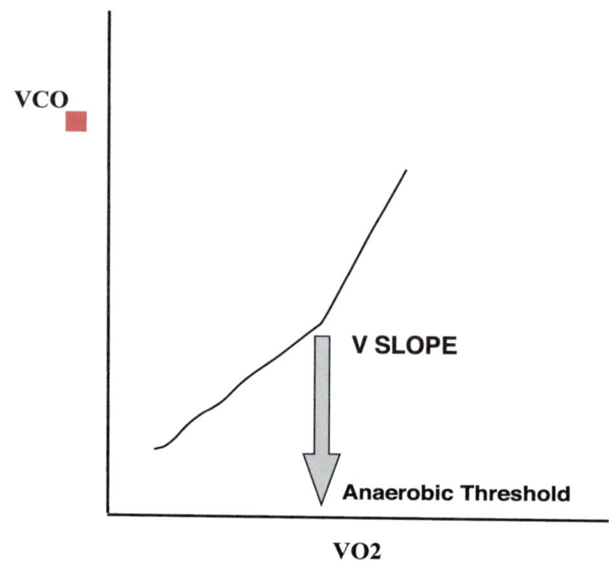

Fig. 12.4 LT measurements. There are several methods to estimate lactate threshold. The V-slope method is determined by break in linearity of the VCO_2–VO_2 graphical relationship

effort that a task represents and its tolerability to the patient are affected by whether the work is above or below lactate or anaerobic threshold. Therefore, Lactate threshold (LT) is a level of effort that is relevant to exercise tolerance or intolerance and the ventilatory threshold is a physiologic change in CO_2 elimination that approximates LT. The rate of rise in lactate is also dependent upon the type of muscle fiber activated (type I—slow oxidative or type II—fast glycolytic) along with power need. In other words, the intensity and load duration can hasten the emergence of anaerobic metabolism. This concept is very important when testing children and adolescents, especially those in sporting activities. Specific sports and age groups often exercise in a burst patterns and performing a graded CPET may not be an adequate representation of their activity patterns and need for power to perform a sport or other ADLs [24].

Lactate is the product of anaerobic glycolysis and is an available source of ATP, but is an inefficient energy source for sustained exercise as the energy produced is small compared to full aerobic oxidation. There is much confusion regarding the physiologic role of lactate. During anaerobic glycolysis the cofactor nicotinamide adenine dinucleotide (NAD) is regenerated during the conversion of pyruvate to lactate. The accumulation of lactic acid cannot be sustained; however, lactate is not what solely causes the muscle to fatigue. There are a multitude of reasons that muscle fatigues (i.e., pH drop due to Hydrogen ion accumulation) [25]. Lactic acidosis is also important for exercise performance as the fall in pH causes rightward shift of the oxy-hemoglobin dissociation curve facilitating the release of oxygen from hemoglobin (Bohr Effect; Fig. 12.5). In summary, muscular fatigue is not reflected

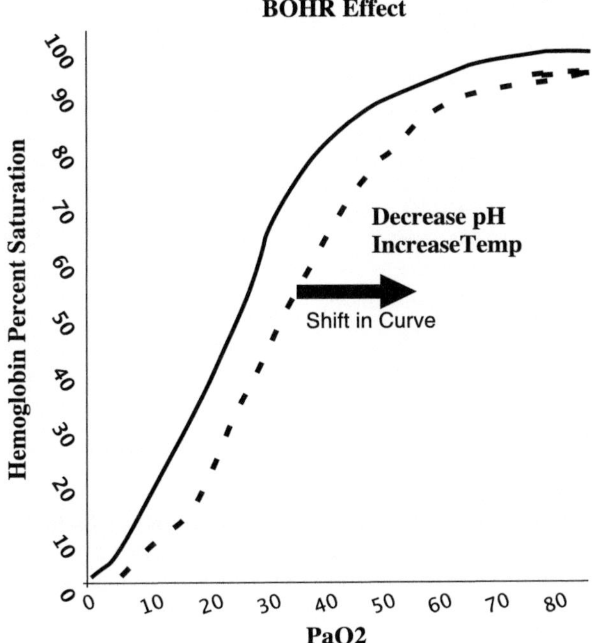

Fig. 12.5 Bohr Effect. An effect by which an increase of carbon dioxide in the blood and a decrease in pH results in a reduction of the affinity of hemoglobin for oxygen. At the muscle level the combination of heat and lower pH increases oxygen delivery to the mitochondria of contracting muscle

alone on lactate level, but is a signal when energy sources have changed and fatigability (muscle inefficiency) is present. But muscle fatigue begins before the onset of anaerobic glycolysis (VO_2 max).

Purpose of Exercise Testing

The purpose of exercise testing is to assess cardiopulmonary, metabolic musculoskeletal power, and motivation/effort during physical stress. Physical stress magnifies the pathophysiology and physical limits, thus allowing the clinician to diagnose and develop interventions which are sport or activity specific. By considering time dimensions, the faster the heart and respiratory rate, the more samples available for analysis. The concept that a classical laboratory based CPET is needed is not necessarily true as exercise intolerance should also be addressed to include the biomechanics which trigger the event. The core of this evaluation is to determine functional capacity of the cardiopulmonary system and power of metabolic-muscular activity while reproducing symptoms or signs of the complaint. This process and the adaptations that occur with training or any exercise are listed in Table 12.6.

Table 12.6 Adaptations that occur with training or any exercise

Parameter	Result	Magnitude	Variable measured CPET
Cardiac output	Increase	4–5	Pulse O_2
Heart rate	Increase	3	HR
Stroke volume	Increase	2	Pulse O_2
Oxygen extraction	Increase	3	$P(A-a)O_2$
O_2-Hgb dissociation	Increase	–	
BP systolic	Increase	1.5	BP
BP diastolic	Minimal change	1.1	BP
Pulse pressure	Increase	1.3	BP
PVR	Decrease	4.5	–
MVO_2	Increase	4	ECG

The goal of laboratory based exercise testing is to address four key issues; (1) cardiovascular limitations, (2) ventilatory limitation, (3) metabolic or musculoskeletal limitation (biomechanics of activity) and (4) motivation or effort limitations or perceptions. The psychological aspects and expectations associated with exercise by the patient, and parents or coaches, can be a major contributor to the complaint [26].

Activity Intolerance and Exercise-Activity Fitness

Activity intolerance and exercise-activity fitness in the pediatric population and evaluation of those components is very age defined and can be difficult. Use of static volumes, resistances, and flows derived from conventional pulmonary functions, even if performed pre and post exercise, tell us little in regard to function during periods of increased physical demand (i.e., exercise). This includes newer modalities involving impulse oscillometry. Importantly, the younger the population the more difficult is the technique for measurement. In addition, some of the techniques presently used in the infant population are technologically challenging and require significant technical skills. There are relationships between classical pulmonary function tests and functional capacity, but there is no predictive consistency as these measurements do not take into account the individuals power needs. Evaluation of cardiac function by ECG and echocardiogram in a non-exercise study do not give us a clear depiction of higher level dynamics and functional risks. These cardiopulmonary measurements lack specific enough information to assess impairment or risk when the system is placed under stress. The absence of this data limits a clinician's ability to fully assess the effectiveness of pharmacologic and or physical therapies designed to promote health and encourage activity.

Intolerance to exercise may have nothing to do with the cardiopulmonary system but may reflect muscle fatigue, fatigability, or incomplete recovery. The delivery of oxygen and elimination of carbon dioxide is most the time normal for the pediatric patient's capacity. The associated dyspnea with exertion is really a reflection that the system is working well and that the problem is more related to power efficiency which is being perturbed by intrinsic muscle inefficiency or neurologic/psychological causes. The measurement of VO_2 provides the clinician with information at a very fundamental level representing only a pathway into asking if the cause of activity intolerance is neuropsychological, nonneurologic (cardiopulmonary), or peripheral (muscle or local neural adaptations).

Evaluation and Assessment of the Infant and Pre-school Child with Observed Activity Intolerance

Infants and pre-school children are active in various ways and the activity intensity is dependent upon their neurodevelopmental age. Simple evaluation of child's neurodevelopment may be a valuable starting point for infants and toddlers and ultimately determines in many cases the activity capacity, power needs, and ability for future participation at any level. Physical evaluation can identify issues related to musculoskeletal abnormalities and dysplasia which in exercise-activity evaluation involves either (1) muscle strength (hypo or hypertonia), (2) skeletal development of the limbs especially including skeletal dysplasia of the chest wall, extremities and/or spine and (3) cardiopulmonary performance. These three areas of exercise physiology are determined by muscular strength, endurance, power and leverage, and ability to provide cardiopulmonary aerobic and anaerobic output to meet power requirements. In reality, the efficiency of performance is the result of metabolic-mitochondrial biochemistry where energy is produced to meet power needs. The first objective data to be gathered is the cardiopulmonary exam. When examining the infant or toddler it is best to think in terms of the following physiologic concepts; (1) neurodevelopmental level of ability and agility, (2) chronotropy, (3) inotropy, (4) strength, (5) anatomy/anomaly, (6) chest wall kinetics, and (7) breathe sounds-airflow (gas exchange). While this may seem to be obvious, the evaluation often times is under-appreciated and key predictors of present and possibly future activity tolerance are missed. When a parent complains that their child cannot keep-up, the provider can use these concepts to follow and discuss the issue in an organized fashion. This also provides a base for longitudinal evaluations regarding activity/exercise tolerance.

Chronotropy is not only about the heart rate appropriate for age and activity level, but is the heart rate variability that is expected to meet the changing metabolic demand at all levels of activity [27–34]. The autonomic nervous system function can be assessed in clinical settings by measuring resting heart rate (HR), heart rate variability (HRV), or heart rate recovery-reserve (HRR) following exercise. During the last decade, heart rate variability (HRV), that is, a marker of parasympathetic heart rate (HR) modulation has also been used in exercise physiology to evaluate the fitness level and the physiological responses to physical activity. Regulating cardiovascular function to satisfy the metabolic demand of working muscles, the autonomic nervous system has been investigated during recovery after physical exercises performed at different intensities. Low heart rate variability, especially during sleep suggests lack of autonomic input or responsiveness resulting in decreased cardiac output and places burden for activity on inotropic response [35]. Chronotropic and cardiopulmonary inefficiency in general may be elucidated in part by a sleeping overnight oximetry study. Some information can also be derived from holter monitors. Overnight oximetry can identify periods of poorly compensated hypoxemia and or excessively high or low heart rate variability. Overnight oximetry may also provide information about autonomic modulation as periods of sleep require activation of the sympathetic and parasympathetic systems. Inefficiencies in this output especially in the face of transient hypoxemia-desaturations can demonstrate chronotropic demand problems. When desaturations occur, the auto-resuscitation response should consist of increase heart rate and minute ventilation. In addition, there should be an arousal response to hypoxemia-desaturation. Absence of any these responses is a sentinel for possible abnormal or immature autonomic loop-gain processes and these mechanisms are important for development of activity tolerance. Increased oxygen consumption associated with activity requires modulation of heart rate and changes in vascular resistances. Failure of these mechanisms results in decreased perfusion to areas most involved in the activity and decreased functional capacity. While seemingly simple, overnight oximetry and especially polysomnography is a physiologic window into the capacity for activity-exercise as sleep is not a period of energy storage or biophysical restoration, but a period of reorganization and growth that requires energy consumption and strategic delivery by changing vascular flows to specific areas of the body [34]. These simple techniques are easily performed (especially overnight-sleeping oximetry) but are not well understood and interpreted by clinicians. The difficulty in interpretation is really made more challenging by the quality of the recording and this is very dependent on the type of pulse oximeter used. The signal-to-noise ratio and signal variance and toleration of movement are important to consider in regards to obtaining an optimal signal for study. This is especially true of probe and placement on the body. For example, placement of digits may not be the best choice and often times the headband probe delivers a more consistent signal. In summary, there are no gold standard assessments of activity intolerance in infants and toddlers with the exception of observation, examination, and vital signs. There are pulmonary functions that can provide some information that are discussed in other chapters of this text book. Measurement of HRV by overnight oximetry and polysomnography may be of some value but there are no studies to provide any evidence based recommendations. The most important part of this evaluation is to potentially identify those children with the potential for activity intolerance and at risk for long-term sedentary behavior. This allows the clinician to develop a long-term strategy for evaluation and intervention which ultimately can impact the future health of these patients.

Early School Age

School-age children become much more "in tune" with their exercise or activity based symptoms and can give some age level description of potential problems. One technique that can be used in 5–6 year olds is to have them draw or select an illustration or picture of what happens when they participate in exercise or activity [36]. We use an I-pad or other tablet with a standard stylus when possible, but paper and pen work as well (Fig. 12.6). Use of an I-pad or tablet device allows us to annotate on the picture and makes it easy to import pictures into a report. Child participation allows the clinician to begin probing into more specifics and may also trigger responses from parent(s) which can add to or create confusion regarding the true issue. Well meaning parents can present their biases into the symptoms and signs which can often lead the clinician to a conclusion that the parent is in part facilitating the complaint or may have push levels of activity and skill (training) upon the child which is not age appropriate. The opposite may also occur where parents limit the child's activity for fear of inducing or triggering an event or the assumption that the child cannot be active. In a way, the parent may be indirectly participating in the limitation or they may just be uninformed or have been given incorrect information by others. Pushing children and adolescents to unachievable levels of physical activity occurs at all ages and is the most common cause of exercise intolerance and avoidance of exercise in pediatrics [37]. Sports specific specialization with development of skill really occurs during teenage years. The amount of practice in early age groups does not necessarily increase the probability a child will become a performance level athlete in a particular sport. Furthermore, teens that participate later in sport specialization can make up for less practice time and experience [38].

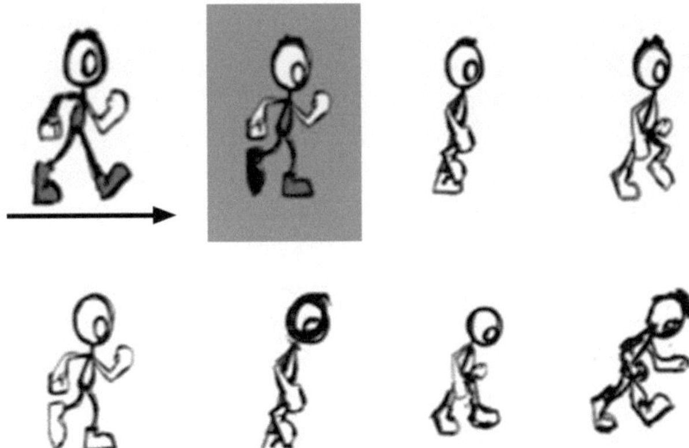

Fig. 12.6 PCET. Pictorial exercise intolerance screening using an tablet device. The child pick the animation that best describes how they feel during exercise. Which one is you when chasing your friend. The top (*green*) pictures show the animation increasing in power while the lower panel is consistent with decreasing power.

Unfortunately, the clinician cannot often openly express their concern that the patient-child is being asked to participate at a level far above (overtraining) or below their physical age. This conclusion requires clinicians to investigate all physical causes first which may require some objective testing (CPET or ACPET) which can show parents that biomechanics and physiology of exercise at their child's age level are very intact and the child is capable of engaging in some form of physical activity. The opposite may occur where pathology is demonstrated as previously reviewed. This also allows clinicians to develop a prescription plan which involves parental participation. This objectified evaluation and prescription is the core principle which allows us to promote healthy development in our children.

Initial Evaluation to Determine the Study Type and Procedure in School Age Children, Adolescents; Including those Participating in Organized Sports

The initial evaluation of a child or adolescent and/or caregiver complaining of physical activity intolerance is to define the characteristics of the observed or perceived events. This physical activity history assists in the study design and directs a purpose for the evaluation. The indications for CPET or other types of field exercise capacity testing (ACPET) are listed in Tables 12.7 and 12.8. Once again, the ultimate goal is to provide the patient with an individualized exercise evaluation, plan, medical intervention, psychological counseling, and educational training to counterbalance their limitations and/or pathology. Secondary goals are to assist in longitudinal planning for interventions by assessing functional capacity at intervals to provide information about exercise training or disease progression. Longitudinal exercise evaluations are often used to (1) assess the effectiveness of exercise training programs, (2) plan surgical interventions (transplantation-lung volume reduction-bariatric surgery), (3) assist in evidence based interventions for chronic diseases, (4) evaluation of occupational injury and (5) for research development of new therapies or training modalities. CPET can be used to reassure the patient and/or parent that the biomechanics and cardiopulmonary systems are functioning well or demonstrate pathophysiology. CPET is also used to assist the patient and family toward developing healthy attitudes about the quantity and quality of the patient's physical activity/exercise program (i.e., frequency, intensity, time, and type (Table 12.9). Reassuring the parents and patients that the physiological systems are working efficiently will allows the clinician to investigate deeper into the physical activity/sport execution-performance, attitudes of physical activity, and sport-specific movements and expectations. Addressing these issues can be challenging and our laboratory asks the will often ask parents to not be present during the study, CPET or other challenges are performed. Video recording the study can be helpful allowing the laboratory technicians and clinicians to review the events (or the absence of events) with parents and concerned coaches and trainers. We also ask

Table 12.7 Indications for cardiopulmonary exercise testing

Evaluation of exercise tolerance check sheet (check all that apply)
☐ Determination of functional impairment or capacity (peak VO_2)
☐ Determination of exercise-limiting factors and pathophysiologic mechanisms
☐ Evaluation of undiagnosed exercise intolerance
☐ Assessing contribution of cardiac and pulmonary etiology in coexisting disease
☐ Symptoms disproportionate to resting pulmonary and cardiac tests
☐ Unexplained dyspnea when initial cardiopulmonary testing is nondiagnostic
☐ Evaluation of patients with cardiovascular disease
☐ Functional evaluation and prognosis in patients with heart failure
☐ Selection for cardiac transplantation
☐ Exercise prescription and monitoring response to exercise training for cardiac rehabilitation
☐ Special circumstances; i.e., pacemakers
☐ Evaluation of patients with respiratory disease
☐ Functional impairment assessment (see specific clinical applications)
☐ Chronic obstructive pulmonary disease
☐ Establishing exercise limitation(s) and assessing other potential contributing factors, especially occult heart disease (ischemia)
☐ Determination of magnitude of hypoxemia and for O_2 prescription
☐ When objective determination of therapeutic intervention is necessary and not adequately addressed by standard pulmonary function testing
☐ Interstitial lung diseases
☐ Detection of early (occult) gas exchange abnormalities
☐ Overall assessment/monitoring of pulmonary gas exchange
☐ Determination of magnitude of hypoxemia and for O_2 prescription
☐ Determination of potential exercise-limiting factors
☐ Documentation of therapeutic response to potentially toxic therapy
☐ Pulmonary vascular disease (careful risk–benefit analysis required)
☐ Cystic fibrosis
☐ Exercise-induced bronchospasm
☐ Specific clinical applications
☐ Preoperative evaluation
☐ Lung resectional surgery
☐ Lung volume resectional surgery for emphysema
☐ Exercise evaluation and prescription for pulmonary rehabilitation
☐ Evaluation for impairment–disability
☐ Evaluation for lung, heart–lung transplantation
☐ Evaluation of performance athletes or sports participants
☐ Other ___________________________________
Signature:

parents and observers to video events they observe in real time at sporting events or during physical activity events. The team trainer and or physician should also be asked to record their observations. Video is a valuable tool and in some circumstances, we provide relatively inexpensive video cameras for home if smart phones

Table 12.8 Contraindication review checklist

Absolute (adult) checklist (check all that apply)
☐ Changed resting ECG suggestive of ischemia—recent
☐ Infarction in past 48 h
☐ Unstable angina-chest pain
☐ Uncontrolled arrhythmias
☐ Known coronary artery anomaly or disease
☐ Severe aortic stenosis
☐ Uncompensated CHF
☐ Pulmonary embolus or infarction in past 3 months
☐ Dissecting aneurysm
☐ Acute infection
☐ Hyperthyroidism
☐ Anemia
☐ Myocarditis or pericarditis
☐ Uncooperative patients
☐ Neuromuscular, musculoskeletal, or rheumatoid disorders (fall risk)
Relative contraindications (adult)
☐ Left coronary artery stenosis
☐ Stenotic valvular disease mild-moderate
☐ Severe hypertension
☐ Asymmetrical septal thickening
☐ Uncontrolled metabolic disease
☐ High degree AV block
☐ Tachy or brady arrhythmias
☐ Inability to be safe or follow directions
Confounders
☐ Beta blockers
☐ Calcium channel blockers
☐ Digoxin effects
☐ Tricyclic antidepressants
☐ Diuretic induced electrolyte disturbance
☐ SSRI
☐ ACEI lower BP without HR response
☐ Medications used for erectile dysfunction
☐ Supplements
Signature:

Table 12.9 FITT principle

Frequency	Sessions per week	Minimum 3–5 times per week
Intensity	Level of difficulty	Target 60–80 % target heart rate
Time	How long	Minimum 30 min
Type	Training method	Preference or training need

are not available. The videographer is asked to share the files by uploading the movie to a secure site or we download the device in the office or lab. In some difficult high profile cases or circumstances clinicians should try if possible to attend the sporting event to make observations and perhaps plan interventions. Coaches are usually very willing to grant access to sidelines and welcome input. This is especially true in performance athletes whom are candidates for scholarships, participate in professional or collegiate athletics or are Olympians. Most training sessions and events (competitions) at this level are recorded and with permission the videographers that film these events are happy to provide footage of the observations. It is important the exercise team obtains written consent from the participant, parent or guardian, coaches, and institution. Patient confidentiality and consent must be followed as the ramifications of disclosure of this information can have significant monetary and psychosocial consequences. One of the most important aspects when dealing with any competitive athlete is to be positive when addressing the issues. Instilling confidence that the exercise limitation is solvable or self-limiting is extremely important for the success of any intervention. Performance athletes are often suspicious and susceptible to negative thoughts or demeanor. Negativity will not be received well by the patient and definitely not by good coaches. Persistence of negativity by the coaching staff and/or parents may in itself be a cause of perceived exercise limitation from overtraining or sports related anxiety. Always ask the coaches, parents or guardians, and patient about recent head injury or symptoms of sports related concussion regardless of the sport. While these recommendations may seem excessive, the purpose for collecting data in this manner is to be thorough, to instill confidence in the patient and family and be positive that exercise is possible in anyone with the right modifications.

Study Set-Up Preparation and Evaluation

The execution of exercise studies is clearly dependent upon the history and physical exam, and the study designed should include age appropriate functional studies like CPET, but also studies specific to the triggering activity. The study should address the characteristics of the individuals exercise intolerance. There are biomechanical characteristics of the incident event that should be reproduced when possible. The power requirement for an activity depends on the exercise, exercise intensity, and which muscle groups and fiber types are activated or recruited to perform the exercise. For CPET or ACPET, the incremental changes in work load and time interval may need to be adjusted depending upon the ability and motivation of the subject. For example, patients with complaints of exercise intolerance should be evaluated performing movements and intensity similar to their sport specific activity. This requires the clinician to have some fundamental knowledge or resource of which muscle groups are activated and the tempo of movement required to perform. For instance, a; volleyball participant may need to be evaluated doing repetitive jumps from a semi-static position at specific frequencies similar to that occurring in competition.

Table 12.10 Muscle groups predominately activated during exercise by specific field testing

Exercise	Field test	Muscle group
Running	Running, burpee, stationary cycle-wingate	Quadriceps, hamstrings, glutes, calves, and iliopsoas
Swimming	Rowing, burpee	Core, gluteal muscles, rectus femoris, quadriceps, and hamstrings
		Entire arm, including triceps and biceps, shoulders, hands, neck, chest, abdominals, all parts of your upper back, glutes, hips, and the majority of your leg muscles
Volleyball	Box jumps, burpee	Bicep tricep and shoulder muscles, quads, gluteus shoulder muscles, pectorals, and the abdomen-core
Basketball	burpee	Biceps brachii, triceps brachii, deltoid, hamstrings group (biceps femoris, semitendinosus and semimembranosus), and quadriceps group (rectus femoris, vastus lateralis, vastus medialis, and vastus intermedius)

Table 12.10 depicts the type of activity/sport, the muscle groups activated, and type of exercise challenge test that may be used to evaluate the patient. The specifics some techniques will be described later in this chapter. The biomechanics of these activities can be scaled down to address intolerance to activities of daily function like climbing stairs. The facilities, supplies, information, and equipment needed to perform comprehensive activity and sport specific evaluations are listed in Table 12.11.

The performance of these tests will be described in the next section. Once again the patient should be evaluated without external stressors and parents and coaches should ideally not be present during the study. Safety is also important and the technique should be modified and closely supervised. An emergency cart should be immediately available and all technicians are BLS (basic life support), ACLS (advanced cardiac life support) and PALS (pediatric advanced life support) certified. A physician should be immediately available during all studies.

A technician and monitoring provider pre-challenge checklist is always needed, as nothing is more distressing than performing a study wand not being prepared to extract all the information possible; especially when you meet the parent(s) for the post study review. A pre-study checklist is provided and it is the responsibility of the technician/scheduler and ultimately the provider to review and check-off each item relevant to the study (Table 12.11). The pre-test evaluation and clearance is most important as any contraindications or perceived risks should be described to the patient when age of assent and definitely the parent.

Questionnaires are important additions to the development of a comprehensive laboratory. There are many validated instruments available, but the most common used questionnaire is the Modified Borg Dyspnea Scale [39]. There are a few instruments used in children like the Dalhouise Dyspnea Scale and the Pictorial Children's Effort Rating Scale (PCERT) similar to that illustrated in Fig. 12.6 [40, 41]. We recommend using the scale that best works with the patient's neurodevelopmental

Table 12.11 Pre-challenge checklist for technician and provider

H and P Checklist
☐ Activity type and experience level notation
☐ Environment (indoors–outdoors)
☐ Temperature during testing
☐ Humidity and barometric pressure
☐ Time of event symptoms occur (circadian and during event)
° Early morning
° Mid-exertion
° Late night
° Light
° Dark
☐ Intensity level (exercise load) description
☐ Symptom description
☐ Activity history
☐ Trained (frequency, duration, and techniques)
☐ Performance athlete
☐ Weekend activity
☐ New participant
☐ Prior evaluations
☐ Medications
☐ Supplements
☐ Diet log (if indicated)
☐ Anthropomorphics
☐ Height
☐ Weight
☐ Age
☐ Vital signs
☐ Past medical history
☐ Psych history
☐ Surgical or disability history
☐ Family history of metabolic or cardiovascular problems
Demographics and pre-certifications
☐ Patient identification
☐ Insurer
☐ Responsible party
☐ Referring provider
☐ Order for studies
☐ Scheduler
Equipment and space
☐ Stop watch
☐ Metronome
☐ Marker cones
☐ Oximeter

(continued)

Table 12.11 (continued)

H and P Checklist
☐ BP cuff
☐ Towels and disinfectant
☐ Hand sanitizer
☐ Sink and restroom facilities
☐ Potable water
☐ Stethescope
☐ Pedometer–accelerometers–actigraphs
☐ Heart rate monitor
☐ Spirometer
☐ Plethysmograph (optional recommendation)
☐ Cardiopulmonary exercise equipment
☐ Cycle ergometer
☐ Adjustable pedals
☐ Large treadmill
☐ Vertical boxes
☐ 7 in
☐ 12 in
☐ 24 in
☐ Tilt table
☐ Airway reactivity challenge (optional)
☐ Audio–video capabilities
☐ Resuscitation equipment (crash cart)
☐ Bronchodilators
☐ Naso-pharyngoscope
☐ Ultrasound-echocardiography
Data instruments
☐ Chest pain/angina scale
☐ Health quality questionnaires
☐ Pittsburg sleep quality indicator
☐ HIPPA disclosure
☐ Consent
☐ Dyspnea scale
☐ Rate perceived exertion scale (RPE)
☐ Pain scale
Standard operating procedure protocols
☐ EMS protocol plan
☐ Beep test instructions
☐ Box jump instruction
☐ Burpee instruction
☐ EAC protocol
☐ Protocols-data collection instruments
☐ Technique briefing videos or explanation demonstrations for patient

(continued)

Table 12.11 (continued)

H and P Checklist
☐ Study termination protocol
☐ Technician directed
☐ Patient directed
FTE available at study
☐ Medical director or physician
☐ Lab director-technician
The physician responsibilities and checklist are as follows:
MD responsibilities
☐ Pre-test evaluation and clearance
☐ Informed consent
☐ Selection of protocol
☐ Performance of test
☐ Patient preparation
☐ Patient monitoring
☐ Test termination
☐ Test recovery
☐ Interpretation
Protocol selection
☐ Maximal vs submaximal
☐ Termination protocol (standard)
☐ Dyspnea
☐ BP
☐ SaO$_2$
☐ Leg pain
☐ Chest pain
☐ Dizziness
☐ Blood pressure decrease
☐ Abnormal rhythm
☐ ST or T wave changes
☐ Brugada pattern
☐ Incremental
☐ Nonincremental
☐ Treadmill or ergometer
☐ CPET or ACPET or both
MD-provider pre-test check list
☐ Equipment safety
☐ Check informed consent
☐ Pre-test H and P on reviewed and on chart
☐ Plethysomographic or other pulmonary function test available
☐ Record patient demographics (repeat check)
☐ Examine skin for electrodes and other apparatus correctly and safely
☐ Connected devices in place

(continued)

Table 12.11 (continued)

H and P Checklist
☐ BP cuff correct size
☐ Supine resting ECG and BP are completed and in expected pattern or range (prestudy-reading resting)
☐ Stand (treadmill) or sitting (bike) with ECG and BP completed
☐ Patient instructions
☐ Study termination sign review
☐ Emergency stop instructions
☐ Use hand rails to stop-dismount
☐ Remind that BP will be checked during study
☐ Remind dyspnea scale (place in view of patients to review during study (point to level thumbs-up or down)
☐ Remind patient when last minute of maximal protocol has started
☐ Check other tests blood glucose others, etc. (diabetics or glucose regulation issues suspected)
☐ Last meal or fluid intake
☐ Pulse oximeter (two sites)
☐ FEV_1 post procedure reminder
☐ Final questions
☐ Mouthpiece or face-mask in place and fits
☐ Summary of results with patient and family immediately afterwards

abilities to comprehend the questions. Often we use both the Borg and in addition either a Dalhousie or PCERT in case there is some level of understanding issues. Visual analog scales seem to be the most understood of all the methods. Exercise symptoms can be related to anxiety disorders of the patient or parent. We also recommend the Physical Activity and Sport Anxiety Scale (PASAS) and The Parental Beliefs About Anxiety Questionnaire (PBA-Q) for anxiety related issues, and the Perceived Symptoms and Disability in Asthma Questionnaire (PSDAQ) for questions regarding asthma and exercise participation [42–44]. Age appropriate pain scales can also be utilized if needed.

Cardiopulmonary Testing—CPET

CPET can be performed with any commercially available equipment of which there are over 25 manufacturers. Not all of the devices are pediatric friendly, so the choice depends upon the age group and adaptability of the devices. The equipment should be able to collect at a minimum the data listed in Table 12.4 and be modifiable to allow different age groups and exercise abilities to be tested. The pedals and foot cage straps on cycle ergometer should be adjustable and the treadmill needs to have adjustable child bars and those for adults as depicted in Fig. 12.7. The treadmill should also be wide and long enough for track or performance level running. Protective padding and an auto-stop lanyard should be available should a patient

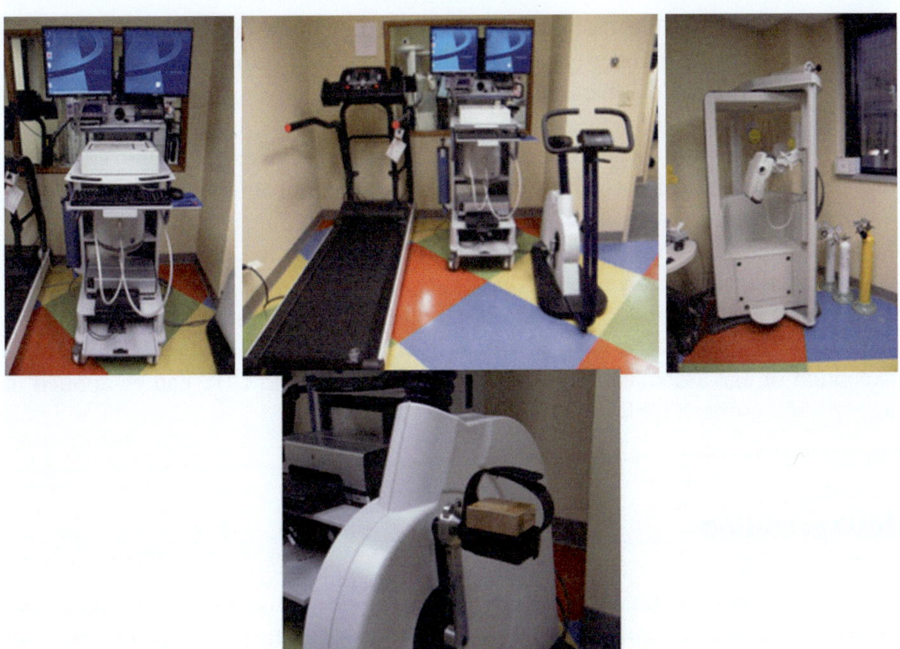

Fig. 12.7 CPET equipment. The treadmill should be long enough to allow runners to reach a comfortable stride length and the side rails must be adjustable for different age groups. The instructionsfor dyspnea and stopping are posted on the front wall or periodically held up by the technician. The bicycle pedals are adjustable in length as is the seat to accommodate different ages. Blocks can be used if the pedal length does not adjust completely to their leg length. Static pulmonary functionsincluding DLCO should be performed before the CPET preferably on the same day

have a syncopal event or just stop running while the belt is in motion. A sign should be in front of the patient demonstrating a safe dismount from the treadmill. During evaluation of a running athlete, a short length treadmill may cause the patient to step over the front or rear of the device as the stride length is different in those trained for such events. Keep in mind that the CPET will more times than not be normal or demonstrate anxiety or poor effort. It can also demonstrate physical *noncardiopulmonary* limitations or challenges like musculoskeletal and mechanical issues (physical ability or coordination). Evaluation of the biomechanics of running should be addressed. The true value of testing is to determine the functional level and efficiency of the body to sustain age appropriate activity/exercise. In children and adolescents it is more likely that the study will not show any cardiopulmonary or metabolic problems and will be more of an indicator of ability, effort, and fitness. The most important finding is to use these techniques as a diagnostic tool as to why a pediatric or adolescent patient cannot exercise or participate in activity like their peers or complains of exercise intolerance.

The contraindications for cardiopulmonary exercise testing in pediatric patients are mostly age and ability defined. The adult criteria are well published and are listed later in this section. These types of contraindications usually do not apply uniformly to pediatric and adolescent patients. The agility and ability from a biomechanical basis are the major limiting factors for children and adolescents. Thusly, safety is the number one concern. The need for treadmill and ergometer fitting is most important (handrails, speed, and pedal adjustments). Patients with sickle cell disease and pulmonary hypertension can be tested, but there needs to be a good reason for the test. Appropriate hydration is very important in both sickle cell and sickle cell trait patients. Other complex hemoglobinopathies can also be relative contraindications, not absolute. Patients with complex congenital heart disease can be tested, but it is advisable to discuss the challenge with a pediatric cardiologist beforehand if there is any doubt. Absolute and relative testing contraindications in adults that can be applied to pediatric and adolescent patients are listed in Table 12.8. Indications for CPET are well described in both adults and children and with the exception of age associated coronary artery syndrome and CHF can be applied in age specific groups (Table 12.9).

Interpretation

This initial interpretation is to determine the presence or absence of signs and symptoms of exercise intolerance. Questionnaires are utilized to examine the level of dyspnea, intensity of pain and attitudes towards exercise; specifically anxiety. Once the CPET is complete, the primary screen consists of determining effort and quality/consistency of the study. This is followed by an initial interpretation of normal versus abnormal values. The normal values in children are an area of interest and we recommend using some internal controls and frequent analysis of prior studies. There should be a documented internal reliability program. Normal controls for each age group should be performed yearly at a minimum and ideally every 6 months. High level athletes or trained individuals should also be added to the quality assurance internal review. If possible, patients with known limitations should be tested annually (if safe and willing) to maintain some quality assurance measures. Once the study effort is determined to be of good quality, a review of abnormal and normal tabular values is performed and the data transcribed to a form. Table 12.12 provides some indicators of effort which can be used to screen the initial quality of the CPET session. Table 12.13 and Figs. 12.8 and 12.9 are then used in our lab to identify the pathophysiologic mechanism that is causing exercise/ activity intolerance. The nine panel graph (Fig. 12.10) should then be examined for any patterns of exercise inefficiencies and the tabular results should be consistent with the graphics in the nine panel display. There are many references available that provide normative data that can be used in the interpretation. Table 12.14 is used in our CPET lab for the pre-teen age groups. There are similar published values for the teenagers [18, 23].

Table 12.12 Effort indicator worksheet to determine quality of the CPET

Effort indicators	Yes	No
VO$_2$ greater than 80 % of MVV,		
Heart rate within ten beats/min (one standard deviation) of predicted maximum,		
Plateau of VO$_2$ or heart rate in the face of increasing work rate		
Exercise in the very-heavy-intensity range, that is, well beyond the lactate threshold		
Peak exercise respiratory exchange ratio (RER) values above 1.10 or 1.15 imply significant lactic acidosis		
Peak VO$_2$ that exceeds the anaerobic threshold by 80 % or more (supports a high degree of effort)		

Table 12.13 Sample interpretation worksheet table

Variable	Y	N	H	L	Not apply
VO$_2$ max predicted attained or					
Maximum VO$_2$ reached?					
Work load predicted from equations attained?					
Oxygen use high for work level					
Plateau of VO$_2$ or heart rate with increasing work rate?					
RER maximal test (1.15)?					
Maximum HR predicted achieved?					
Max HR to low (sick heart-chronotropy)?					
Max HR too high (sick heart-inotropy)?					
ST segment displaced?					
Cardiac arrhythmias?					
Echocardiogram result					
Was the breathing reserve low (<20)?					
Was the breathing reserve normal or high?					
Dead space ventilation increase or decrease (VD/VT)?					
Oxygenation by (SaO$_2$) normal					
Obese?					
Effort reason for stopping (if patient stopped)					
Blood pressure increase appropriately?					
Is the patient a performance athlete?					
HRR normal?					
HR1 (1 min postexercise)?					
HR2 (2 min postexercise)?					
Pulse O$_2$ normal (rise and plateau)?					
VAT percent of VO$_2$ (V-slope)?					
VE to high or VE too low?					

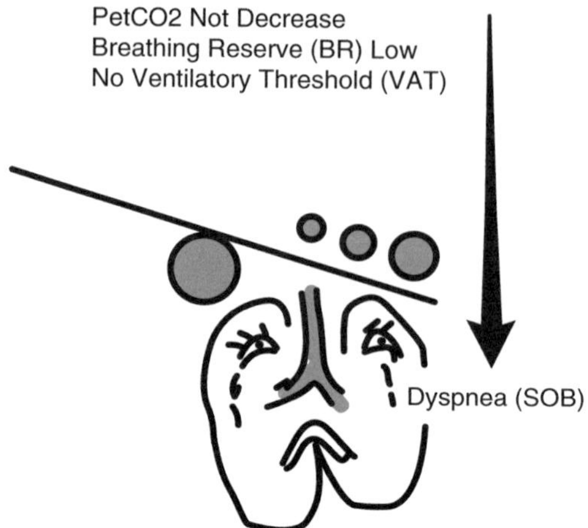

Fig. 12.8 Ventilatory limitation. Ventilatory limitation is suspected when the PETCO$_2$ does not decrease, the breathing reserve is low and there is no ventilatory threshold. The clinical result isdyspnea or shortness-of-breath (SOB). Children may describe SOB and chest pain

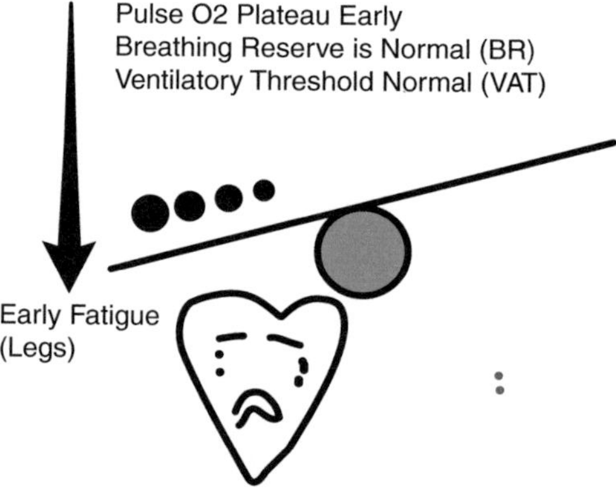

Fig. 12.9 Cardiac limitation. Cardiac limitation is best represented as the pulse O$_2$ plateaus early while the breathing reserve and ventilatory threshold is normal. Clinically the patient cannot meet the expected work level because of leg fatigue (hurting). The cause is inefficient oxygen delivery to the muscles. If there is both cardiac and ventilatory limitation then peripheral vascular disease with pulmonary hypertension is a likely cause of the decrease performance

Explaining the Pathophysiology of the Study for the Final Interpretation

Any cardiovascular, pulmonary, or muscle metabolic disorder can cause abnormalities of oxygen delivery, so attribution of the findings to a particular condition involves consideration of history, physical findings, ECG, and blood pressure responses. Abnormalities of oxygen delivery and/or utilization during CPET are reflected in the responses listed in Table 12.13. An absence breathing reserve

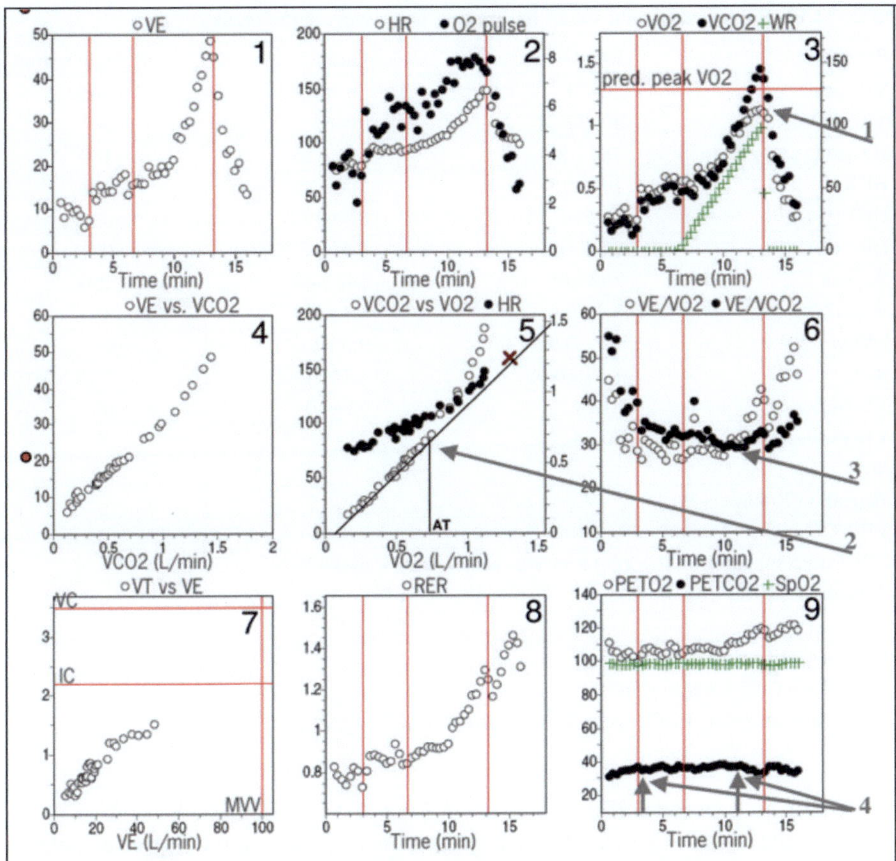

Fig. 12.10 Nine Panel. Graphical relationship of variable from a CPET. These relationships depict interactions between the cardiopulmonary and musculoskeletal systems in the development of power. Limitations of any of these systems can be determined from these plots. Arrow 1 points to the peak VO$_2$ in panel 3 (branch-point 1). Arrow 2 points to the AT in panel 5 (branch-point 2). Arrow 3 points to the VE/VCO$_2$ at the AT in panel 6 (branch-point 3). Arrow 4 points to the changing PETCO$_2$ from start of exercise to AT in panel 9

indicates ventilatory limitation, and a low reserve (<20 % of MVV) is suggestive of the same. However, long distance runners and other highly aerobic trained athletes can push the BR close to zero. If changes in breathing mechanics occurring during exercise are not reflected in the calculated breathing reserve, then findings on the flow-volume loop or physical examination, such as inspiratory stridor or reduction of inspiratory (IC) and inspiratory reserve volume (IRV), indicate potential ventilatory limitation. This may be true even if the even if breathing reserve appears normal. Erratic patterns of tidal volume and frequency suggest hyperventilation or malingering. The fraction of tidal volume to inspiratory capacity used in breathing (VT/IC) is high when lung compliance is decreased (restrictive physiology).

Table 12.14 Published normal values for exercise parameters in pre-teens

Parameter	Boys	Girls	Lab norms
VO_2 peak	40–54	36–48	>35
VAT % VO_2	50–72	49–63	60
HR peak	184+12	186+10	180
HRR	104+15	100+13	100
HR1 (%)	0.35+0.13	31+0.11	0.30
HR2 (%)	0.54+0.11	0.51+0.12	0.50
W peak	162±65	142±44	150
W peak/kg	3.4+0.6	3.1+0.5	3
DVO_2/DWR	9.9+0.9	9.3+1.0	9
RER	1.13±0.08	1.14±0.09	1.12
VE/AET	61+11	62+10	60
VE/VCO_2	30+4	31+4	30
Boys			
W peak = $(20 \times age) - 94$			
VE/VCO_2 = $(-0.64 \times age) + 38$			
HR01 percentage = $(-2.16 \times age) + 63$ VO_2 peak = $(0.66 \times age) + 38.6$			
W peak/kg = $(0.11 \times age) + 2.04$			
Girls			
W peak = $(13 \times age) - 23$			
VE/VCO_2 = $(-0.64 \times age) + 38$			
HR01 percentage = $(-1.84 \times age) + 55$ W peak/kg = $(0.07 \times age) + 2.16$			

VD/VT is a nonspecific indicator of lung V/Q mismatch. P(a-ET) CO_2 is measures the high V/Q mismatch within the lung and suggest the degree of pulmonary circulation impairment or low perfusion of well ventilated alveoli (alveolar ventilation). P (A-a) O_2 is a measure of low ventilation to perfusion matching. This variable best describes decrease diffusion or shunting right to left resulting from decrease oxygen transport from a decrease in available lung-alveolar surface area or diffusion for oxygen transfer. The rate (slope) of the VO_2 curve is an indicator of increase pulmonary blood flow by recruitment and distention of the capillary beds. The higher the slope (especially in phase one of a study) indicates the ability to increase pulmonary blood flow.

Inefficiency of oxygenation is identified by abnormally low arterial PaO_2 or high P (A-a) O_2. These measures are based on analyses of exercise arterial blood gases. Inefficiency of CO_2 elimination by failure of dead space ventilation (VD/VT) to decrease as expected. Inefficient gas exchange may alternatively be inferred from pulse oximetry findings of desaturation by more than 3 % or by abnormally high relative to work performed. Because noninvasive oximetry is not always precise and high relationships can reflect acute or chronic hyperventilation (e.g., due to anxiety or compensation for chronic metabolic acidosis), an exercise arterial blood gas can be useful in confirming or excluding defects in gas exchange when the noninvasive measures are unexpectedly abnormal. A capillary blood gas is not a good substitute for an ABG.

Peripheral processes can also impair the response to exercise. Muscle symptoms are typical of both myopathies and peripheral arterial disease. Metabolic myopathies may be suggested by a history of rhabdomyolysis, use of myotoxic drugs, or family history compatible with mitochondrial disorder. Confirmation ultimately depends on histological and biochemical analysis of a muscle biopsy specimen. Impairments in blood flow distribution to exercising skeletal muscle can contribute to exercise intolerance and is evidenced by autonomic dysfunction (e.g., heightened sympathetic vasoconstriction) and/or peripheral vascular dysfunction. These types of autonomic dysfunction occur in both autoimmune disorders and cardiomyopathies.

Alternative (Field) ACPET

ACPET or field evaluation of activity/exercise intolerance is best accomplished by using techniques which are similar in the context of muscle activation as related to the complaint. The techniques vary depending on the time symptoms occur and at what load or work level. Evaluation of the sprint type complaint is much different from the endurance track athlete. Different muscle groups, fiber types, and energy resources are used depending on the activity (Table 12.10). The power requirement (especially rate of production) changes depending on the exercise and which muscle groups are activated and the sequencing of activation. These power requirements change at different stages of exertion and as a result the fuel source changes. It is important to remember that the cardiopulmonary system changes to meet the metabolic demand for power. Metabolic demand changes with the work needed and that depends on phasic activation of different muscle types and these activations are load and frequency dependent. The utilization of each type of skeletal muscle depends upon the activity, the load or resistances being moved, intensity and the duration. The testing should attempt to ideally simulate all of these components and be of sufficient duration to achieve the work level at which symptoms occur. The rate-of-load change and duration place demands on the cardiorespiratory and musculoskeletal system that most times cannot be reproduced in a conventional incremental CPET evaluation. At times the classical CPET technique activates and accomplishes the desired workload and technique. At other times, CPET only provides information on the capacity and positive function of the patient's cardiopulmonary and musculoskeletal systems. When the CPET does not activate the rate of workload or is normal but the intolerance persists, exercise specific evaluation is definitely warranted. For example, volleyball participants engage in explosive vertical and lateral movements followed by brief periods of rest (5–10 s). The endurance component of volleyball is how long (or how many) the participant can engage in these explosive movements at the needed level until fatigue, dyspnea, or true symptoms occur. A portable spirometer and pulse oximeter-blood pressure cuff should always be available to determine if exercise induced bronchospasm (EIB) and other symptoms have been triggered. This type of evaluation consists of muscle strength endurance and sustained aerobic metabolism. Volleyball type exercise is performed at sub-maximal levels. Box jumps and or combination box jumps and burpees are very similar to the actions of volleyball, soccer, and swim participants. Figs. 12.11a, b depict

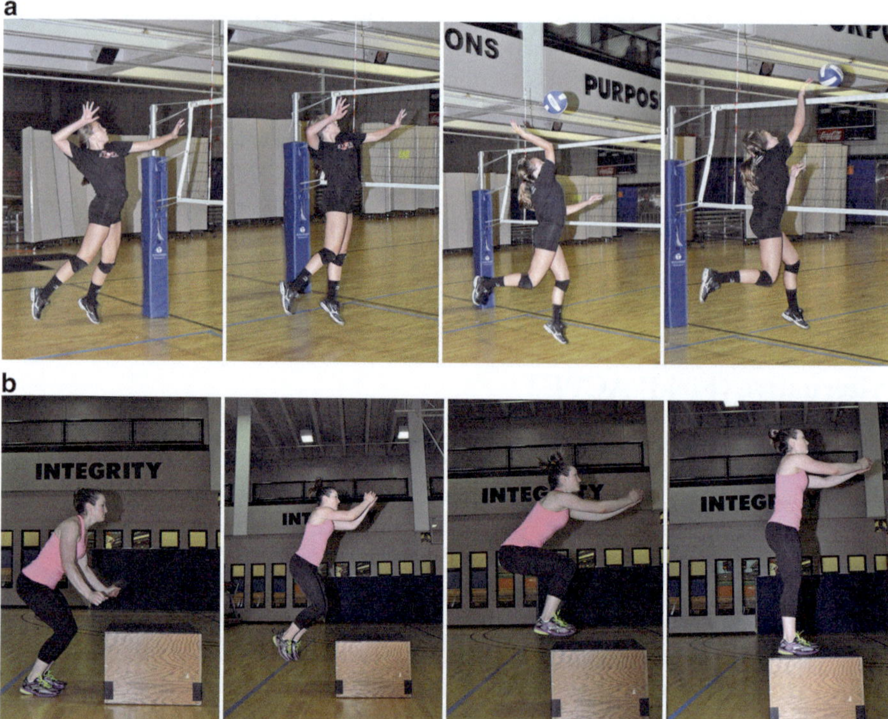

Fig. 12.11 (a) Volleyball biomechanics. The mechanics of a volleyball spike are similar to that of a plyometric box jump. (b) Plyometric box jumps. Box jumps are exercises that develop both explosiveness and endurance. The boxes range from 6 increase to 42 in. in height. The jumper performs a 130° squat and jumps using and upward motion of the arms landing in squat position followed by a vertical stand. The jumper should then step down for safety. The frequency of jumps can be increased depending on the need to increase work to simulate specific exercises. This technique works well for volleyball and other explosive type activities (gymnastics and others) as it activates

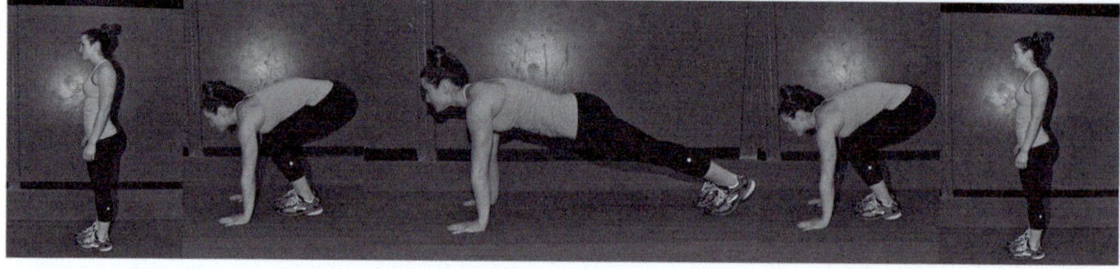

Fig. 12.12 Burpee. The burpee, also known as the squat thrust, is a full body exercise used in strength training and as aerobic exercise. It is performed in four steps, and was originally knownas a "four-count Burpee": (1) Begin in a standing position. (2) Drop into a squat position with your hands on the ground (count 1). (3) Extend your feet back in one quick motion to assume the front plank position (count 2). (4) Return to the squat position in one quick motion (count 3). (5) Return to standing position (count 4)

Table 12.15 Advantages and disadvantages of field test vs laboratory test

1. Cheap to administer
2. Easy access
3. Potentially less threatening depending on the intensity and skill required to participate
4. No expensive equipment necessary
5. Specific expertise is not required to conduct
6. Potentially more threatening to young children (ability to perform is dependent upon activity maturational age
7. Useful in large population studies
8. Difficult to perform in large research studies
9. Limited long-term validity data
10. Utility in diagnosing problems depends upon the symptom description
11. Valid assessment short- and long term
12. Useful clinical diagnostic test for specific complaints
13. Good physiological ventilation measures (rate of work load development more real life)
14. More challenging to measure VO_2

examples of inexpensive techniques that can provide valuable information. It is important to time the test and sometime utilize a metronome/timer or similar to set the pace consistent with the exercise activity in an effort to elevate the work load increased cardiopulmonary requirements. Specific data is collected as represented by various forms and this should include a dyspnea scale (if applicable) and spirometry post-testing. Video recording is a valuable tool as well and allows the reviewer to count the number of repetitions and can be a gauge to effort. An accelerometer (pedometer) and be used as well and the device can be placed on the arm, ankle, or waist. Situation or exercise-specific muscle group activation testing is always done after CPET (but not on the same day) and specific cardiovascular risk factors have been assessed and participation clearance and consent provided by the subject and/or parent-guardian. Safety is always important and close supervision with the technician standing immediately next to the patient is mandatory to prevent injury from falls and similar mishaps. Other activities and situation simulations are noted in the tables, figures and diagrams. The advantages and disadvantages of ACPT are listed in Table 12.15.

The Harvard Step Test is a type of cardiac stress test for detecting and/or diagnosing cardiovascular disease. It also is a good measurement of fitness, and your ability to recover after a strenuous exercise. The more quickly your heart rate returns to resting, the better conditioned is the subject. It is kind of a cardiovascular endurance test. The test computes the capability to exercise continuously for extended intervals of time without tiring. The subject (person who is taking the test) steps up and down on a platform at a height of about 45 cm. at a rate of 30 steps per minute for 5 min or until exhaustion. Exhaustion is the point at which the subject cannot maintain the stepping rate for 15 s. The subject immediately sits down on completion of the test, and the heartbeats are counted for 1–1.5, 2–2.5, and 3–3.5 min. Spirometry and pulse oximetry along with BP are also important. This is an example of just one of many step-test variations. The most well known is the classical 6 min walk test. The

6 min walk test is a well standardized tool that can be used to evaluate functional capacity. The indications, technical requirement, execution, and evaluation of the data can be reviewed in the American Thoracic Society Statement [3].

Other ACPET techniques include Plyometric Box Jumps, Burpees, Beep test (shuttle run), and Interval Sprints (suicides). The numbers of repetitions achieved during these tests have been compared to VO_2 aerobic capacity and are good interval methods to detect improvements in treatments and training. Plyometric Box Jumps are exercises that develop both explosiveness and endurance. The boxes range from 6 to 42 in. in height. The jumper performs a 130° squat and jumps using and upward motion of the arms landing in squat position followed by a vertical stand. The jumper should then step down for safety. The frequency of jumps can be increased depending on the need to increase work to simulate specific exercises. This technique works well for volleyball and other explosive type activities (gymnastics and others) as it activates similar muscle groups (Fig. 12.11).

The Burpee, (Fig. 12.12) also known as the squat thrust, is a full body exercise used in strength training and as aerobic exercise. It is performed in four steps, and was originally known as a "four-count Burpee":

1. Begin in a standing position.
2. Drop into a squat position with your hands on the ground (count 1).
3. Extend your feet back in one quick motion to assume the front plank position (count 2).
4. Return to the squat position in one quick motion (count 3).
5. Return to standing position (count 4).

This is a good exercise for football of all types and is used and was developed for military training. Therefore; it is a good screen for patients that are being considered for admission to military training schools and or enlistment in the military. Burpees can also be used for secondary complaints of exertion intolerance. The workload to perform a Burpee is substantial.

The Beep Test (Fig. 12.13) involves continuous running between two 20 m apart in time to recorded beeps. For this reason the test is also often called the "beep" or "bleep" test. The test subjects stand behind one of the lines facing the second line, and begin running when instructed by the CD or audio. The speed at the start is quite slow. The subject continues running between the two lines, turning when signaled by the recorded beeps. After about 1 min, a sound indicates an increase in speed, and the beeps will be closer together. This continues each minute (level). If the line is not reached in time for each beep, the subject must run to the line turn and try to catch up with the pace within two more "beeps." Also, if the line is reached before the beep sounds, the subject must wait until the beep sounds. The test is stopped if the subject fails to reach the line (within 2 m) for two consecutive ends. There are several versions of the test, but one commonly used version has an initial running velocity of 8.5 km/h, which increases by 0.5 km/h each minute. Another version starts at 8.0 km/h, then up to 9.0 km/h for level 2 and then increases by 0.5 km/h. The suicide drill is a basic drill to develop footwork and stamina or aerobic endurance. The subject lines up at the baseline and as the whistle sounds, sprint to the free

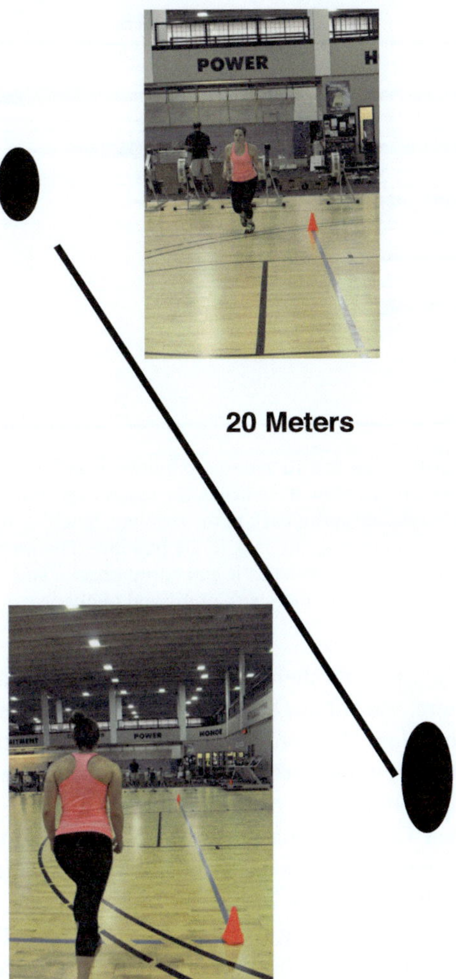

Fig. 12.13 This test involves continuous running between two 20 m apart in time to recorded beeps. For this reason the test is also often called the 'beep' or 'bleep' test. The test subjects stand behind one of the lines facing the second line, and begin running when instructed by the cd or audio. The speed at the start is quite slow. The subject continues running between the two lines, turning when signaled by the recorded beeps. After about one minute, a sound indicates an increase in speed, and the beeps will be closer together. This continues each minute (level). If the line is not reached in time for each beep, the subject must run to the line turn and try to catch up with the pace within 2 more 'beeps'. Also, if the line is reached before the beep sounds, the subject must wait until the beep sounds. The test is stopped if the subject fails to reach the line (within 2 meters) for two consecutive ends. There are several versions of the test, but one commonly used version has an initial running velocity of 8.5 km/hr, which increases by 0.5 km/hr each minute. Another version starts at 8.0 km/hr, then up to 9.0 km/hr for level 2 and then increases by 0.5 km/hr

SUICIDE SPRINTS

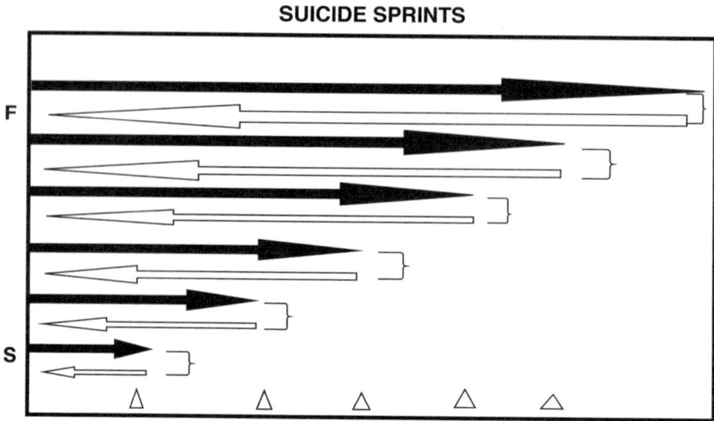

Fig. 12.14 The suicide drill is a basic drill to develop footwork and stamina or aerobic endurance. Line up at the baseline. When you blow the whistle, the subject sprint to the free throw line. They touch the line with their hands and sprint back to the baseline, touching it. From there, they run to the half court line, touch it and then sprint back to the baseline. The process continues until each player reaches the opposite baseline, touches it and sprints back. This is a good evaluation for basketball, baseball, soccer, football (American), rugby and track

throw line, touches the line with their hands and sprint back to the baseline, touching it again. From there, the subject runs to the half court line, touches it and then sprints back to the baseline. The process continues until each player reaches the opposite baseline, touches it and sprints back. This is a good evaluation for basketball, baseball, soccer, football (American), rugby and track.

Suicides or Interval Drills is a basic drill to develop footwork and stamina or aerobic endurance. The subject lines up at the baseline and when the whistle blows, the subject sprints to the free throw line. They touch the line with their hands and sprint back to the baseline, touching it. From there, they run to the half court line, touch it, and then sprint back to the baseline. The process continues until each subject reaches the opposite baseline, touches it, and sprints back (Fig. 12.14). This is a good evaluation for basketball, baseball, soccer, football (American), rugby, and track.

Summary

Exercise testing either formally in the lab or in alternative (field) scenarios is use to determine power or aerobic power and anaerobic persistence or toleration. The need for power and persistence can be limited by cardiopulmonary, musculoskeletal, metabolic, or neurologic inefficiencies. There are also psychological influences on exercise or activity capacity. Aerobic power for activity is reflected by patient's VO_2 max or peak VO_2. However, it is important to remember that the VO_2 may be increased but the amount of work performed may be low as seen in overweight

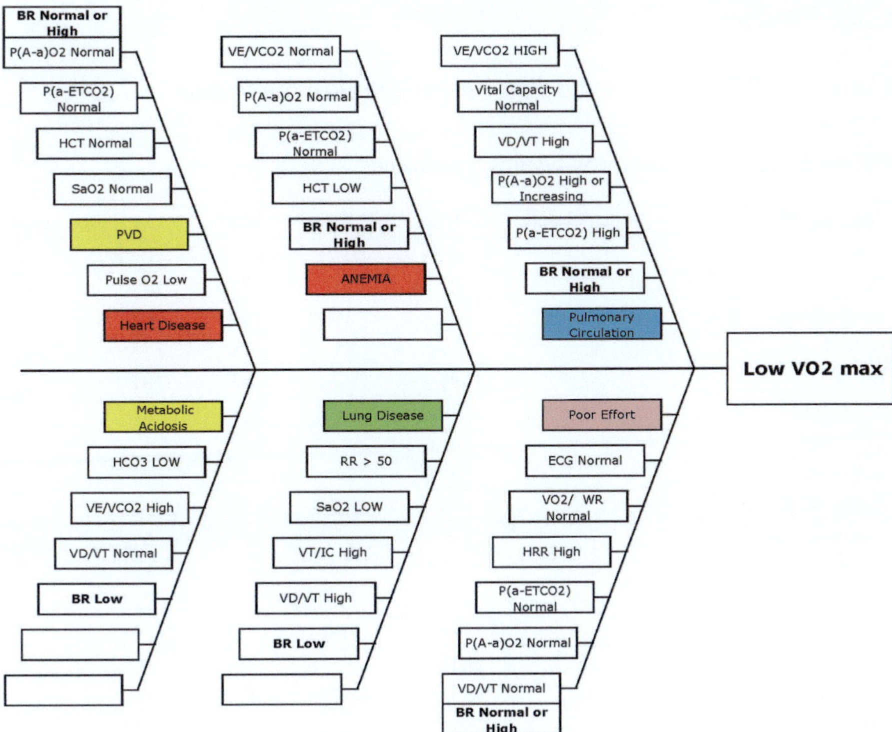

Fig. 12.15 Causes and Effect of low VO_2 can be determined by highlighting or checking which variable results apply. The causal line with the most checked or highlighted treat is the likely cause of the plow VO_2

subjects. When aerobic metabolism switches to anaerobic, the increase in metabolic acid (lactate) requires the respiratory system the decrease $PaCO_2$ by increasing the minute ventilation (MV). This increase in MV is reflected by an increase in VCO_2 and a reduction in $PaCO_2$ or $PETCO_2$. When compared to VO_2, the deflection of the VO_2–VCO_2 curve is identified as the ventilatory threshold. Patients with decrease ventilatory capacity will use more of their breathing reserve and increase their RR, but the $PaCO_2$ or $PETCO_2$ with not decrease as normally expected or may possibly increase and the ventilatory threshold (VAT) is not achieved; thus, the subject has a respiratory limitation to exercise. If the breathing reserve is normal and VAT is achieved, then the limitation to exercise is cardiac if the pulse O_2 plateaus early in the study. If the exercise limitation is not explained by either of these mechanisms, the cause may be related to peripheral vascular disease including pulmonary hypertension, metabolic disorders including muscle and mitochondrial disorders or oxygen carrying capacity (anemia or hemoglobinopathies). The cause-and-effect diagram (Fig. 12.15) can assist is guiding the provider in developing a differential diagnosis and evaluation resulting in development of a treatment plan.

Case Studies

Case 1: *CPRT Performed Pre-pectus Repair Nuss Bar*

Patient 17 year old with Erlos-Danlos Syndrome.

Test variable	Predicted max	Rest	AT	AT2	VO_2 max (peak)
RER		0.89	0.92		0.98
Pulse O_2	18	2	5	7	9
Work (Watts)	306		34	60	62
HHR%		100	85	78	75
BR%		95	92	87	81
HRR (bpm)		109	93	85	82
VO_2 slope	–	–	–	–	–
VO_2 pred (%)		*6*	*14*	*22*	*32*
HR pred (%)		*47*	*55*	*59*	*60*
Exer time (min)			2	4	6
BP systolic		122			121
BP diastolic		81			75
$PETO_2$		108	106	105	108
$PETCO_2$		34	37	39	39
VO_2 ml/kg/min	>35	3.6	8.2	12.9	18.9
HR bpm	205	96	112	120	123
$VECO_2$		32	28	27	28
Vd/VT (estimated)		0.26	0.2	0.18	0.17
RR (br/min)					

Variable checklist used to identify the pathophysiologic mechanism resulting in activity/exercise intolerance (N for normal range)

Variable	Y	N	H	L	Other
VO_2 max predicted attained or		x			
Maximum VO_2 reached?		x			
Work load predicted from equations attained?		x			
Oxygen use high for work level		x			
Plateau of VO_2 or heart rate with increasing work rate?		x			
RER maximal test (1.15)?		x			
Maximum HR predicted achieved?		x			
Max HR to low (sick heart-chronotropy)?		x			
Max HR too High (sick heart-inotropy)?		x			
ST segment displaced?		x			
Cardiac arrhythmias?		x			
Echocardiogram result		x			

(continued)

(continued)

Was the breathing reserve low (<20)?		x		
Was the breathing reserve normal or high?	x			
Dead space ventilation increase or decrease (VD/VT)?		x		
Oxygenation by (SaO_2) normal		x		
Obese?		x		
Effort reason for stopping (if patient stopped)				Dyspnea fatigue
Blood pressure increase appropriately?		x		
Is the patient a performance athlete?		x		
HRR normal?				
HR1 (1 min postexercise)?				x
HR2 (2 min postexercise)?				x
Pulse O_2 normal (rise and plateau)?		x		
VAT percent of VO_2 (V-slope)?				x
VE too high or VE too low?		x		

Variable	Result
$PETCO_2$ (no change) or $VECO_2$ (increase)	Normal
Breathing reserve low	No (high)
VAT (ventilatory threshold) present	Yes low
Pulse O_2	low
Breathing reserve normal	High (normal)
VAT present	low

Cause-and-Effect Diagram Result (Case 1: Check All That Apply)

- **Conclusion: (check or circle)**
- **Cardiac Limitation.**
- Respiratory Limitation.
- Peripheral Vascular Limitation (PVD).
- Pulmonary Hypertension (Circulation).
- Metabolic Limitation.
- Muscle Limitation.
- **Deconditioned.**
- Poor Effort.

Summary:

CPRT performed pre-pectus repair Nuss Bar.
   Patient with Erlos-Danlos Syndrome.

The PETCO$_2$ did not decrease, but VAT was achieved. The BR was normal. PaETO$_2$ and VD/VT were normal as well. The pulse O$_2$ was significantly low as was the VO$_2$ max at levels seen in cardiomyopathies. The Echo results note a normal structured heart with good ejection fraction. Cardiac limitation likely from decrease left ventricular filling at higher (nonresting) level due to abnormal chest wall dynamics and decrease LV filling and stroke volumes at higher work levels. The patient is not physically fit.

Case 2: 14-year-old female complaints of dyspnea and inability to run cross country recent onset last 2 months.

Variable	Result
PETCO$_2$ decrease or VECO$_2$ increase	Normal yes
Breathing reserve low	Normal
VAT (ventilatory threshold) present	Yes (early)
Pulse O$_2$	Low
Breathing reserve normal	Normal
VAT present	Yes

Suggest Cardiac Limitation

Other data:

VO$_2$ max low
SaO$_2$ low at max exercise
RR less than 50
HRR normal
Basal HR Slightly High for Age and Fitness Level (Runner)
Normal Chronotropic Response (80% of predicted maximal HR)
Hemoglobin 5.9

Cause-and-Effect Diagram Result (Case 2: Check All That Apply)

Conclusion: (check or circle)
° Cardiac limitation
° Respiratory limitation
° Peripheral vascular limitation (PVD)
° Pulmonary hypertension (circulation)
° Metabolic limitation
° Muscle limitation
° Deconditioned
° Poor Effort
° **Anemia**

Summary:

Good Effort (RER . 1.15)

Additional History:

Complaints of dyspnea and inability to run cross country recent onset last 2 months.

Complete study with dyspnea at end, stopped complaining of fatigue, leg cramps, and dizziness. BP increase appropriately and the HRR reserve was normal though basal HR was increased. Leg Cramps likely from early VAT and low peripheral oxygen extraction at muscle level.

Pre-study same day pulmonary function tests pending calculation of DLCO

CBC reviewed (low hemoglobin)

SaO_2 decrease likely secondary to increase oxygen extraction.

Exercise Intolerance secondary to anemia.

Additional History—teen with dysfunctional uterine bleeding menorrhagia for 4 months.

Diet vegetarian.

Sent to adolescent to reproductive health and iron indices ordered. sports nutrition discussed.

Primary care informed for follow-up.

Case 3: 22 year old prior 28 week premie born 1,088 g and did not receive surfactant. Bronchopulmonary dysplasia (BPD), intraventricular hemorrhage, osteopenia, and retinopathy of prematurity. College Student Masters Program Psychology.

Test variable	Predicted max	Rest	AT	AT2	VO_2 max (peak)
RER			0.85	1.04	1.28
Pulse O_2	8	2	3	6	9
Work (Watts)					
HHR%		100	101	30	28
BR%		92	91	50	37
HRR	105	106	32	30	39
VO_2 slope					
VO_2 pred (%)		13	15	62	91
HR pred (%)					
Exer time		2	7	15	16
BP systolic					
BP diastolic					
$PETO_2$		106	107	124	121
$PETCO_2$		34	33	24	25
VO_2 ml/kg/min	38	5.1	5.7	23	34
HR bpm	198	92	116	168	172
VE/VCO_2	42	44	45	44	46
Vd/VT (estimated)		0.22	0.22	0.13	0.14
RR (br/min)		20	24	40	68

Variable	Result

PETCO$_2$ decrease or VECO$_2$ increase	+
Breathing reserve low	Normal
VAT (ventilatory threshold) present	+
Pulse O$_2$	Normal
Breathing reserve normal	Normal
VAT present	+

Other data

VO$_2$ ml/kg min^{-1} (normal).
RR > 50 at VO$_2$ max.
FEV1 105 % predicted.
FVC 98 % predicted.
EKG normal during study.

Cause-and-Effect Diagram Result (Case 3: Check All That Apply)

Conclusion: (check or circle)

- Cardiac limitation.
- Respiratory limitation.
- Peripheral vascular limitation (PVD).
- Pulmonary hypertension (circulation).
- Metabolic limitation.
- Muscle limitation.
- Deconditioned.
- Poor effort.
- **None**

Summary

Complains of chest pain with exercise

22 year old prior 28 week premie born 1,088 g and did not receive surfactant. Bronchopulmonary dysplasia (BPD), intraventricular hemorrhage, osteopenia, and retinopathy of prematurity. Gymnastics and Cheerleading at local university runs for exercise complaining of chest pain. Problems with cervical and thoracic scoliosis with secondary neuropathy manifest as pain, restless leg syndrome, and periodic limb movement disorder of sleep. Anxiety disorder and ADHD. Good student on medications

Medications:

1. Pregbalin.
2. Vyvanse.
3. Adderall 7.5 mg prn once daily.
4. Dulera two puffs twice a day.

Results:

There is no evidence of cardiopulmonary limitation. The VO_2 max is normal and the cause-and-effect diagram is not valid in this case. The spirometry data shows no pre–post difference. However, the use of the *cause-and effect-diagram* does point out an interesting finding, at maximal work the RR was greater than 50 breaths-per-minute. If the VO_2 was low and $PETCO_2$ did not decrease and dead space ventilation not decrease, then respiratory limitation would be likely if the breathing reserve was low. The breathing reserve was normal and with the clinical history of BPD and prematurity pulmonary vascular disease should be considered. The dynamics of chest wall movement should also be considered due to the longstanding cervico-thoracic scoliosis. Exercise associated anxiety should also be entertained as the patient has a known issue.

Recommendations:

1. Close follow-up and yearly CPET- Echo/EKG monitoring for evidence of pulmonary hypertension.
2. Cognitive behavioral therapy for anxiety. Monitor scoliosis and associated neuropathy with sleep problems.

References

1. Cooper DM, Radom-Aizik S, Shin H, Nemet D. Exercise and lung function in child health and disease. Kendig and Chernick's disorders of the respiratory tract in children. Saunders 2012; Chapter 13, pp. 234–50.
2. Wasserman K, et al. Principles of exercise testing and interpretation. Williams & Wilkins: Lippincott; 2012.
3. Weisman IM, Marciniuk D, Martinez FJ, Sciurba F, Sue D, Myers J, et al. ATS/ACCP statement on cardiopulmonary exercise testing. Am J Respir Crit Care Med. 2003;167(2):211–77. http://www.ncbi.nlm.nih.gov/pubmed/12524257.
4. Pina IL, Balady GJ, Hanson P, Labovitz AJ, Madonna DW, Myers J. Guidelines for clinical exercise testing laboratories. A statement for healthcare professionals from the Committee on Exercise and Cardiac Rehabilitation, American Heart Association. Circulation. 1995;91(3):912–21. http://circ.ahajournals.org/content/91/3/912.full.
5. Morton AR. Exercise physiology. In: Pediatric respiratory medicine. 2nd edn. Elsevier Inc. 2008; p. 89–99. http://dx.doi.org/10.1016/B978–0–323–04048–8.50012–8.
6. Guazzi M, Adams V, Conraads V, Halle M, Mezzani A, Vanhees L, et al. EACPR/AHA Joint Scientific Statement. Clinical recommendations for cardiopulmonary exercise testing data assessment in specific patient populations. Eur Heart J. 2012;33(23):2917–27. http://www.ncbi.nlm.nih.gov/pubmed/22952138.
7. Roca J. Exercise testing (chapter 10). In: Clinical respiratory medicine. 4th ed. Elsevier Inc. 2010;143–53. http://dx.doi.org/10.1016/B978–1–4557–0792–8.00010–6.

 8. Teoh OH, Trachsel D, Mei-Zahav M, Selvadurai H. Exercise testing in children with lung diseases. Paediatr Respir Rev. 2009;10:99–104.
 9. Lipnowski S, LeBlanc CMA, Bridger TL, Houghton K, Philpott JF, Templeton CG, et al. Healthy active living: Physical activity guidelines for children and adolescents. Paediatr Child Health. 2012;17:209–10.
10. Han JC, Lawlor DA, Kimm SYS. Childhood obesity – 2010: progress and challenges. 2011;375(9727):1737–48.
11. Lattavo A, Kopperud A, Rogers PD. Creatine and other supplements. Pediatr Clin North Am. 2007;54:735–760 xi.
12. Maughan RJ, Greenhaff PL, Hespel P. Dietary supplements for athletes: emerging trends and recurring themes. J Sports Sci. 2011;29 Suppl 1:S57–66.
13. Samuels C. Sleep, recovery, and performance: the new frontier in high-performance athletics. Neurol Clin. 2008;26:169–80 ix–x.
14. Dement WC. Sleep extension: getting as much extra sleep as possible. Clin Sports Med. 2005;24:251–268 viii.
15. DeHass DM. NCAA study of substance use of college student-athletes. National Collegiate Athletic Association. 2006.
16. Tomporowski PD. Cognitive and behavioral responses to acute exercise in youths: a review. Pediatr Exercise Sci. 2003;15(4):348–59. http://journals.humankinetics.com/pes-back-issues/pes-back-issues/cognitiveandbehavioralresponsestoacuteexerciseinyouthsareview.
17. Ramos RP, Alencar MCN, Treptow E, Arbex F, Ferreira EM V, Neder JA. Clinical usefulness of response profiles to rapidly incremental cardiopulmonary exercise testing. Pulm Med. 2013;359021. http://www.pubmedcentral.nih.gov/articlerender.fcgi?artid=3666297&tool=pmcentrez&rendertype=abstract.
18. Ten Harkel ADJ, Takken T, Van Osch-Gevers M, Helbing WA. Normal values for cardiopulmonary exercise testing in children. Eur J Cardiovasc Prevent Rehabil. 2011;18:48–54.
19. Lucía A, Fleck SJ, Gotshall RW, Kearney JT. Validity and reliability of the Cosmed K2 instrument. Int J Sports Med. 1993;14:380–6.
20. Skootsky SA, Abraham E. Continuous oxygen consumption measurement during initial emergency department resuscitation of critically ill patients. Crit Care Med. 1988;16:706–9.
21. Schrack JA, Simonsick EM, Ferrucci L. Comparison of the Cosmed K4b2 portable metabolic system in measuring steady-state walking energy expenditure. PLoS ONE. 2010;5:5.
22. Duffield R, Dawson B, Pinnington HC, Wong P. Accuracy and reliability of a Cosmed K4b2 portable gas analysis system. J Sci Med Sport. 2004;7:11–22.
23. Rowland TW. Oxygen uptake and endurance fitness in children: a developmental perspective. 1989.
24. Fisher M. Children and exercise: appropriate practices for grades K-6. JOPERD. 2009;80:18–23.
25. Hargreaves M. Fatigue mechanisms determining exercise performance: integrative physiology is systems biology. J Appl Physiol. 2008;104:1541–2.
26. Baker J, Côté J, Hawes R. The relationship between coaching behaviours and sport anxiety in athletes. J Sci Med Sport. 2000;3:110–9.
27. Birch SL, Duncan MJ, Franklin C. Overweight and reduced heart rate variability in British children: an exploratory study. Prev Med. 2012;55:430–2.
28. Walter LM, Foster AM, Patterson RR, Anderson V, Davey MJ, Nixon GM, et al. Cardiovascular variability during periodic leg movements in sleep in children. Sleep. 2009;32(8):1093–9. http://www.pubmedcentral.nih.gov/articlerender.fcgi?artid=2717200&tool=pmcentrez&rendertype=abstract.
29. Sookan T, McKune AJ. Heart rate variability in physically active individuals: reliability and gender characteristics. Cardiovasc J Afr. 2012;23(2):67–72. http://www.pubmedcentral.nih.gov/articlerender.fcgi?artid=3721889&tool=pmcentrez&rendertype=abstract.
30. Millar PJ, Rakobowchuk M, McCartney N, MacDonald MJ. Heart rate variability and nonlinear analysis of heart rate dynamics following single and multiple Wingate bouts. Appl Physiol Nutr Metab. 2009;34:875–83.

31. Gui-Ling X, Jing-Hua W, Yan Z, Hui X, Jing-Hui S, Si-Rui Y. Association of high blood pressure with heart rate variability in children. Iran J Pediatr. 2013;23(1):37–44. http://www.pubmedcentral.nih.gov/articlerender.fcgi?artid=3574990&tool=pmcentrez&rendertype=abstract.
32. McCain GC, Knupp AM, Fontaine JL, Pino LD, Vasquez EP. Heart rate variability responses to nipple feeding for preterm infants with bronchopulmonary dysplasia: three case studies. J Pediatr Nurs. 2010;25(3):215–20. http://www.ncbi.nlm.nih.gov/pubmed/20430282.
33. Yiallourou SR, Sands SA, Walker AM, Horne RSC. Maturation of heart rate and blood pressure variability during sleep in term-born infants. Sleep. 2012;35(2):177–86. http://www.pubmed-central.nih.gov/articlerender.fcgi?artid=3250356&tool=pmcentrez&rendertype=abstract.
34. Lammers AE, Munnery E, Hislop AA, Haworth SG. Heart rate variability predicts outcome in children with pulmonary arterial hypertension. Int J Cardiol. 2010;142:159–65.
35. Scrogin K, Henze M, Hart D, Samarel A, Barakat J, Eckert L. Persistent alterations in heart rate variability, baroreflex sensitivity, and anxiety-like behaviors during development of heart failure in the rat. Am J Physiol Heart Circ Physiol. 2008;295:H29–38.
36. Ehrlén K. Drawings as representations of children's conceptions. Int J Sci Educ. 2009; 31:41–57.
37. Lau J, Engelen L, Bundy A. Parents' perceptions of children' s physical activity compared on two electronic diaries. Pediatr Exerc Sci. 2013;7:124–37.
38. Lau PWC, Fox KR, Cheung MWL. An analysis of sport identity as a predictor of children' s participation in sport. Pediatr Exerc Sci. 2006;415–25.
39. Borg G. Borg's perceived exertion and pain scales. Champaign: IL: Human Kinetics. 1998; 104. Available from The Free Library. http://www.thefreelibrary.com/Borg's+Perceived+Exertion+and+Pain+Scales.-a053509933. Accessed 01 Sep 2014.
40. McGrath PJ, Pianosi PT, Unruh AM, Buckley CP. Dalhousie dyspnea scales: construct and content validity of pictorial scales for measuring dyspnea. BMC Pediatr. 2005;5:33.
41. Roemmich JN, Barkley JE, Epstein LH, Lobarinas CL, White TM, Foster JH. Validity of PCERT and OMNI walk/run ratings of perceived exertion. Med Sci Sports Exerc. 2006;38:1014–9.
42. Norton P, Hope D, Weeks J. The physical activity and sport anxiety scale (PASAS): Scale development and psychometric analysis. Anxiety Stress Coping. 2004;17:363–82.
43. Francis SE, Chorpita BF. Parental beliefs about child anxiety as a mediator of parent and child anxiety. Cogn Ther Res. 2009;35:21–9.
44. Powell CV, Primhak RA. Asthma treatment, perceived respiratory disability, and morbidity. Arch Dis Child. 1995;72:209–13.

Chapter 13
Imaging for the Pediatric Pulmonologist

Mantosh S. Rattan and Alan S. Brody

Abstract This chapter provides an overview of the different modalities that are used to image the pediatric chest. The chapter is organized by imaging modality and includes the advantages, limitations, and uses of the different imaging studies. Sections on chest radiographs, fluoroscopy, computed tomography, magnetic resonance imaging, ultrasound, nuclear medicine, and interventional radiology are included. An additional section on radiation risk and one on which test to order for specific indications provide additional practical information for the pediatric pulmonologist.

Keywords Diagnostic imaging • Radiology • X-ray • Chest radiographs (CXR) • Computed tomography (CT) • Ultrasound (US) • Magnetic resonance imaging (MRI) • Nuclear medicine (NM) • Fluoroscopy

Introduction

Imaging is an integral part of the evaluation and care of the child with respiratory disease. It is unlikely that any child who has been referred to a pediatric pulmonologist will not have had at least one imaging study. There have been dramatic changes in imaging. Digital images have replaced hard copies. The commonly used term "chest film" is now an anachronism. New modalities are available including positron emission tomography (PET) scanning, and magnetic resonance imaging (MRI) using hyperpolarized gas. New uses are being found for long standing modalities, such as the use of ultrasound imaging to evaluate the lung parenchyma for pathology including pneumonia and interstitial lung disease.

It is not possible to fully address thoracic imaging in a chapter, or in a single book. In this section, we hope to provide background information and a framework to help the pediatric pulmonologist when choosing an imaging study and when

M.S. Rattan, M.D. (✉) • A.S. Brody, M.D.
Cincinnati Children's Hospital and the University of Cincinnati College of Medicine,
Cincinnati, OH, USA

Department of Radiology, Cincinnati Children's Medical Center,
MLC 5031, 3333 Burnet Ave, Cincinnati, OH 45229, USA
e-mail: Mantosh.Rattan@cchmc.org

© Springer Science+Business Media New York 2015
S.D. Davis et al. (eds.), *Diagnostic Tests in Pediatric Pulmonology*,
Respiratory Medicine, DOI 10.1007/978-1-4939-1801-0_13

interpreting the results. By "interpreting the results," we refer to results obtained from a dedicated imager. Many pediatric pulmonologists are very comfortable reviewing imaging studies, but due to the complexity of current imaging and the need to provide the best care to our patients an imager should be involved. It is our hope that what follows will help the pediatric pulmonology care team to provide the best possible care through imaging.

Radiation Risk

CT scanning, PET scanning, other nuclear medicine studies, fluoroscopy, and chest radiography all use ionizing radiation. The dose for a chest radiograph is so low that there is no demonstrable risk, but other studies, particularly CT and PET scanning, may carry a risk of later cancer from the ionizing radiation used. Cancer risk from diagnostic imaging has been an area of increased interest and concern since 2001 when Brenner and colleagues estimated later cancer deaths in children who had had CT scans. They used data from then recent reports of atomic bomb data that evaluated the cancer risk from radiation in the same range as that from CT scanning [4].

Since that time, there have been many additional studies on radiation risk and on methods of decreasing radiation dose from diagnostic imaging. CT scanning has been the major focus of these efforts because CT scanning is frequently performed and uses a relatively high radiation dose. Data continue to support that there is a small risk of later cancer from the radiation exposure from CT scanning [15, 20]. Due to this concern and with improvements in CT technology the dose required for a CT scan has decreased dramatically since 2001 with new techniques likely to result in a dose reduction of as much as 90 % when compared to 2001 doses.

For pulmonologists and families it is important to understand that the estimated risk is extremely low, while the benefit from an indicated CT scan should be high. Current estimates of later cancer are in the range of 1 fatal cancer later in life for every 5,000 children scanned, so it is correct to tell a family that in regard to radiation risk the odds are 99.8 % that the CT scan will not result in a later cancer. In almost all cases the benefit from the information gained from the CT scan will greatly outweigh the possible risk. If this is not clearly the case, the CT scan should probably not be done. Of all the methods of decreasing radiation exposure the most effective is to not perform an unnecessary CT scan, as this is the only method that reduces the risk 100 %. Table 13.1 lists radiation dose estimates for some commonly performed imaging studies.

Table 13.1 Radiation dose estimates for common thoracic imaging procedures in a 5-year-old child

Procedure	Effective dose (mSv)
Chest PA	0.003
Chest PA/Lat	0.009
Upper GI series	0.04
Lung perfusion scan	2.6
Chest CT	3.6
Whole body PET/CT	15
Chest MRI	0.0
Chest US	0.0

Chest Radiographs

The chest radiograph (CXR) is the most frequently obtained study in the diagnostic imaging department. CXRs are also one of the least expensive imaging studies. CXRs can be obtained portably with an easily transported system, making them available in all parts of the hospital for patients who cannot be transported. The CXR is the starting point for almost every indication for thoracic imaging. CXRs are sufficient for many tasks, and are often useful in planning further imaging.

CXRs are obtained by sending X-rays from an X-ray tube through the patient to a detector. Until the 1990s this detector was usually radiographic film. Current systems use a reusable detector plate that is either permanently connected to a digital imaging system (digital radiography), or a free standing imaging plate that is scanned by a reader after the CXR has been obtained (computed radiography). The reader digitizes the image recorded on the plate (computed radiography). CXRs use ionizing radiation, but the dose, approximately 0.01 mSv, is low enough that here is no measurable radiation risk.

CXRs are routinely obtained at the end of a normal inspiration. Maximal inspiration by a cooperative patient may simulate severe air trapping. Expiratory CXRs are obtained at the lowest lung volume that can be easily obtained. If cooperation is not possible, the CXR can be obtained during breathing by timing the exposure to end expiration. This requires a skilled technologist, and will still not be successful in all cases.

For many indications, the value of a CXR can be increased by obtaining the study with the patient in different positions. A standard CXR series includes upright frontal and lateral images. A frontal film can be obtained with the X-ray beam passing from posterior to anterior with the detector in front (posteroanterior or PA). If the beam passes from anterior to posterior with the detector behind the patient this is referred to as an anteroposterior or AP projection. PA projections are used almost entirely when an upright CXR is obtained using a dedicated chest imaging system in the radiology department. This is the "gold standard" and in particular provides better evaluation of heart size. AP positioning exaggerates heart size somewhat and is more sensitive to positioning, but is the only practical approach for portable CXRs. Lateral radiographs are usually obtained with the patient upright, with the X ray source on one side of the patient and the detector plate on the opposite side. The standard lateral projection is a left lateral with the detector plate on the patient's left side. There is usually little difference between a right and left lateral projection. A cross-table lateral is obtained with the patient supine. The X-ray beam thus passes across the examination table. This can be useful when evaluating air fluid levels, pneumoperitoneum, and to a lesser extent, pneumothorax. A decubitus CXR is an AP projection obtained with the patient lying on the right or left side. A right decubitus CXR, for example, refers to a CXR obtained with the right side down. Decubitus CXRs are useful for evaluating pneumothoraces, pleural effusions, and air/fluid levels. Decubitus images can also be used to evaluate for air trapping. In the decubitus position the volume of the normal dependent ("down") lung is decreased compared to the nondependent ("up") lung. If there is air trapping, the dependent lung, or a portion of the lung will remain lucent and similar in volume to the

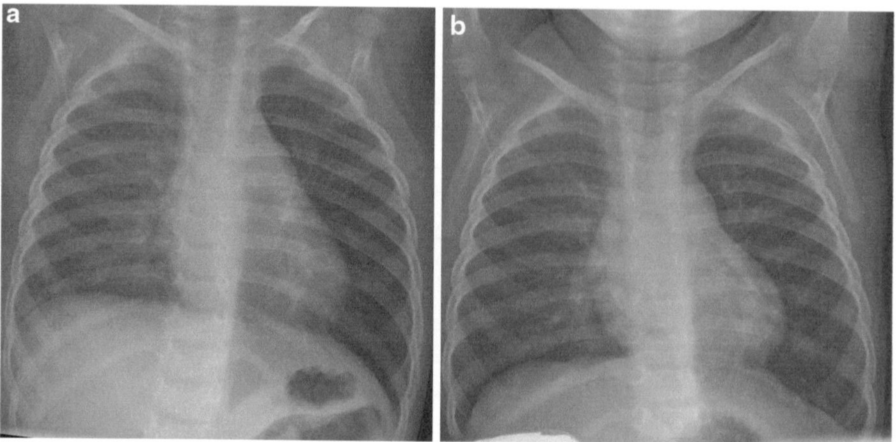

Fig. 13.1 Left main bronchus foreign body shown by bilateral decubitus radiographs. With the patient lying on the right side (**a**) the volume of the right lung has decreased and the density increased compared to the left lung. This indicates that the volume of air in the right lung has decreased due to compression by the heart and mediastinum. With the child lying on the left side (**b**) the left lung has not decreased in volume or increased in density. This indicates obstruction of the left main bronchus, trapping the air in the left lung

nondependent lung (Fig. 13.1). Both decubitus images are often obtained to allow additional comparison between the two lungs. In infants and young children, supine CXRs are much easier to obtain than upright studies, and are commonly used for both frontal and lateral images.

CXRs accurately identify and quantitate extraparenchymal air. Upright or decubitus positioning provides the greatest accuracy for pneumothoraces, as air will rise to the highest point in the pleural space. In a supine patient pleural air is more difficult to detect. Neonatal supine radiographs are particularly difficult, as the protuberant abdomen of the infant will result in air located at the lung bases, often adjacent to the cardiac margin. A pneumomediastinum can be identified by air dissecting between tissue planes in the mediastinum usually with a linear appearance (Fig. 13.2). Structures such as the outside margin of the trachea or main bronchi, or the space between the aorta and pulmonary artery become visible. Air in the anterior mediastinum above the diaphragm can separate the inferior margin of the heart from the diaphragm allowing the superior margin of the diaphragm to be traced completely across the chest, the "continuous diaphragm" sign. Mediastinal air frequently dissects into the neck in young children and adults, but is less common in infants. Small quantities of pleural fluid can be detected when fluid blunts the usual sharp angles of the diaphragm with the chest wall. The posterior costophrenic sulcus on lateral view is the first to show the presence of fluid.

The trachea and main bronchi are also well seen on CXR. The trachea should be visible throughout its length on both frontal and lateral CXR. Imaging technique can make the trachea less visible, but it usually can be identified. In addition, it is rare for tracheal abnormalities to affect the entire cervical and thoracic trachea. If part of the

Fig. 13.2
Pneumomediastinum.
Air in the mediastinum
separates the azygous vein
from surrounding structures
(*asterisk*). Air is seen
between the heart and the
diaphragm (*arrows*), and
extending into the upper
mediastinum and the soft
tissues of the neck

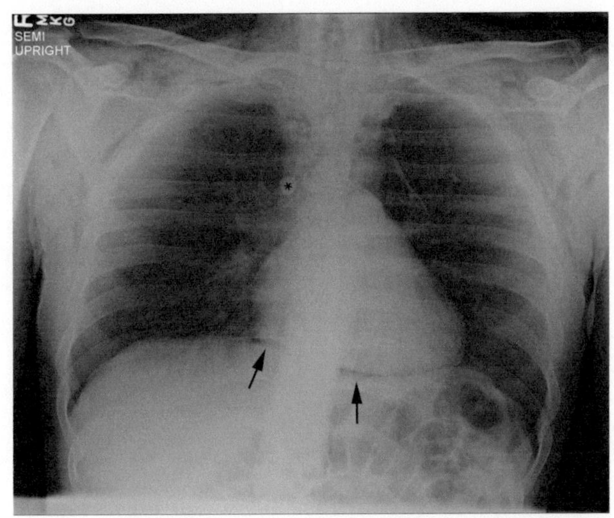

Fig. 13.3   Normal tracheal
buckling. In expiration and
with neck flexion the trachea
buckles to the right. This is a
normal finding and should
not be mistaken for evidence
of a mass. The trachea
buckles away from the side of
the aorta, so buckling to the
left suggests a right-sided
aortic arch

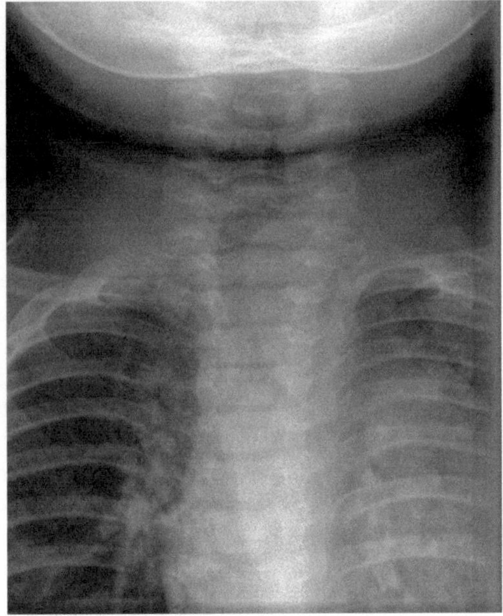

trachea is seen and part is not, tracheal narrowing, tracheomalacia, or a foreign body
(the "missing segment" sign) should be considered. The trachea should be to the
right of the midline at the level of the aortic arch. In the upper chest and lower neck
the normal trachea can buckle dramatically in children (Fig. 13.3). This buckling
should always be to the right due to the position of the aortic arch on the left.
A midline or left of midline trachea suggests a right sided or double aortic arch.

The bony thorax is well evaluated by CXR. Rib and spine fractures or anomalies are well demonstrated. Pectus excavatum, when moderate or marked, is identified on lateral view when the anterior ribs project anterior to the sternum. While cross-sectional imaging is most often used to quantitate the severity of the pectus, CXRs have been shown to provide similar information.

Diffuse (interstitial) lung disease is not well evaluated on CXR. The CXR may be normal, or the appearance may simulate viral airways disease. The CXR is still useful in suspected diffuse lung disease by excluding other entities such as focal lung disease or mass, central airway narrowing, or an abnormal appearance of the heart suggesting a cardiac abnormality.

Fluoroscopy

Fluoroscopy uses X-rays to obtain real time video images. As with all imaging equipment that uses ionizing radiation, reducing radiation dose has been a major goal of equipment manufacturers and radiologists. Pulse fluoroscopy is a technique that turns the X-ray source on and off at operator determined intervals, usually between 7.5 and 30 pulses per second. At 7.5 pulses per second, the dose is less than 1/3 that of continuous fluoroscopy. The operator remains the most important single factor in radiation dose. Limiting the area exposed to X-rays and avoiding excess fluoroscopy time can markedly reduce fluoroscopy dose. In the evaluation of the GI tract, contrast material is used. Barium is most commonly used. Barium is inert and does not cause allergic reactions, although flavoring elements and other components may rarely cause allergic reactions. Barium is not absorbed, and can remain for prolonged periods of time if aspirated into the lung or spilled into the mediastinum or peritoneal cavity. Water soluble contrast material is used when there is a concern for aspiration or perforation. Many formulations are available. These differ largely in cost and in osmolarity, with less expensive formulations often sufficiently hyper-osmolar to cause fluid shifts in young children. Isosmolar formulations that are sufficiently radiodense to be seen easily under fluoroscopy are available, and are the contrast materials of choice when either perforation or aspiration is a concern [5, 8].

Multiple different studies use fluoroscopy. Respiratory system evaluations include fluoroscopic evaluation of the airway, from the oral and nasal cavities through the mainstem bronchi. Laryngomalacia and tracheobronchomalacia can be assessed over multiple breaths using fluoroscopy. No airway instrumentation is required and the patient can usually be made sufficiently comfortable to be observed during normal respiration. Redundant soft tissues in young children can simulate a retropharyngeal abscess or a pharyngeal mass. Fluoroscopic observation of multiple breaths will often demonstrate that suspected abnormalities resolve at some point in the respiratory cycle. A process such as a retropharyngeal abscess would not resolve intermittently, and so the apparent mass can then be attributed to soft tissue variation during respiration. Fluoroscopy provides the most complete evaluation of diaphragmatic motion and contour. While ultrasound can accurately evaluate diaphragmatic motion, only a portion of the diaphragm can be seen. Ultrasound is useful when the patient cannot be transported, but provides a less confident assessment of overall diaphragmatic contour and motion. Eventration can be distinguished from paralysis in many cases. Differentiation of eventration from diaphragmatic hernia is more difficult and may be impossible with any imaging modality.

Gastrointestinal studies include the swallowing study, esophagram, and upper GI. A swallowing study evaluates the swallowing mechanism by placing the patient in the lateral position, limiting the X-ray beam to the nasopharynx, oropharynx, and upper trachea, and observing all phases of swallowing with different foods. This is the modality of choice for the evaluation of swallowing and for detecting small volume aspiration.

An esophagram evaluates esophageal appearance and motility by placing the patient in multiple positions and observing swallowed material, usually thin barium, pass from the mouth to the stomach. An esophagram is the imaging modality of choice for the evaluation of esophagitis, strictures, dysmotility, and suspected impacted material in the esophagus. In pediatric institutions it is common to follow the barium past the ligament of Treitz to exclude malrotation. This is not universal, and at some institutions an upper GI series should be ordered if evaluation for malrotation is required. A swallowing study and an esophogram or upper GI may require two separate visits. If performed together the upper GI series must be performed first to allow evaluation for malrotation. This study is likely to agitate the child who will be less likely to cooperate with the swallowing study.

The upper GI examination includes evaluation of the esophagus, although less time is usually spent evaluating the esophagus when compared to a dedicated esophagogram. The upper GI examination includes evaluation of the stomach and duodenum, with documentation of passage of contrast material into the jejunum. The upper GI series can be useful in evaluating suspected aspiration as gastroesophageal reflux and gastric outlet obstruction, both treatable factors in aspiration, can be detected.

Computed Tomography (CT)

CT scanning provides the most complete evaluation of the chest of any imaging modality. CT scanning provides the best evaluation of the lung parenchyma, airways, lung nodules, masses, the bones, and the pulmonary vessels (Fig. 13.4). MRI provides better soft tissue characterization, but CT is sufficient in most cases. MRI is more sensitive to bone lesions, but CT is usually more definitive. Central vascularity can be well evaluated with both CT and MRI (Figs. 13.4 and 13.5). CT angiography provides better vascular detail than MR angiography of heart and great vessels. Both CT and MRI can be used for functional evaluation of the heart, but MRI is usually chosen because MRI does not use ionizing radiation and CT techniques require a relatively high radiation dose.

Current CT scanners can complete a chest CT scan in less than 10 s and produce contiguous sections less than a millimeter thick. Isotropic imaging, in which the resolution is the same in all three dimensions, divides the imaged volume into cubical voxels that allowing reformatting in any plane without loss of detail.

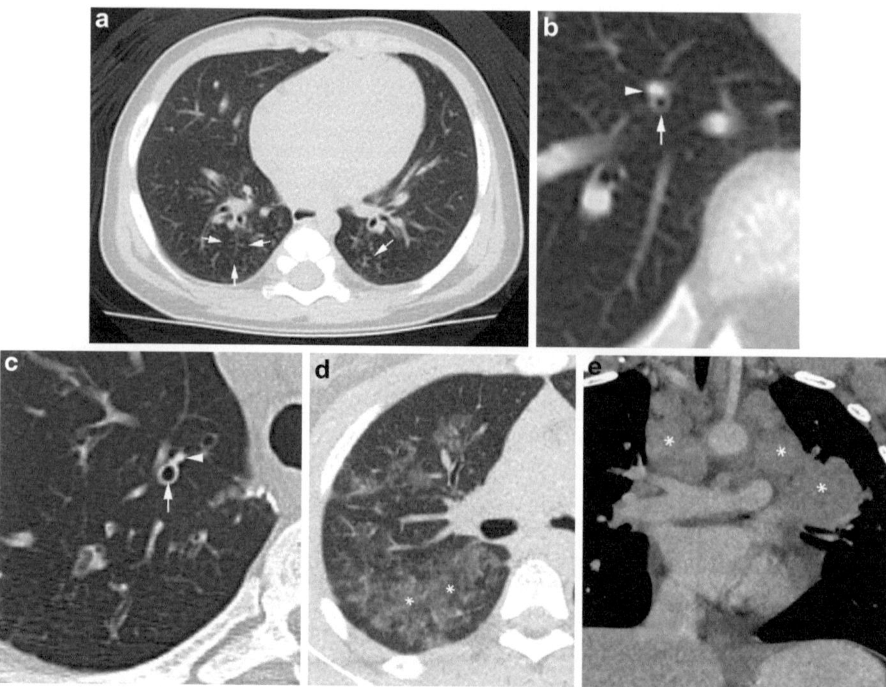

Fig. 13.4 Chest CT scanning can demonstrate a broad range of abnormalities. Tree in bud opacities (*arrows*) have the appearance of *short lines* with *small circles* at the ends (**a**). This appearance is due to material filling the distal bronchioles and acini. In children the most common causes are aspiration and indolent infection, although many other entities can produce this appearance. Bronchiectasis is identified when the airway lumen is larger than the accompanying pulmonary artery branch. In a normal child the lumen (*arrow*) is smaller than the vessel (*arrowhead*) (**b**). In a patient with bronchiectasis the airway is dilated and the lumen (*arrow*) is larger than the accompanying vessel (*arrowhead*) (**c**). When lung density is increased so that it is greater than the density of normal lung, but less than the density of non-enhanced vessels (*asterisks*), the term ground glass is used (**d**). The appearance is nonspecific with causes including any process that thickens alveolar walls or the interstitium, or that partial fills alveoli. Adenopathy is easily detected when large nodular non-enhancing masses are present (**e**). Less striking adenopathy is much more difficult to identify without the use of intravenous contrast material and knowledge of cross-sectional anatomy

CT uses X-rays, as does fluoroscopy and CXR. The radiation dose required is similar to fluoroscopy dose and much greater than a CXR dose. The X-rays are produced by an X-ray tube that is larger, but otherwise similar to the tubes used for fluoroscopy and CXR. The patient lies on a table that moves through a "doughnut" that contains the X-ray tube and a series of detectors that surround the patient. The X-ray tube moves around the patient and the radiation that passes through the patient is measured by the detectors. The data recorded by each of the detectors is sent to a computer that constructs the image. This recorded data is called raw data. The raw data is a multiple gigabyte file that is usually stored for a limited time and then discarded. The CT images are produced by the computer as digital files.

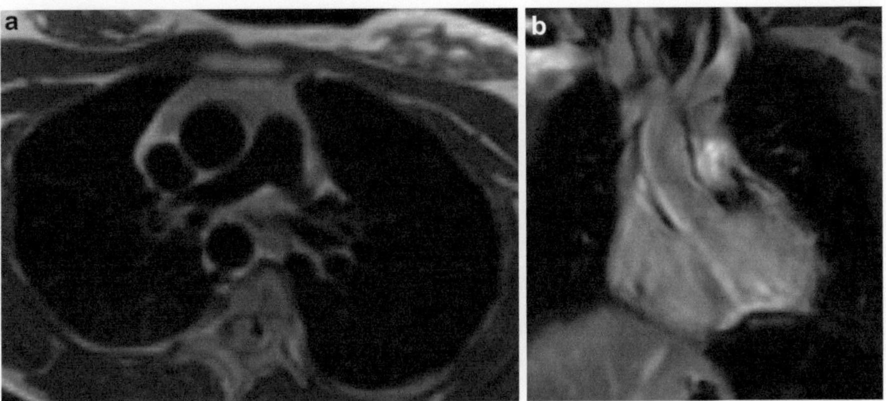

Fig. 13.5 MRI can be performed in ways that dramatically change the appearance of the tissues of the chest. Here an axial image shows the blood vessels as black voids (**a**). Using a different technique, the coronal images shows the vessels with more variable, but generally light *gray* or *white* appearance (**b**)

These are megabyte rather than gigabyte files and are maintained as a permanent part of the patient's medical record. This distinction is important because advanced image manipulation usually requires the raw data, which is only available for a day to a few weeks.

Most CT scanning moves the patient through the CT scanner as the X-ray tube is rotating and emitting X-rays. The X-ray beam forms a helix, and this technique is called helical or spiral CT. When someone refers to a "regular CT" this probably refers to a helical CT. Two situations do not use helical CT. CT scanners that use a very wide X-ray beam can cover most of the lung in a single rotation. This type of CT scanner is commercially available and is currently in use in numerous hospitals. Sixteen centimeter of the chest can be imaged by rotating the X-ray tube once around the patient without table motion. The table can then be moved by the width of the X-ray beam and the process repeated, allowing complete coverage of the child's chest, usually in one or two rotations. The second technique that does not use helical imaging is high resolution CT. This technique is a source of such frequent confusion that it is addressed in the following section.

Most CT scanning is performed during quiet breathing or at full inspiration. Expiratory images are very useful when identifying air trapping is important. This includes the interpretation of mixed attenuation where either the area of high attenuation can represent a parenchymal abnormality or low attenuation can be due to air trapping. There are often indications of air trapping on inspiratory images, but expiratory images may identify air trapping not seen on inspiratory images and will almost always increase confidence when evaluating air trapping (Fig. 13.6).

With their high speed, motion artifact is rarely a problem on current CT scanners. It is still necessary for the child to lie still on the CT scanner table and breathe quietly. In infants, feeding and swaddling are usually sufficient. In older infants and toddlers, a "child friendly" environment and distraction techniques usually work well.

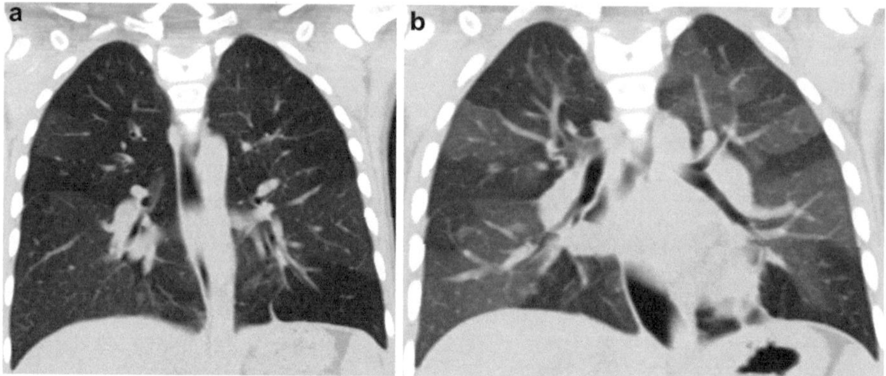

Fig. 13.6 Air trapping may be very difficult to detect on inspiratory CT scans. In this case an inspiratory image shows well-defined areas higher and lower density are seen in both lungs (**a**). An expiratory image shows a marked increase in the difference in density (**b**), with normal areas increased in density due to a decrease in the volume of air while the less dense areas do, not due change because of air trapping

CT scanning in young children can usually be performed during quiet breathing, so few instructions are needed. In children who can follow directions, inspiratory CT scans should be obtained during suspended respiration after a deep breath, ideally at or near total lung capacity (TLC). Total breath hold time will usually be less than 10 s. Most children older than 5 years can cooperate for an inspiratory CT scan. Expiratory breath holds are often difficult for children less than 7 years old. It is often difficult to assess the degree of expiration in the CT scan room. Lung volumes for expiratory CT are far less reliable than for inspiratory CT. Spirometer controlled CT can be used with cooperative patients to provide optimal lung volumes and reproducibility, but this capability is not widely available.

For children who cannot cooperate and for whom high quality inspiratory and particularly expiratory image are needed, sedation or anesthesia can be used. General anesthesia with rapid acting agents such as Propofol allows rapid induction and recovery with total time in the imaging department of an hour or less. Lung volume can be controlled by administering positive pressure for inspiratory images and allowing the child to passively exhale toward functional residual capacity (FRC) for expiratory images. The development of atelectasis, however, often limits the quality of CT scans done under general anesthesia. Specific anesthesia protocols can minimize atelectasis. Beginning assisted ventilation with deep sigh breaths as soon as possible, and giving multiple prolonged deep inspirations immediately before imaging have been effective [19]. Atelectasis is less of a problem with sedation, but sedation without lung volume control is rarely needed. If lung volume control is needed, the controlled ventilation technique, which uses sedation and mask ventilation, is very effective, but the technique is difficult to learn and is not widely available.

High Resolution CT (HRCT)

The HRCT technique was developed in the 1980s to provide a high quality survey of the lung parenchyma using the technically limited CT scanners available at that time. At that time each CT slice was obtained independently, and required approximately two seconds for tube rotation and 4 s to move the table. A 300 slice thin section CT, as commonly obtained today, would have required 1,800 s or 30 min. In addition, the radiation dose for each of these sections was much higher than it is today, and the CT scanners could not produce more than 10–20 images before the X-ray tube heated to a point that scanning had to be interrupted to allow the tube to cool.

HRCT uses a sampling technique, and indeed would be more accurately described as a "limited sample parenchymal evaluation CT." The sample is obtained by imaging one thin section at much wider intervals, commonly 1 mm each 10 mm apart. This reduces the radiation dose and the number of slices. Pausing to allow the patient to take a breath before each slice provides sufficient time for tube cooling without additional pauses.

Current CT scanners have none of the limitations that require the use of the sampling technique described above. Current CT scanners can provide contiguous 1 mm sections through the chest in less than 10 s. The radiation dose is no higher than for a CT with thicker slices, and in some cases the dose is less for contiguous sections than for the one in ten sample. Tube heat capacity is sufficient so that pauses for tube cooling are no longer required.

For these reasons there is currently little indication for traditional HRCT. The helical technique allows the chest to be imaged in a single very short breath hold rather than one very long or several shorter breath holds. Contiguous imaging improves assessment of the airways and mediastinum. Comparison between serial CTs is much easier as well. For nearly all cases there is little or no difference between an inspiratory HRCT and a routine non-contrast CT.

Contrast Material

Intravenous contrast material may be helpful in most situations when obtaining CT scans of the chest. Exceptions are largely limited to the evaluation of diffuse lung disease and in follow-up of lung nodules or lung metastases. The use of intravenous contrast material is necessary to evaluate the heart and great vessels. Distinguishing normal hilar vessels from adenopathy is much more difficult in children than in adults, so contrast material markedly increases confidence when evaluating the mediastinum or hila. Contrast is necessary to identify aberrant vessels including those that supply sequestrations. Contrast enhancement can distinguish atelectasis from pneumonia, and can help distinguish solid from cystic masses. Contrast material is very safe, with major complications seen in less than 1 in 40,000 uses. Contrast material is mildly nephrotoxic, and it should be used with care in children with suspected or known renal insufficiency.

Chest MRI

MRI uses strong electromagnets and radio frequency energy to form images. Conventional, proton based, MR image signal is based on the physicochemical behavior of protons contained in tissues and liquids. This behavior produces images that emphasize different characteristics of the imaged tissue depending on the specific series of magnetic field changes and radio frequency transmissions used (a pulse sequence). By using multiple pulse sequences, MRI can provide excellent contrast between different tissues, and can often provide information on the type of tissue such as fat, muscle, or fluid. MRI also offers functional imaging capability such as perfusion and ventilation quantification through a wide range of different techniques that include using MRI signal changes to track oxygen saturation, the use of intravenous paramagnetic contrast material ("MRI contrast"), and inhaled hyperpolarized gases. The lack of radiation makes MRI of the lungs particularly desirable in pediatrics. While MRI provides superb demonstration of the soft tissues of the body, technical limitations are posed by the low proton density in the lungs and MR signal loss caused by magnetic field inhomogeneities at air/soft tissue interfaces. This has made lung imaging a challenge, and lung parenchymal and airway detail remain lower than the detail provided by CT scanning.

MRI studies usually require 30 min or more, with most individual sequences lasting several minutes during which the child must lie very still. In addition, the child must be completely within the central tube of the MRI scanner, which is noisy and can be claustrophobic or disorienting. For these reasons the quality of MR images is highly dependent on patient compliance, more so than with radiography or CT. Sedation or general anesthesia is often needed when scanning infants and young children but technologic improvements in motion compensation may reduce this requirement in the future.

Pathological conditions in the lung result either in an increase or decrease in lung density. Atelectasis, fluid accumulation in the alveolar spaces and/or interstitium, and soft tissue masses increase density and can be detected because of the increased number of protons present [3]. Diseases resulting in decreased lung attenuation including air trapping, over-inflation, and lung destruction cause a decrease in proton density. Because the proton density of normal lung is so low, these entities are more difficult to detect. Recent improvements in image quality have clearly shown areas of air trapping as low signal areas on expiratory images. It is likely that areas of decreased density will be confidently identified on inspiratory images in the near future.

Pulmonary diseases resulting in alveolar filling are well depicted on MRI using T2/fluid sensitive sequences due to the localized increase in proton density. Examples include pneumonia, pulmonary edema, and less common entities such as alveolar proteinosis (Fig. 13.7). Early interstitial processes are not as conspicuous as those that cause alveolar filling [9]. Intravenous contrast can be used to characterize complications in the setting of pneumonia such as parenchymal abscess, necrosis/gangrene, and empyema.

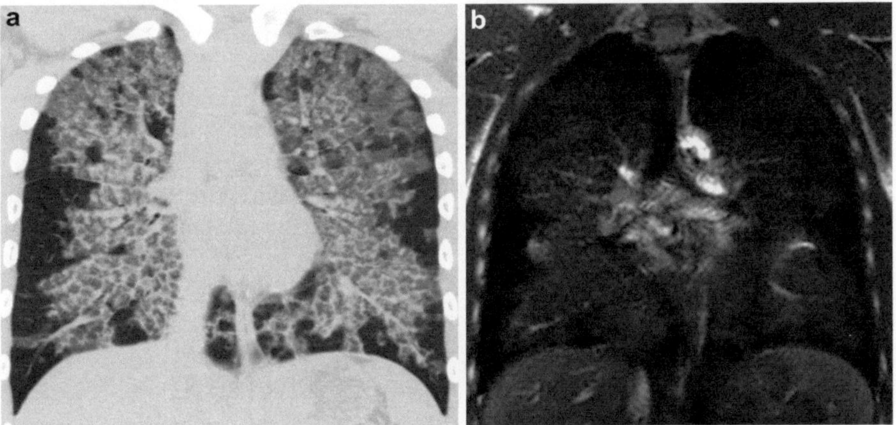

Fig. 13.7 The areas of alveolar proteinosis are well seen on this coronal CT image (**a**). An MRI image shows less detail, but the central abnormal lung can be easily distinguished from the peripheral areas of normal lung (**b**)

Using MR signal characteristics the composition of the material causing increased density can often be suggested. Fluid is easily distinguished from solid tissue. Hemorrhage has distinct patterns that relate to the acuity of the hemorrhage. Tissues with high cellularity have higher signal on water sensitive sequences than tissues that have a large fibrous or osseous component. The use of MRI contrast material can distinguish perfused from non-perfused tissue.

Imaging of the Soft Tissues of the Chest

Chest MRI is widely utilized for chest wall and mediastinal mass evaluation, especially when there is posterior mediastinal and/or paraspinal involvement. MRI is by far the imaging modality of choice when there is a concern for intraspinal involvement by a mass. MRI, after an initial plain radiograph, is also the modality of choice for the evaluation of suspected bone or cartilage abnormalities.

Cardiac Imaging

Cardiac imaging will only be mentioned briefly. Both CT scanning and MRI scanning can be used to provide morphologic and functional imaging of the heart and great vessels. Cardiac CT and MRI can both provide useful morphologic information, with CT providing better detail. Functional cardiac CT often requires a relatively high radiation dose, so MRI is often preferred when functional evaluation is required.

Vascular Imaging

Both CT and MRI can provide excellent imaging of the pulmonary or systemic arterial and venous systems. CT scanning provides higher resolution, and is the modality of choice for the assessment of pulmonary embolism, small bronchial arteries and the coronary arteries. When contrast material is contraindicated, MRI can produce high-quality vascular images using the MRI properties of non-opacified blood.

Cystic Fibrosis

Children with Cystic fibrosis may require frequent imaging and MRI is an attractive option in order to decrease cumulative radiation exposure. MRI is comparable to CT in detection of mucous plugging, central bronchiectasis, and consolidation. MRI can provide superior functional assessment of the lungs and vessels [2, 7, 22, 23].

The use of contrast material is currently being studied as a means to differentiate morphologic findings and to detect active inflammation and altered perfusion related to reflex hypoxic vasoconstriction. MRI is less accurate than CT in the detection of peripheral bronchiectasis and air trapping. CT scanning can be completed in seconds rather than tens of minutes, making the study much easier for the patient.

Pulmonary Neoplasms

Primary lung neoplasms are rare in children and there is scarce literature regarding the use of MRI in this setting [10]. Pulmonary metastases can be reliably diagnosed when larger than 3 mm in size [9, 25]. CT continues to be the gold standard for initial diagnosis with MR potentially being performed to evaluate metastatic disease during therapy.

Ultrasound

Ultrasound uses high frequency sound waves to generate images. It is a robust technique with exciting potential in the chest. No ionizing radiation is used and ultrasound machines are portable, facilitating bedside evaluation. Ultrasound can be used on essentially any patient in any setting. This is particularly useful for critically ill patients in the intensive care setting.

While commonly utilized for detection and characterization of pleural effusion and as guidance for percutaneous intervention, ultrasound is now being recognized as a method to identify parenchymal lung disease including pneumonia, interstitial lung disease, and pulmonary edema.

Normal Appearance

The normal lung shows a diffusely echogenic appearance. Normal lung has specific echogenic lines and the absence of other findings. The large difference in acoustic impedance between the normally aerated lung and adjacent pleura results in sound reflection and produces repeating posterior echoes (A lines). A lines appear as several well-separated thin transverse lines that parallel the pleural surface (Fig. 13.8a) "Comet tails" are lines that originate at the pleural surface and extend a variable distance into the lung, usually not to the deepest margin of the image The lung can be seen to move up and down relative to the chest wall at the pleural surface during normal respiration. This normal sliding motion of the lung is an important confirmation that the visceral and parietal pleura are contiguous.

Pleural Effusion

The pleural space is superficial to normally echogenic aerated lung and is well visualized by US. While pleural fluid collections are often suspected from radiography, US is more sensitive in detecting pleural fluid [12]. This is particularly true in the critically ill, in whom decubitus and upright radiography is not possible.

The appearance of pleural fluid is dependent on its composition and may range from anechoic (usually transudative) to collections with mobile echogenic debris (hemorrhage, infection), to septated or solid in appearance (empyema, organizing infection) (Fig. 13.9).

Simple, non-loculated pleural collections will change shape with changes in positioning or breathing. As infected pleural collections progress and organize, fibrinous strands form, initially mobile and thin, eventually maturing with

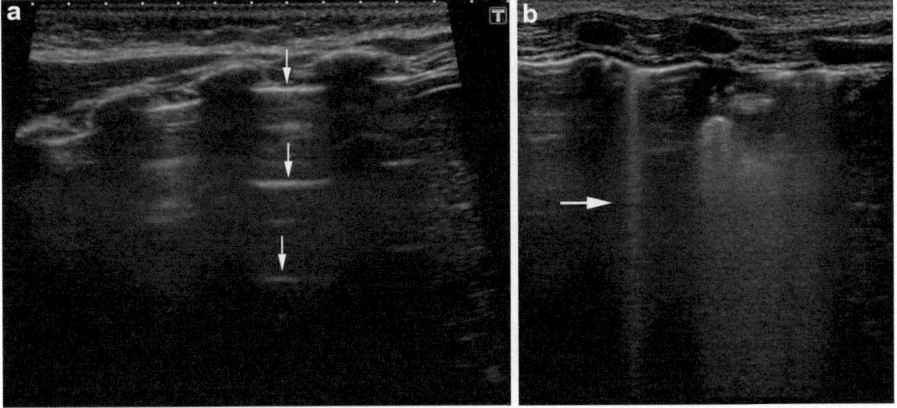

Fig. 13.8 (**a**) Ultrasound image of normal lung show multiple lines (*A lines*) that parallel the chest wall (*arrows*). (**b**) An image of a child with interstitial fluid shows a *thicker line* perpendicular to the chest wall (*B line*) that extends to the deepest part of the image (lung rocket)

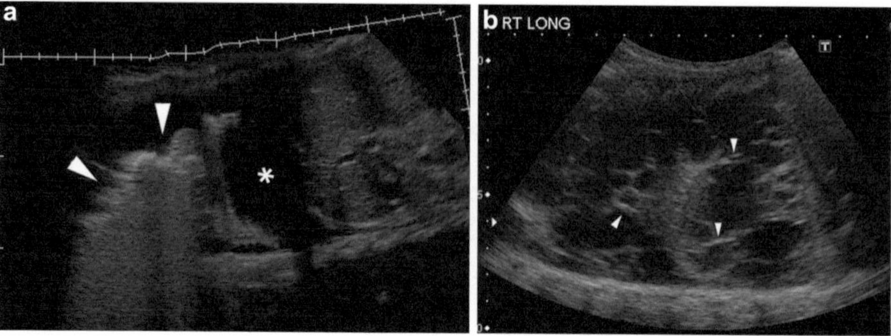

Fig. 13.9 (**a**) An ultrasound image of a simple pleural effusion shows anechoic fluid (*asterisk*) with dependent collapsed lung. (**b**) An image in a different patient with an empyema shows multiple echogenic bands throughout the pleural space (*arrowheads*). These bands cause loculation of the pleural fluid. Simple drainage is unlikely to evacuate this collection

progressive thickening and an increased number of strands resemble a honeycomb. Loculation and increase tenacity of the fluid results in fluid that does not change shape with changes in position and respiration. The pleural layers may thicken and infected pleural collections may eventually solidify into a homogenous echogenic mass encasing the lung (fibrothorax).

US has proven superior to CT in the characterization of pleural fluid collections and is very useful in guiding percutaneous drainage.

Pneumothorax

With air in the pleural space, the normal contact between the visceral and parietal pleura is lost and with it the normal transmission of sound into the lung. The sliding of the lung against the chest wall is no longer seen, and normally visualized artifacts are lost (comet tails). The margin of the air in the pleural space can be identified at the point where the normal features of the lung, particularly lung sliding are seen. This "lung point sign" increases confidence that a pneumothorax is present. A recent meta-analysis suggests a higher sensitivity and equivalent specificity of sonography for pneumothorax compared to radiography [6].

Parenchymal Consolidation

As alveolar gas is replaced by the products of disease it becomes sonographically visible due to changes in acoustic impedance in which it resembles hepatic parenchyma (hepatization). The internal architecture is preserved, allowing for differentiation from masses. Branching linear echoes can be seen representing gas within airways (air bronchograms) [11, 28]. Fluid or mucoid material trapped within bronchi in necrotizing or postobstructive pneumonias produces hypoechoic branching structures, the sonographic fluid bronchogram [16].

Parenchymal perfusion is preserved in simple pneumonic consolidation and is easily seen with color Doppler [16]. With atelectasis, air bronchograms are also present, with evidence of volume loss often with crowding of blood vessels resulting in a parallel orientation. Their orderly and linear branching pattern is preserved, allowing distinction from the irregular vasculature seen in neoplasms [29].

Studies have suggested that US can be more specific than radiography in distinguishing pneumonic consolidation from atelectasis. The presence of a "dynamic air bronchogram" (movement of the air within bronchi) usually indicates pneumonia whereas the air bronchograms in atelectasis are most often static [14].

In progressive lung infection, areas of parenchymal necrosis can develop. These are seen as hypoechoic areas within consolidated lung without color Doppler flow. As the area of necrosis enlarges a lung abscess forms often with a thick wall. With cavitation and communication with the airway, an air fluid level can be seen. US has been shown to be as accurate as CT in detecting complications of pneumonia (necrosis/abscess) [13].

Interstitial Lung Disease

Although aerated pulmonary parenchyma is not directly visualized with US the analysis of various artifacts produced from the surface of aerated lung can provide diagnostic information. The interaction of the sound beam with abnormal lung, likely due to thickening of the interlobular septa can produces the so called B lines (aka lung rockets). These lung rockets can be distinguished from comet tails by the deep extension of B lines to the deepest margin of the image (Fig. 13.8b). While a few B lines can be normal, multiple B lines can indicate pathology, which thickens the interlobular septa (edema, fibrosis, cellular infiltrate, etc.). B lines have been subdivided into B7 lines (7 mm apart), indicating thickened interlobular septa, and B3 lines (3 mm apart), indicating the equivalent of ground glass opacity seen at CT. The presence of B lines has been shown to correlate accurately with other imaging, pulmonary artery pressure, and fluid status [27].

Though experience in children is limited, surfactant deficiency disease produces variable appearances ranging from multiple B lines to a diffusely echogenic lung. It has been suggested that the progression of US findings from surfactant deficiency to BPD may appear earlier than chest radiographic findings.

Nuclear Medicine

Nuclear medicine offers a broad range of functional and metabolic imaging evaluations. Of particular interest to the pediatric pulmonologist are ventilation perfusion (V/Q) studies, positron emission tomography (PET) scanning, and radionuclide

GI studies including GE reflux, gastric emptying, and salivagrams for pulmonary aspiration. Radionuclide lung imaging most commonly involves the evaluation of pulmonary perfusion using Tc-99 m macroaggregated albumin (technetium 99 m MAA), which is trapped in the pulmonary capillaries. Only a small number of capillaries are blocked, so there is no impact on respiratory function. Ventilation is assessed using an inspired radioactive inert gas (usually Xenon) [17]. In a patient without other respiratory disease and clear lungs, the perfusion scan can be performed without the ventilation scan as any defects in perfusion are far more likely to be due to vascular occlusion, than due to decreased perfusion of an underventilated area without an infiltrate, or due to non-acute abnormality of the pulmonary vessels. This is particularly useful in younger children who cannot cooperate with breathing instructions and cannot reliably hold a mouthpiece tightly to maintain a closed system for the radioactive gas. In older children and in those with abnormal chest radiographs the diagnosis of PE is further confirmed by demonstrating a disassociation between ventilation and perfusion secondary to obstruction of segmental pulmonary artery blood flow by an embolus. MAA is unable to enter the capillary bed distal to the occlusion and thus appears as perfusion defect outlined by the adjacent normally perfused parenchyma. Because ventilation is generally unaffected, the ventilation images are normal in the same distribution. The most typical appearance of PE is as a wedge shaped perfusion defect with preserved ventilation, the segmental ventilation-perfusion mismatch [17]. While this principle is simple, great expertise is often needed to accurately interpret V/Q scans.

While data is sparse in pediatric patients regarding V/Q vs. CT pulmonary angiography V/Q studies in adults are highly sensitive and specific for pulmonary embolism with a reduced radiation exposure compared to CT. CTPA is more commonly performed due to widespread availability, rapid image acquisition, experience in image interpretation, and ability to evaluate for other causes of the patient's symptoms. In adults the "triple rule out," a CT scan to exclude pulmonary embolism, coronary artery disease, and aortic dissection is commonly performed. This should be discouraged in children in whom aortic and cardiac disease is extremely rare. At centers with available equipment and expertise, V/Q scans can be performed as the primary evaluation for PE in children. While V/Q scans have been criticized for frequent indeterminate results, these most commonly occur in the setting of underlying lung disease or focal parenchymal opacities, suggesting that V/Q scans may be particularly useful in children with normal chest radiographs. V/Q scans should be performed rather than CTPA in patients who have contrast allergies, renal failure, abnormal vasculature or cardiac physiology that might influence bolus timing, or who are too large for the CT-scanner gantry [17].

Perfusion scanning can also be used to determine the relative blood flow to different parts of the lungs. In patients with congenital anomalies, for example, the amount of function of a lung or lobe can be assessed. Percentage blood flow of similar areas of the right and left lung can be calculated.

Nuclear medicine studies can be useful in the evaluation of suspected aspiration. Aspiration can occur as a result of dysfunctional swallowing (usually diagnosed by fluoroscopy), food and/or acid in the stomach may be refluxed to the pharynx and aspirated, or aspiration of saliva may occur. Both GE reflux and gastric emptying can be assessed using orally administered liquid containing a radiotracer such as Tc-99 m. Gastric emptying can be measured at different time intervals and compared with normative data. Reflux can be observed over much longer periods of time than with fluoroscopy, and both the frequency and severity of reflux may be assessed. Aspiration of oral secretions is very difficult to identify. Radionuclide salivagrams can be used to detect aspiration of oral secretions, which is extremely difficult to detect otherwise. Salivagrams are moderately sensitive when performed in the appropriate patient populations (swallowing problems) [1]. The scan utilizes a small aliquot of Technetium-99 m sulfur colloid placed along the buccal mucosa or under the tongue with planar imaging subsequently performed while the patient is supine for 45 min to 1 h. Pulmonary aspiration is detected by visualizing radionuclide activity in the airway or lungs.

PET (positron emission tomography) is a recently developed, but now widely used imaging modality that provides functional evaluation of tissue by showing tissue localization of a specific marker. The most commonly used marker is fluorine isotope (^{18}F) containing fluorodeoxyglucose (^{18}F-FDG or FDG) which is a glucose analog. FDG is taken up by metabolically active cells, but cannot be metabolized and so remains within the cell. Accumulation of FDG on PET scans indicates the presence of metabolically highly active cells and is useful in both infection and neoplasms. The specific uptake value (SUV) indicates how much activity is present and can be useful in distinguishing different causes of increased uptake. PET is frequently combined with CT (PET-CT). Adding CT allows better estimation of the FDG uptake in tissue by measuring the overlying soft tissue, and improves the anatomic localization of abnormalities. The quality of these CT scans is lower than that of a standard CT scan because a lower dose technique is used. PET scanning takes many minutes and does not allow breath hold imaging, so images are obtained at resting lung volume, which further limits the images. It is important to understand that PET and especially PET-CT require a relatively high radiation dose, higher than for a standard CT.

Interventional Radiology

Image guided techniques offer a minimally invasive option for both diagnosis and treatment in a myriad of clinical settings. Expertise in pediatric interventional radiology varies between centers, and part of care planning involving interventional radiology should include a frank discussion of the complexity of the procedure and the experience of the interventional radiologist. A wide range of procedures are available to address different diseases, and new tools and procedures are continually being developed. A few of the more common procedures are presented here.

Pleural space interventions are the most common thoracic interventional procedures at most institutions. At sites with the necessary expertise, placement of small-caliber thoracostomy tubes has become the primary method of treating pleural effusions and pneumothoraces. Small-caliber thoracostomy tubes are less painful than larger surgical tubes and provide more accurate positioning when compared with tubes placed without image guidance [21, 24]. Guidance for these procedures is most commonly performed with ultrasonography. CT is useful when US is technically difficult and when multiple catheters are needed for multifocal and/or complex collections [26]. A combined approach can be used using ultrasound to access the pleural space followed by fluoroscopy to monitor the position of the guide wire and catheter within the pleural space. Two plane fluoroscopy, commonly used in interventional and cardiac catheterization suites, allows the fluoroscopy tube to be rotated around the patient to provide the optimum view of the area of abnormality. Seldinger technique is commonly used, where the target is entered with a needle and a guide wire is placed through the needle. Further instrumentation, either with dilators or drainage catheters is placed over the wire. In addition to evacuating pneumothoraces and draining simple pleural effusions, the guide wire can be used to disrupt loculations in complex effusions, allowing improved drainage. Fibrinolytic agents for treatment of loculated pleural fluid collections (most commonly complex parapneumonic effusions and empyema), can be easily delivered through the catheter. Sclerosing agents can be introduced into the pleural space for treatment of persistent or recurrent pleural collections including pleural effusions, chylothoraces, and pneumothoraces.

Biopsies of the lung, chest wall, and mediastinum can be performed less invasively by interventional radiology than by thoracotomy or thoracoscopy. Multiple biopsy techniques are available. Fine needle aspiration uses very thin needles, usually 18 G or less. These needles can be placed with minimal trauma including a much smaller risk of pneumothorax or bleeding when compared to larger needles. The limitation of this technique is that only a small amount of tissue can be obtained for pathologic evaluation. In addition, this technique disrupts the architecture of the lesion, providing groups of cells rather than a true tissue sample. This limits pathologic evaluation in many cases. Differentiating the type of "small blue cell" tumor, for example, is very difficult with fine needle aspiration samples. Unlike adults, a specific tissue diagnosis is usually required, and "small blue cell" tumors are common. This has limited the use fine needle aspiration in children. Core biopsies use larger needles, usually several millimeters in diameter. Core biopsies provide a larger sample and largely preserve the architecture of the sampled tissue. If additional tissue is required, multiple biopsies can be performed. Although more traumatic than a fine needle biopsy, core biopsies remain a safe and effective biopsy method.

Interventional radiology can also be used to localize difficult to identify sites for subsequent surgery. Parenchymal lung nodules can be difficult to identify at thoracotomy or thoracoscopy. A needle can be placed adjacent to a nodule and a hook type wire can be deployed or dye such as methylene blue injected with surgery performed immediately afterward to resect the nodule.

The use of diagnostic angiography has decreased due to the high quality images that can be obtained with CT angiography. Both conventional pulmonary angiography for pulmonary emboli and aortography to evaluate for traumatic aortic injury have been almost entirely replaced by CT. Catheter based angiography is now primarily performed as a therapeutic modality. Examples include embolization of bronchial arteries and intra-arterial pulmonary arterial thrombolysis.

New interventional equipment and techniques are developing at a rapid pace. These current examples will likely be joined by many new indications in the future.

Continuing dialogue between the direct care team and interventional radiologists will allow patients to benefit from continuing advances.

Which Test Should I Order?

Pneumonia

A CXR is usually all you need. A CT will almost never show consolidation sufficient to diagnose pneumonia if a CXR is normal. In complicated pneumonia, a contrast CT is the next step. Ultrasound can detect pneumonia, but has not been shown to add information on the parenchymal disease.

Pleural Effusion

CXRs are sensitive to very small amounts of pleural fluid, with blunting of the posterior costophrenic sulcus on lateral view, usually the earliest finding. Decubitus views will confirm a free flowing effusion by showing layering parallel to the ground. Ultrasound shows clear fluid in simple effusion and debris or septations in complex fluid. CT provides a better overview of the fluid, with medial and subpulmonic fluid in particular that is often difficult to detect on US.

Nodules

CT scanning is the test of choice. One contrast-enhanced CT scan makes sense to exclude mediastinal and hilar abnormalities, follow-up CTs can be done without contrast material. Contrast material is not useful in evaluating nodules in children, except in the very rare case when vascular lesions, such as AVMs are suspected. Cavitary nodules are also well evaluated with non-contrast CT.

There are no guidelines on how to follow up incidental nodules detected on CXR or CT. Adult guidelines have been specifically developed for patients over 35 years and cannot be extrapolated to children.

Cavitary Lesions

Even the worst looking cavities and necrotic lung will usually resolve without surgery, due to excellent blood supply and drainage. A contrast enhanced CT scan early in the course allows comprehensive evaluation. Progression can be monitored with chest radiographs. CTs performed to evaluate complications should also be performed with contrast.

Congenital Lung Lesions

Either contrast enhanced CT or contrast enhanced MRI can be used. CT scanning provides a better evaluation of the rest of the lung. Because it is important to identify any feeding or draining vessels, intravenous contrast should be used. These vessels may originate or terminate in the upper abdomen and including the upper abdomen when performing the chest CT scan should be considered.

Diffuse Lung Disease

Noncontrast CT is the primary modality. Expiratory images are used to show air trapping and have been regarded as an important component of HRCT. In CF and suspected bronchiolitis obliterans, expiratory images remain an important part of CT evaluation. In most other diseases, the presence or absence of air trapping is not of primary importance. Some sites use ventilation control, usually with general anesthesia, to obtain images at full inspiration and at approximately FRC. A thin section CT, which can be obtained on any current CT scanner, can be performed without sedation during quiet breathing. Image quality is not quite as good, but the difference does not usually limit the ability to make a diagnosis.

Bronchiectasis

Noncontrast CT is the modality of choice, with no other modality approaching CT in the identification and characterization of bronchiectasis. Expiratory images are not required to evaluate bronchiectasis.

Suspected Vascular Abnormality

Contrast CT shows vascular lesions well and also provides a full evaluation of the lung parenchyma. MRI can also show vascular lesions, and better defines the chest wall, but lung evaluation is limited. Most lesions are well seen without the use of CT angiography, but complex vascular lesions may be better evaluated with CT angiography.

Mediastinal Abnormalities

Contrast CT and MRI with or without contrast can be used. If lung information is important, do CT. If soft tissue characterization is important, do MRI.

A Few Final Tips on CXRs and CTs

CXRs

CXRs do not provide the detail of CT, but there is much useful anatomic information (Fig. 13.10) Low lung volumes make the lungs dense and often heterogeneous due to crowding of normal vessels. On the other hand, well expanded lungs with

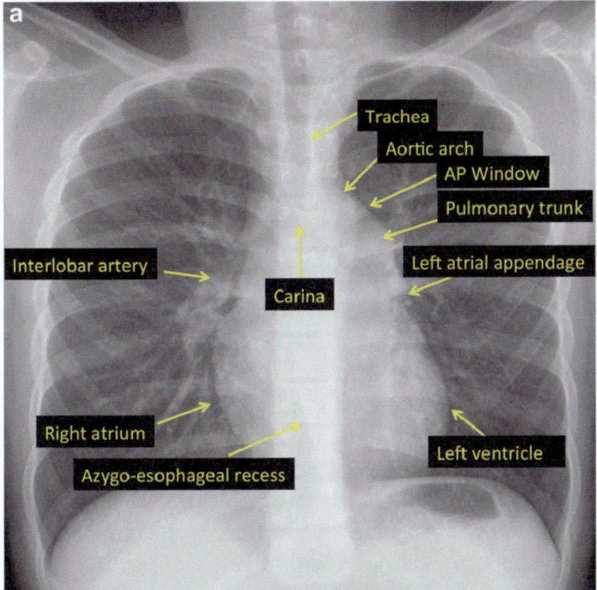

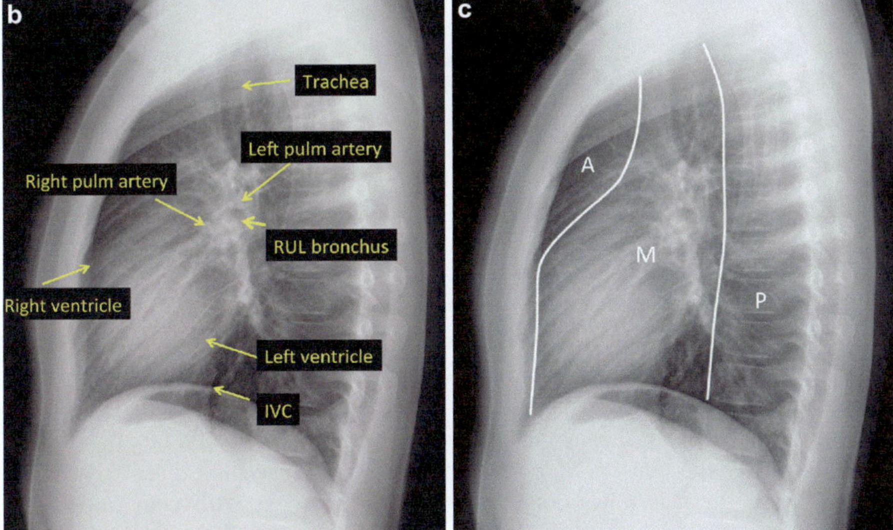

Fig. 13.10 Normal structures are labeled on a frontal (**a**) and lateral (**b**) CXR. The mediastinal divisions, anterior (*A*), middle (*M*), and posterior (*P*), which are useful in suggesting the etiology of a mediastinal abnormality, are shown on this lateral CXR (**c**)

marked peribronchial thickening or increased vascularity can look like an expiratory film. Evaluate the lung volume by counting anterior ribs. The sixth anterior rib should be the first to cross the diaphragm. Below five ribs is low volume, over seven ribs is high volume. In between it is a judgment call. This method is not perfect, but it is easy and it probably works as well as any.

The medial right middle lobe has been called "the fool's triangle." Vessels from the inferior hilum cause increased density and the heart obscures this area on the left so right to left comparison is impossible. Two tricks for evaluating this area are to look at the lateral for any abnormality in the right lung base. If necessary, a left side down decubitus CXR will hyperinflate this area and make artifactual density go away.

In infants and young toddlers up to about 2 years old, superior mediastinal masses are almost always due to a prominent or unusually shaped thymus. The thymus is soft so it is indented by the anterior rib ends at its periphery on frontal CXR. It is also denser anteriorly and gradually decreases in density posteriorly on lateral views which is unusual for pneumonia. Remember that the thymus is soft, so compression of airways or vessels should strongly suggest that the "mass" in question is a mass and not the thymus. Ultrasound is a good way to confirm that a "mass" is actually thymus. CT and MR are also excellent, but US is quick and less expensive.

Pneumonias in the posterior lung bases can be hard to see. The posterior lung base extends well below the diaphragm on frontal view. Look for a change in density over the spine on lateral view. The spine should become increasingly dark moving from the upper thoracic spine to the lung bases. Any vertebral body that is denser than the one above suggests the possibility of a superimposed infiltrate.

Everyone forgets how to name decubitus films. They are named for the side that is down, but do not worry about it. Order "left side down decubitus or "right side up decubitus" and you will get the same, and hopefully the correct film. If you want to see an effusion layer, put that side down. If you want to see a pneumothorax, or hyperinflate the lung, put that side up.

CT

The anatomic detail seen on CT is similar to that seen on gross anatomic sections. Figure 13.11 shows some of the structures that can be identified. Atlases are available that show detailed annotations of bronchial and vascular branching as well as mediastinal anatomy [18].

A high-resolution chest CT (HRCT) is a misnomer. It is not a more detailed CT. It is a technique that was developed when it was not possible to scan the entire chest with the thin sections that are needed to best evaluate the lung parenchyma. A typical HRCT scan images 1 mm then skips 10 mm and repeats this through the chest. That means that an almost 9 mm nodule could be missed. Use HRCT scans of the chest ONLY when evaluating diffuse lung disease, where a missed focal lesion is not a concern. Better yet, discuss with your radiologist prior to performing the image. Current techniques have made true HRCT of the chest nearly obsolete at many centers.

Should I get my CT with and without contrast? You should order one or the other, not both. For parenchyma evaluations, only choose non-contrast. For evaluation of soft tissues or vessels, choose contrast. Very subtle calcifications can be missed with contrast, but it is almost always possible to distinguish contrast enhancement from calcification.

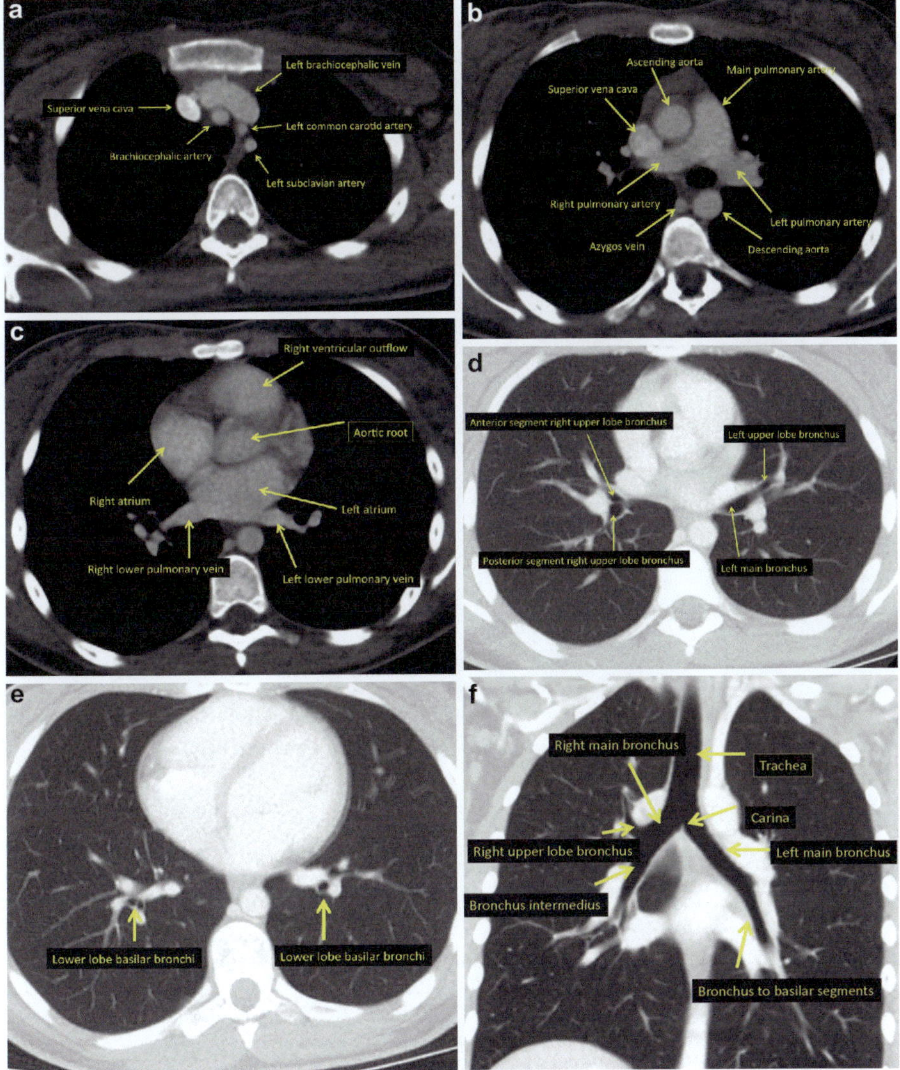

Fig. 13.11 Normal structures seen on axial (**a–e**), coronal (**f, g**), and sagittal (**h, i**) CT images

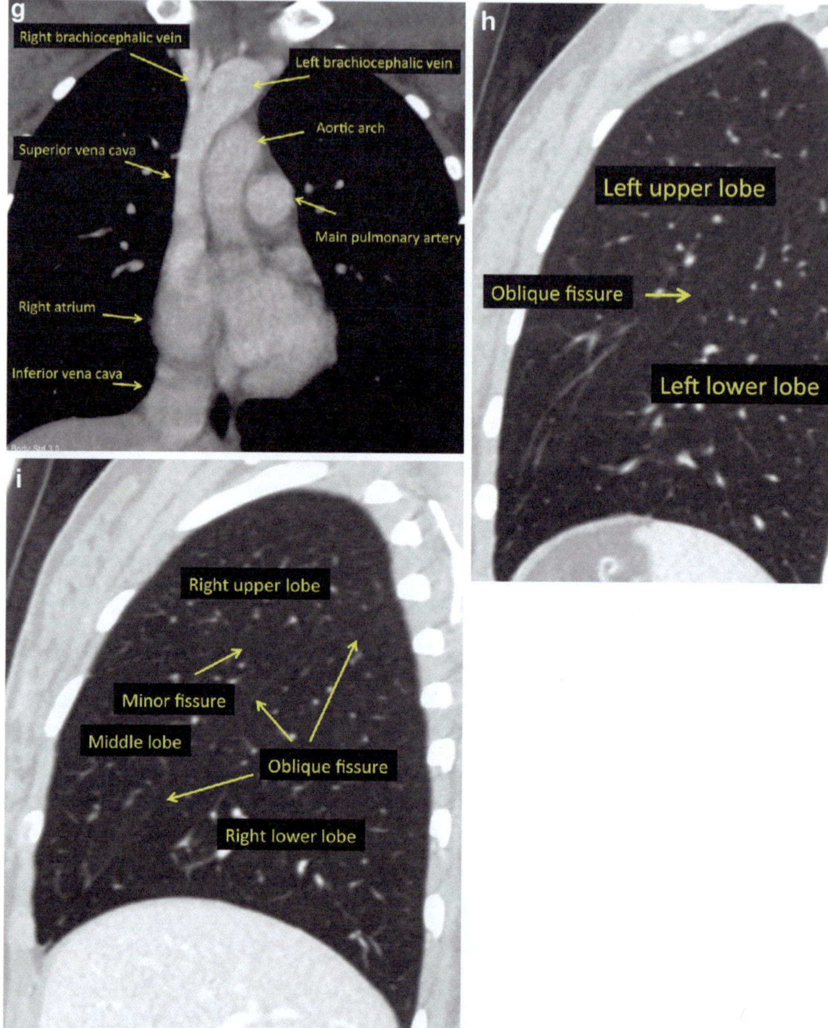

Fig. 13.11 (continued)

References

1. Akbunar AT, Kiristioglu I, Alper E, Demiray H. Diagnosis of orotracheal aspiration using radionuclide salivagram. Ann Nucl Med. 2003;17(5):415–6.
2. Bauer R, Atke A, Danielsen E, Marcussen J, Olsen CE, Rehfeld J, et al. The potential of perturbed angular correlation of gamma rays as a tool for dynamic studies of peptides/proteins. Int J Rad Appl Instrum A. 1991;42(11):1015–23.
3. Biederer J, Beer M, Hirsch W, Wild J, Fabel M, Puderbach M, et al. MRI of the lung (2/3). Why … when … how? Insights Imaging. 2012;3(4):355–71.

4. Brenner D, Elliston C, Hall E, Berdon W. Estimated risks of radiation-induced fatal cancer from pediatric CT. AJR Am J Roentgenol. 2001;176(2):289–96.
5. Cohen MD. Choosing contrast media for the evaluation of the gastrointestinal tract of neonates and infants. Radiology. 1987;162(2):447–56.
6. Ding W, Shen Y, Yang J, He X, Zhang M. Diagnosis of pneumothorax by radiography and ultrasonography: a meta-analysis. Chest. 2011;140(4):859–66.
7. Failo R, Wielopolski PA, Tiddens HA, Hop WC, Mucelli RP, Lequin MH. Lung morphology assessment using MRI: a robust ultra-short TR/TE 2D steady state free precession sequence used in cystic fibrosis patients. Magn Reson Med. 2009;61(2):299–306.
8. Friedman BI, Hartenberg MA, Mulroy JJ, Tong TK, Mickell JJ. Gastrografin aspiration in a 3 3/4-year-old girl. Pediatr Radiol. 1986;16(6):506–7.
9. Gorkem SB, Coskun A, Yikilmaz A, Zurakowski D, Mulkern RV, Lee EY. Evaluation of pediatric thoracic disorders: comparison of unenhanced fast-imaging-sequence 1.5-T MRI and contrast-enhanced MDCT. AJR Am J Roentgenol. 2013;200(6):1352–7.
10. Hirsch W, Sorge I, Krohmer S, Weber D, Meier K, Till H. MRI of the lungs in children. Eur J Radiol. 2008;68(2):278–88. Epub 2008/09/06.
11. Iuri D, De Candia A, Bazzocchi M. Evaluation of the lung in children with suspected pneumonia: usefulness of ultrasonography. Radiol Med. 2009;114(2):321–30.
12. Kocijancic I, Vidmar K, Ivanovi-Herceg Z. Chest sonography versus lateral decubitus radiography in the diagnosis of small pleural effusions. J Clin Ultrasound. 2003;31(2):69–74. Epub 2003/01/23.
13. Kurian J, Levin TL, Han BK, Taragin BH, Weinstein S. Comparison of ultrasound and CT in the evaluation of pneumonia complicated by parapneumonic effusion in children. AJR Am J Roentgenol. 2009;193(6):1648–54.
14. Lichtenstein D, Meziere G, Seitz J. The dynamic air bronchogram. A lung ultrasound sign of alveolar consolidation ruling out atelectasis. Chest. 2009;135(6):1421–5.
15. Mathews JD, Forsythe AV, Brady Z, Butler MW, Goergen SK, Byrnes GB, et al. Cancer risk in 680,000 people exposed to computed tomography scans in childhood or adolescence: data linkage study of 11 million Australians. BMJ. 2013;346:f2360.
16. Mathis G. Thoraxsonography–part II: peripheral pulmonary consolidation. Ultrasound Med Biol. 1997;23(8):1141–53. Epub 1997/01/01.
17. Mettler FA, Guiberteau MJ. Essentials of nuclear medicine imaging. Philadelphia, PA: Saunders/Elsevier; 2006.
18. Naidich DP. Computed tomography and magnetic resonance of the thorax, vol. xi. 3rd ed. Philadelphia, PA: Lippincott-Raven; 1999. p. 772.
19. Newman B, Krane EJ, Gawande R, Holmes TH, Robinson TE. Chest CT in children: anesthesia and atelectasis. Pediatr Radiol. 2014;44(2):164–72.
20. Pearce MS, Salotti JA, Little MP, McHugh K, Lee C, Kim KP, et al. Radiation exposure from CT scans in childhood and subsequent risk of leukaemia and brain tumours: a retrospective cohort study. Lancet. 2012;380(9840):499–505.
21. Protic A, Barkovic I, Bralic M, Cicvaric T, Stifter S, Sustic A. Targeted wire-guided chest tube placement: a cadaver study. Eur J Emerg Med. 2010;17(3):146–9.
22. Puderbach M, Eichinger M, Gahr J, Ley S, Tuengerthal S, Schmahl A, et al. Proton MRI appearance of cystic fibrosis: comparison to CT. Eur Radiol. 2007;17(3):716–24.
23. Puderbach M, Eichinger M, Haeselbarth J, Ley S, Kopp-Schneider A, Tuengerthal S, et al. Assessment of morphological MRI for pulmonary changes in cystic fibrosis (CF) patients: comparison to thin-section CT and chest X-ray. Invest Radiol. 2007;42(10):715–25.
24. Rahman NM, Maskell NA, Davies CW, Hedley EL, Nunn AJ, Gleeson FV, et al. The relationship between chest tube size and clinical outcome in pleural infection. Chest. 2010;137(3):536–43.
25. Schroeder T, Ruehm SG, Debatin JF, Ladd ME, Barkhausen J, Goehde SC. Detection of pulmonary nodules using a 2D HASTE MR sequence: comparison with MDCT. AJR Am J Roentgenol. 2005;185(4):979–84. Epub 2005/09/24.

26. Sopko DR, Smith TP. Bronchial artery embolization for hemoptysis. Semin Intervent Radiol. 2011;28(1):48–62.
27. Volpicelli G, Silva F, Radeos M. Real-time lung ultrasound for the diagnosis of alveolar consolidation and interstitial syndrome in the emergency department. Eur J Emerg Med. 2010;17(2):63–72. Epub 2010/10/15.
28. Weinberg B, Diakoumakis EE, Kass EG, Seife B, Zvi ZB. The air bronchogram: sonographic demonstration. AJR Am J Roentgenol. 1986;147(3):593–5.
29. Yang P. Applications of colour Doppler ultrasound in the diagnosis of chest diseases. Respirology. 1997;2(3):231–8. Epub 1997/12/24.

Chapter 14
Fractional Exhaled Nitric Oxide: Indications and Interpretation

Young-Jee Kim, Carolyn M. Kercsmar, and Stephanie D. Davis

Abstract Exhaled nitric oxide (NO) is a marker for eosinophilic airway inflammation. The correlations between fraction of exhaled NO (FE_{NO}) and eosinophils in blood, sputum, bronchoalveolar lavage, and mucosal biopsies of the airway have been well studied. A quantitative, noninvasive, and simple methodology has been developed to determine how best to assess FE_{NO} as a measure of airway inflammation. FE_{NO} measurement has been standardized by the American Thoracic Society/European Respiratory Society (Am J Respir Crit Care Med 171(8):912–930, 2005). The gold standard for measuring FE_{NO} is the single-breath online method, which can be performed in young children from the age of 4–5 years. A chemiluminescence-based analyzer or a portable analyzer using an electrochemical sensor can be used to measure FE_{NO}. Many studies have shown that FE_{NO} has potential diagnostic and therapeutic roles in various respiratory diseases, particularly asthma. In asthma, FE_{NO} is useful to diagnose and monitor eosinophilic airway inflammation, and predict steroid responsiveness. It also can be helpful in supporting the diagnosis of asthma and in guiding adjustment of anti-inflammatory medication. ATS Clinical Practice Guidelines have been published for interpretation and clinical applicability of FE_{NO} (Dweik et al., 184(5):602–615, 2011). FE_{NO} can provide additional information on underlying airway inflammation, and is complementary to respiratory symptoms, lung function tests, and bronchial provocation tests for asthma and other respiratory diseases in the clinical setting.

Keywords Exhaled nitric oxide • FE_{NO} fraction of exhaled nitric oxide • Children • Asthma

Y.-J. Kim, M.D. (✉) • S.D. Davis, M.D.
Section of Pediatric Pulmonology, Allergy and Sleep Medicine, Riley Hospital for Children, Indiana University School of Medicine, 705 Riley Hospital Drive, ROC 4270, Indianapolis, IN 46202, USA
e-mail: yk3@iu.edu

C.M. Kercsmar, M.S., M.D.
Pediatrics, Asthma Center, Cincinnati Children's Hospital Medical Center, 3333 Burnet Ave, MLC 2021, Cincinnati, OH 45229, USA

© Springer Science+Business Media New York 2015
S.D. Davis et al. (eds.), *Diagnostic Tests in Pediatric Pulmonology*, Respiratory Medicine, DOI 10.1007/978-1-4939-1801-0_14

Introduction

Nitric oxide (NO) is an important endogenous regulatory molecule and has numerous physiologic roles in the respiratory system [1]. NO is present in the exhaled breath and has been recognized as biomarker for airway inflammation. The measurement of the fraction of exhaled NO concentration (FE_{NO}) has been used in various clinical conditions, and has become particularly valued in asthma. In asthma, FE_{NO} is used as a surrogate measure of eosinophilic inflammation and is suitable for serial monitoring of airway inflammation due to its noninvasive nature and ease of repeat measurements. The measurement of FE_{NO} is especially appealing in children who have difficulties with other routine tests, such as spirometry.

A joint statement of the American Thoracic Society (ATS) and European Respiratory Society (ERS) recommended standardized procedures for measurement of exhaled lower respiratory NO and nasal NO in 2005 [2]. This 2005 statement was a revision and update of the 1999 ATS exhaled and nasal NO recommendations [3]; an ATS workshop proceedings was also published in 2006 [4]. More recently, ATS published the Clinical Practice Guidelines describing how best to use FE_{NO} measurements and interpret results [5]. Pediatric FE_{NO} measurements were reviewed in an ERS/ATS statement [6] and many studies have been published; however, information on FE_{NO} in children is still limited.

Physiological Background

NO is an endogenous regulatory molecule in humans. This gaseous molecule is produced by various resident and inflammatory cells in the airways and alveoli such as airway epithelial cells, airway and circulatory endothelial cells, and trafficking inflammatory cells, and the physiologic roles of NO in the respiratory system are numerous including neurotransmission, vasodilatation, bronchial dilatation, and immune augmentation [1]. When NO is formed in airway tissues, it can diffuse into the airway lumen, thereby allowing this molecule to be detected in the exhaled breath. The synthesis of NO is mediated by NO synthases (NOS). One of NOS isoenzymes is inducible NOS (iNOS) which is not expressed constitutively but is induced by inflammatory stimuli [1]. Only the expression of iNOS in bronchial epithelial cells correlates with FE_{NO} [7]. FE_{NO} correlates with eosinophilic inflammation of the airways, and has been validated against invasive measurements of eosinophilic inflammation, including sputum, bronchoalveolar lavage, bronchial biopsy, and blood [8–14].

Technical Background

A FE_{NO} analyzer was first approved by the FDA in June 2003 for monitoring asthma. This chemiluminescence-based analyzer is based on a photochemical reaction between NO and ozone, and is sensitive and specific for NO. FE_{NO} is measured in parts per billion (ppb). This analyzer has been the one most widely used for many studies. However, the use of this analyzer is restricted by expense and the bulkiness of this large equipment dictates that it must be stationary requiring on-site calibration. With technologic advances, portable, less expensive, smaller, and simple devices have been produced. The handheld device uses an electrochemical sensor to determine the partial pressure and concentration of NO [15]. The measurements of FE_{NO} with handheld devices are comparable to stationary devices [16–18], although the difference between analyzers becomes greater at higher FE_{NO} level [18]. The results of FE_{NO} measurements are reproducible even in young children and the success rate improves significantly with age from 40 % in children 4 years old to very high up to almost 100 % at school age children [19, 20].

FE_{NO} can be measured either online (immediate, real-time, direct sampling of the exhaled breath) or off line (collection of exhaled breath into a reservoir for later analysis). Online measurement was recommended and updated by the ATS/ERS joint statement [2]. Measurement issues (exhalation flow rate, means of controlling flow, airway pressure, FE_{NO} plateau definitions, number of required exhalations, inhalation phase, calibration gases, and normal range of FE_{NO} values) were later revised by an ATS workshop in 2006 [4].

Online measurements are made by a slow, flow-controlled steady exhalation from total lung capacity (TLC) after inspiring NO-free air (<5 ppb). The subject should exhale immediately after inspiring to TLC to avoid a breath-hold. The subject must maintain a constant expiratory flow rate at 50 ml/s during an exhalation of at least 4 s for children <12 years and at least 6 s for children >12 years and adults [2]. During an exhalation, an NO plateau for 3 s is identified [2]. Since FE_{NO} levels are strongly flow dependent [21–23], maintaining a constant expiratory flow during the measurement is important. Biofeedback signals have been used to help children perform constant-flow expiratory maneuvers [2, 6]. An expiratory flow rate at 50 ml/s, at which NO output is derived mainly from airway NO diffusion [24], is recommended by the guidelines [2, 6]. The exhalation is made against a resistance of 5–20 cm H_2O [2, 6] to ensure velum closure and to avoid contamination from the nose and sinuses since the NO concentration of the upper airway is more than 100 times higher when compared to lower airways [25]. Repeated exhalation (three measurements that agree within 10 % or two within 5 %) should be performed with at least 30 s intervals between measurements, and a mean value of FE_{NO} is recorded [2, 6].

Online single-breath techniques of measuring exhaled NO may not be successful in the preschool aged child. Different modified methods such as flow-driven method [26], automatic controlled flow method [27], and controlled tidal breathing method [28] were proposed for better success rate in these younger children.

Off line techniques, with or without exhalation flow control, can be used to measure FE_{NO}. This technique is useful for epidemiological studies and for monitoring levels at home or school [2, 6]. However, variability in the FE_{NO} levels may occur due to difficulties in maintaining a stable expiratory flow rate, and possible contamination by ambient and/or nasal NO.

FE_{NO} can be measured in infants and several studies have been published by both single-breath and tidal breathing methods [29–35]. The raised volume rapid thoracic compression technique was used in single-breath FE_{NO} measurement method, but various expiratory flows were used in the studies. FE_{NO} levels are flow dependent and FE_{NO} level at low flow (11 ml/s) is consistently higher than the level at higher flow (40 ml/s) [35]. Tidal breathing techniques [32–35] might be easier than raised volume rapid thoracic compression technique, and can be used for both online and offline FE_{NO} measurements, but there is no standardized method protocol. In addition, the single-breath method is better than the tidal breathing method in discriminating healthy infants from infants with recurrent wheezing [35]. The limitations of these approaches are requirements of sedation, specialized equipment, possible nasal NO contamination, or the potential effect of ambient NO. However, the difference between nasal and oral FE_{NO} does not appear to be significant [33]. Although nasal FE_{NO} increases with age, there is no association between age and the magnitude of the difference between nasal and oral FE_{NO}, and this finding suggests both nasal and oral FE_{NO} reflecting mixed FE_{NO} [33]. There is a significant difference in FE_{NO} collected while awake and when sedated [33]. FE_{NO} is lower when sedated compared to unsedated, and the intrasubject variation for FE_{NO} is less when asleep. In order to avoid the effect of ambient NO, breathing NO free or scrubbed air during the study is recommended, particularly when ambient NO is above 5 ppb [2].

Measurement of FE_{NO} at multiple flow rates can provide information on alveolar NO concentration (C_{alv}) and bronchial NO flux (J_{NO}), based on the two compartment model proposed by Tsoukias and George [36]. The model divided lung into alveolar (respiratory bronchioles and alveoli) and bronchial (conducting airway) compartments. J_{NO} is described as the quantity of NO transferred from bronchial wall to luminal air per unit time. It depends on NO diffusing capacity of the bronchial wall, and on NO concentration difference between bronchial wall and luminal air that drives the diffusion. FE_{NO} measurement at 50 ml/s mainly reflects NO output in the large central airways, but is not sensitive for possible changes in the lung periphery. Increased J_{NO} with normal C_{alv} has been found in steroid-naïve adults with newly diagnosed asthma [37, 38], while C_{alv} is elevated in newly diagnosed steroid-naïve asthmatic adults with nocturnal symptoms than healthy controls or asthmatic patients without nocturnal symptoms [39]. Measurement of C_{alv} and J_{NO} can be done in children [40–44] although the method is not fully standardized yet. FE_{NO}, C_{alv}, and J_{NO} are all elevated in asthmatic children, compared to normal control [41]. Children with poorly controlled asthma have even higher values of C_{alv} and J_{NO} than children with good symptom control [41]. However, FE_{NO} and J_{NO} are also elevated in non-asthmatic atopic children, and fail to differentiate asthma and atopy. Unlike FE_{NO} and J_{NO}, C_{alv} is elevated only in asthmatics, while no difference in C_{alv} was noted between non-asthmatic atopic children and healthy controls [41]. Therefore, C_{alv} can be considered as a diagnostic or monitoring marker of alveolar inflammation in asthma.

Interpretation

Normal Range of FE$_{NO}$ Values

Many publications have reported reference values of FE$_{NO}$ for children, and more recent publications on reference values in healthy children are listed in Table 14.1 [19, 45–50]. Asian children have higher reference values [48–50] compared to other published values in Caucasian children. However, there is clearly considerable overlap between FE$_{NO}$ levels in healthy and populations with stable asthma [5]. In addition, multiple confounding factors such as measurement technique, exhalation flow rate, the NO analyzer used, current respiratory symptoms, prior diagnosis of airway disease, and other factors listed as follows in this section may affect FE$_{NO}$. The interpretation of FE$_{NO}$ for an individual patient must take into consideration the clinical status (symptoms, prior diagnoses, age, ethnicity, sex) when the measurement is obtained. Therefore, the ATS guidelines suggested the clinical decision cut points rather than reference values to be used in the interpretation of elevated or reduced FE$_{NO}$ value, and strongly recommended accounting for age as a factor affecting FE$_{NO}$ in children <12 years of age [5].

Table 14.1 Studies of FE$_{NO}$ reference values in healthy children

Author and year (reference)	Number	Age range (years)	Race/ ethnicity	Reference values (ppb)	Analyzer
See 2013 [45]	17,249 (2,519 at 6–11 years of age)	6–80	Hispanic, White, Black, and other	5th–95th percentile 3.5–39 (3.5–36.5 for 6–11 year of age)	NIOX MINO (Aerocrine AB, Sweden)
Kovesi 2008 [47, 48]	657	9–12	White, Asian, African	Mean 12.7 for White (22.8 for Asian)	Echo Physics CDL 88sp (Eco Medics AG, Switzerland)
Malmberg 2006 [46]	114	7–15	Caucasian	Range 7–14	NIOX (Aerocrine AB, Sweden)
Burchvald 2005 [19]	405 (332[a])	4–17	Caucasian, Black, Asian, Hispanic	Mean 9.7 (8.8[a])	NIOX (Aerocrine AB, Sweden)
Wong 2005 [50]	291	11–18	Chinese, Caucasian	Median 17 male, 10.8 female for Chinese (11.6 male, 9.1 female for Caucasian)	NIOX (Aerocrine AB, Sweden)
Saito 2004 [49]	176	10–12	Japanese	Mean 15.3	Model 280i (Sievers, USA)

ppb Parts per billion
[a]Subjects without outliers and atopics

While approximately 10 % or up to 4 ppb has been considered as the within-subject variation in healthy subjects [51, 52], higher variation to more than 20 % was noted in subjects with asthma [20, 51]. Therefore, at least a 20 % change is considered a significant rise or fall in FE_{NO} over time or following an intervention [5].

Factors Affecting FE_{NO} Values

ATS/ERS guidelines should be followed carefully to obtain accurate and reproducible measurements [2].

Age, Anthropometric Factors, Sex, Race

In children, FE_{NO} is age dependent [19, 45, 48] with an increase of about 5 % or 1 ppb/year [19, 48]. Besides age, height, body mass index (BMI), gender, and race can affect FE_{NO}. FE_{NO} has been shown to have a positive correlation with height [45, 46, 48], and a negative relationship with BMI [45]. However, no significant correlation with height, weight, BMI, or body surface area is noted after adjusting for gender [50] and another study using BMI z score, which is age-independent and sex-independent, also shows no correlation between BMI and FE_{NO} [53]. Males tend to have higher FE_{NO} than females [8, 45, 50]. Non-white population, particularly Asians, have higher FE_{NO} [45, 48, 50].

Diet

FE_{NO} can be increased by ingestion of nitrate-rich L-arginine containing foods, such as lettuce, spinach, ham, cucumber, potato, and tomato [54, 55]. FE_{NO} increases steadily after nitrate or nitrate-rich food ingestion with a maximum at 120 min, and then decline. However, FE_{NO} at 3 h after ingestion still remains higher than the baseline prior to ingestion [54, 55]. Therefore, nitrate-rich diet should be avoided in 3 h before the measurement. Dietary intake of fats such as butter has a positive correlation with FE_{NO}, while consumption of salad, one of the major sources of antioxidants, is found to be negatively associated with FE_{NO} level [56]. FE_{NO} decreases with drinking water 5–20 s before exhalation maneuver, and water temperature does not affect this effect [57]. FE_{NO} decreases significantly in the first hour after coffee or caffeine consumption, and this drop remains consistently for 4 h after consumption compared to the placebo [58]. Alcohol also decreases FE_{NO} in asthmatic subjects but not in normal individuals [59]. Previously refraining from eating and drinking for 1 h before FE_{NO} measurement is recommended by ATS/ERS [2], but longer hours of refraining might be needed to avoid the dietary effect.

Medications

Many medications can affect FE_{NO} level. Oral or intravenous L-arginine has been shown to increase FE_{NO} in healthy adults [60, 61], but a recent study did not show a significant increase in FE_{NO} after oral arginine administration regardless of history of allergy [62], at the same dose studied in the previous study [60]. The nitrite-reducing conditions in the oral cavity by using antibacterial mouthwash such as chlorhexidine acetate or sodium bicarbonate reduce FE_{NO} [55, 63]. Inhaled and oral corticosteroid reduce FE_{NO} in asthma [32, 64–66] and leukotriene receptor antagonist such as montelukast also decreases FE_{NO} [67]. However, nedocromil does not reduce FE_{NO} in asthmatic children [66]. Omalizumab decreases FE_{NO} and the degree of inhibition of FE_{NO} is similar to that seen for inhaled steroid alone [68]. Bronchodilators like beta-agonists have been shown to increase FE_{NO} in asthmatics [67, 69–71] while low-dose theophylline does not affect FE_{NO} in mild asthma despite reducing eosinophilic inflammation [72]. Bronchoconstriction by methacholine decreases FE_{NO} in healthy volunteers [70]. However, no significant fall in FE_{NO} is observed after allergen or isocapnic cold air challenge in atopic asthma [73]. The reason for these changes is not clear but is believed to be due to neural mechanisms leading to increase in NO release from lower airways or mechanical effect on airway caliber.

Smoking

Cigarette smoking has been shown to reduce FE_{NO} both acutely and on long-term basis [74, 75]. FE_{NO} is also reduced with passive smoke exposure both in adults [45, 76] and in early infancy [34, 77, 78] and school age children [45]. Infants exposed pre- and postnatally to smoke show lower FE_{NO} than infants exposed only after birth and never-exposed infants [77]. However, this is not the case in infants of mother with atopy or asthma, and FE_{NO} increase [78]. Another study done in young children with mean age 51.3 weeks [79] has a different result, showing higher FE_{NO} with exposure to parental smoking. A dose–response relationship between FE_{NO} and the number of smoking parents is also noted [79]. This discrepancy in result could be related to differences in age of subjects, duration of passive smoking exposure, and prenatal environmental factors such as maternal smoking and atopy.

Respiratory Maneuvers and Exercise

Spirometric maneuvers have been shown to transiently reduce FE_{NO} [69, 71, 73, 80, 81], as early as 1 min after spirometry and FE_{NO} returned to baseline over 1 h. It is important to obtain FE_{NO} consistently prior to spirometry. However, FE_{NO} maneuver itself and body plethysmography do not appear to affect plateau FE_{NO} level [69, 81]. Reduction in FE_{NO} with spirometry is blunted by bronchoprovocation with isocapnic cold air hyperventilation or allergen [73]. FE_{NO} is reduced after sputum induction [82, 83]. However, this change occurs with sputum induction by hypertonic saline, not by isotonic saline, and the decreased FE_{NO} is observed over 4 h and returns to baseline after 24 h [83]. A change in FE_{NO} occurs with exercise, and the largest drop in FE_{NO} is noted at 5 min after exercise [80]. Therefore, ATS/ERS recommends avoiding strenuous exercise for 1 h before the measurement [2].

Circadian Rhythm and Seasonal Variation

The effect of circadian rhythm on FE_{NO} is not conclusive. No variation is shown in healthy and asthmatic adults and children as well as infants [52, 84–86] while other studies report the morning levels higher than the evening levels in asthmatic and healthy children [20, 87]. The opposite finding in circadian variation is also noted with FE_{NO} at 4 pm higher than FE_{NO} at 4 am in nocturnal asthma [86]. If possible, it is ideal to perform serial measurements of FE_{NO} in the same period of the day to avoid the effects of circadian rhythm. Seasonal variation in FE_{NO} is reported due to natural pollen exposure in children with seasonal asthma and pollen allergy [88].

Other Factors

FE_{NO} does not alter significantly with gestation during pregnancy although amniotic nitrite concentration decreases after 37 weeks of gestation [89]. Menstrual cycle may affect FE_{NO} results. FE_{NO} is higher before menstruation than after, in women with complaint of premenstrual asthma [90], but no effect of the menstrual cycle on FE_{NO} is noted in other studies [91, 92].

The amount of NO in ambient air can affect FE_{NO} [73, 93]. Ambient NO at the time of each test recorded, and breathing NO free or scrubbed air during the study is recommended.

Underlying disease condition has shown to affect FE_{NO}. FE_{NO} levels in adults with hypertension, particularly male, and in patients undergoing major surgery are significantly lower than healthy volunteers [75]. Renal failure and dialysis do not appear to have a significant impact on FE_{NO} [75]. The application of positive end-expiratory pressure has been shown to increase FE_{NO} in animals [94–96]. High FE_{NO} is also detected in mechanically ventilated patients with septic syndrome [75]. Hypoxia causes a dose-dependent decrease in FE_{NO} in both animal research [94] and human studies [97, 98] while carbon dioxide also causes a dose-dependent reduction in FE_{NO} [94, 95]. Change in pulmonary blood flow did not affect FE_{NO} in humans but the effect of hemodynamic change on FE_{NO} is noted in animal study [94]. Many studies report elevated FE_{NO} in atopy and allergy [30, 31, 33, 99]. Other conditions affecting FE_{NO} are discussed in the clinical practice section.

Exhaled NO in Clinical Practice

Asthma

Many studies have assessed the roles of FE_{NO} in asthma. FE_{NO} can be used to support the diagnosis of asthma, evaluate eosinophilic airway inflammation, assess potential response to anti-inflammatory agents, guide dose titration of anti-inflammatory medications, predict asthma exacerbation, predict asthma relapse, and evaluate adherence to anti-inflammatory medications [1, 4–6].

The official ATS Clinical Practice Guidelines [5] reported a strong recommendation for using FE_{NO} to assess eosinophilic airway inflammation and steroid responsiveness. Other strong recommendations supported by ATS are age as a factor affecting FE_{NO} in children <12 years of age; measures of low FE_{NO} of <20 ppb in children (<25 ppb in adults) indicating less likelihood of eosinophilic inflammation and responsiveness to corticosteroids; cautious interpretation of FE_{NO} values between 20 and 35 ppb in children (25–50 ppb in adults); persistent and/or high allergen exposure as a factor associated with higher levels of FE_{NO}; and the use of FE_{NO} to monitor airway inflammation in asthma. On the other hand, ATS Guidelines provided only weak recommendations for the use of FE_{NO} as supporting the diagnosis of asthma. Recommendations are also weak for identifying proper cut points in interpretation and in quantitating a significant increase or decrease in values between visits.

FE_{NO} is considered as an indirect marker of airway eosinophilic inflammation, and many studies describe the correlation between FE_{NO} and eosinophils measured in sputum, bronchoalveolar lavage, bronchial biopsy, and blood. This relationship was also studied in children [8–14]. In summary, eosinophilic inflammation is unlikely present when FE_{NO} is low.

Airway inflammation in asthma is heterogeneous and is not always associated with eosinophilic inflammation. The use of FE_{NO} for diagnostic purpose has been evaluated. In epidemiologic studies, FE_{NO} can be used as an indicator for allergic airway inflammation in children [14, 49, 99, 100], and performs better than respiratory function measured and bronchodilator responsiveness in identifying preschool children with probable asthma [101], and in predicting subsequent wheezing treated with systemic steroid in infants and toddlers [29]. Sensitivity, specificity, and positive and negative predictive values as diagnostic of asthma are high [101, 102]. However, a cross-sectional survey in adolescent children shows high negative predictive values of FE_{NO} for asthma but positive predictive value is low for the diagnosis of asthma [14]. High FE_{NO} can be also noted in atopic children without asthma [47, 100]. The combination of FE_{NO} and methacholine provocation test may have more diagnostic power in epidemiological studies than FE_{NO} alone for allergic asthma [103].

In children with respiratory symptoms, FE_{NO} in the diagnosis of asthma can be a predictor of asthma [101, 102, 104]. Significant association between FE_{NO} and reported asthma symptoms is also shown [14, 99, 101, 105], while the correlations between symptoms and spirometry are poor [105]. In nonallergic patients, normal FE_{NO} does not exclude the diagnosis of asthma, and in patients who have already been treated with inhaled steroids, is significantly reduced from previously elevated FE_{NO} in inflammatory airway diseases. Overall, the results of studies examining the use of FE_{NO} in the diagnosis of asthma have also been inconsistent in the adult literature. Therefore, FE_{NO} reflects only one aspect of the asthma phenotype, and should be used as a supportive method to other diagnostic tests.

It is well known that not all patients with asthma respond to corticosteroids. High FE_{NO} (>35 ppb) in adults has been shown as a positive indicator that the patient would likely respond to inhaled corticosteroids (likelihood ratio of a positive response, 4.9; 95 % confidence interval, 2.2–10.9) [106]. In children, the response to anti-inflammatory treatment was also found to be correlated with the FE_{NO} [107–109]. High FE_{NO} (median 17.4 ppb) is associated with a good FEV_1 response (>15 % increase) while lower FE_{NO} (median 11.1 ppb) is associated with a poor response (<5 % increase) [107]. FE_{NO} is predictive of steroid responsiveness more consistently than spirometry, bronchodilator response, peak flow variation, or airway hyperreactivity to methacholine [107, 110–112], even when no sputum eosinophilia is demonstrated [113]. The reduction response of FE_{NO} to corticosteroid treatment is both rapid (within 1 week, potentially as early as 48 h) and dose dependent [112, 114, 115]. Anti-leukotrienes also reduce FE_{NO} in asthma, but to a lesser extent [109]. FE_{NO} is also helpful in predicting asthma relapse after clinical remission [116] and in anticipating eligibility for inhaled corticosteroid dose reduction [117, 118]. However, tailoring anti-asthma therapy according to FE_{NO} in comparison to usual care treatment strategies shows no added value of FE_{NO} for clinical symptoms, asthma exacerbations, pulmonary function, β-agonist use, and overall daily dose of inhaled corticosteroid [119–123]. A recent systematic review and meta-analysis [124] also conclude no significant benefit of adding FE_{NO} to traditional treatment algorithms with respect to asthma exacerbations, asthma symptom scores, or forced expiratory flow in 1 s (FEV_1). In children, FE_{NO}-based treatment group received significantly higher dose of inhaled corticosteroid [123], and this finding is opposite to that adult studies [124]. However, pregnant women with asthma [125] may benefit the most from FE_{NO} monitoring, resulting in significant reduction in asthma exacerbation during pregnancy.

A strong positive correlation between the reduction of FE_{NO} and the adherence to anti-inflammatory treatment is noted [126]. Therefore, besides reviewing adequate doses of anti-inflammatory treatment, checking adherence and inhaler technique is needed for children with high exhaled NO who are already being treated with anti-inflammatory treatment.

FE_{NO} may be able to predict long-term outcome. In adults with difficult-to-treat asthma, FE_{NO} predicts accelerated decline in lung function [127]. In infants and toddlers with recurrent wheeze, high FE_{NO} also predicts deterioration in z-scores of forced expiratory volumes and flows, as measured 6 months later [29].

It is important to choose the appropriate cut point in relation to the clinical setting (Table 14.2). Clinical practice strategies for use of FE_{NO} in patients with asthma have been explained in detail in the text and tables of the ATS Clinical Practice Guidelines [5].

Table 14.2 General guideline for interpretation of fraction of exhaled (FE_{NO}) at 50 ml/s flow rate

	FE_{NO} (ppb)		
Children (<12 years)	<20	20–35	>35
Adult	<25	25–50	>50
Eosinophilic inflammation	Unlikely	Mild if present	Likely
No previous diagnosis of asthma and no anti-inflammatory treatment			
Symptomatic	• Neutrophilic asthma • Alternative diagnoses[a]		• Eosinophilic asthma
Response to inhaled corticosteroid (ICS)	Unlikely	Possible	Likely
Previous diagnosis of asthma and on anti-inflammatory treatment			
Symptomatic	• Alternative diagnoses[a]	• High allergen exposure • Infection • Poor adherence or inhaler technique • Inadequate ICS	• High allergen exposure • Poor adherence or inhaler technique • Inadequate ICS dose • Risk of relapse or exacerbation • Steroid resistance
Previous diagnosis of asthma and on anti-inflammatory treatment			
Asymptomatic	• Adequate ICS dose • Good adherence	• Adequate ICS dose • Good adherence	• Poor adherence or inhaler technique
ICS dose	Reduction or withdraw	No change	No change

ppb Parts per billion

[a]Consider cystic fibrosis, bronchopulmonary dysplasia, primary ciliary dyskinesia, immunodeficiency, rhinosinusitis, vocal cord dysfunction, gastroesophageal reflux

Viral Infection

Since NO functions in host defense against viral infections, elevation of FE_{NO} is likely beneficial to the host by inhibiting viral replication. In both healthy and asthmatic adults, higher FE_{NO} was noted during viral respiratory tract infections [128–130]. In contrast, infants with rhinorrhea [131] or acute virus-associated wheezy bronchitis [85] have significantly lower FE_{NO} than healthy infants. With resolution of symptoms, a significant increase in FE_{NO} is noted in some of the infants with rhinorrhea [131]. These findings suggest possible downregulation of NO production, impaired NO diffusion into the airway due to epithelial damage and increased airway secretions, and an inflammatory reaction mostly related to neutrophils. However, a more recent study in children with respiratory syncytial virus bronchiolitis shows FE_{NO} higher (but without statistical significance) than healthy control during the acute phase of illness, and a positive correlation between FE_{NO} and the clinical score (Downes) of bronchiolitis is noted with higher FE_{NO} in children with more distress [132]. The inconsistency of the effect of viral infection on FE_{NO} level is not fully explained but the differences in method, sample size, gender, atopy, allergy, asthma of study subjects, maternal smoking as well as possible virus-specific disease process can be speculated. The infants with future wheezing episodes in 2 years [132], and young children <4 years of age with clinical index for predicting asthma at school age [133] already present elevated level of FE_{NO}. FE_{NO} in young children with history of recurrent wheezing is also higher than healthy control and children with other pulmonary diseases [134], and atopic wheezers show higher FE_{NO} than nonatopic wheezers [134].

Chronic Lung Disease (CLD) of Prematurity

Data on FE_{NO} values for children with CLD of prematurity are inconsistent possibly due to the differences in the age of study subjects, gestational age, definitions and severity of CLD, or measurement techniques. Compared to controls, equal [134–136] or higher [137–139] FE_{NO} was noted in infants and younger children with CLD. FE_{NO} is particularly elevated in infants with moderate or severe CLD [138]. Although FE_{NO} is not elevated in infants with CLD, calculated NO output V_{NO} (nl/min), by multiplying online flow rate (L/min) and FE_{NO} (ppb), is reduced in infants with lower gestational age, higher clinical risk index for babies score, longer duration of oxygen therapy, postnatal treatment with corticosteroids, and more severe CLD [135]. Even at school age, no significant differences are observed in FE_{NO} among children with CLD of prematurity, healthy control, and preterm-born children without CLD, unless atopy is not present [140]. FE_{NO} in prematurely born atopic children is significantly higher than nonatopic children without prematurity [140]. On the other hand, Baraldi et al. [141] reports lower FE_{NO} in school-age children with CLD of prematurity than healthy matched term-born control and preterm-born children without CLD. FE_{NO} in children with CLD is four times lower than children with asthma despite a comparable airflow limitation in FEV_1 in both CLD and asthma groups [141]. The low FE_{NO} in children with CLD is not due to effects of medications such as corticosteroid or leukotriene receptor antagonist, based on study protocol. However, other factors affecting FE_{NO} such as atopy, allergy, smoking exposure, and severity of CLD are not described for the study subjects.

Pulmonary Hypertension (PHN)

NO in airway gases obtained by bronchoscopy, NO reaction products in exhaled breath condensate or bronchoalveolar lavage fluid, FE_{NO}, and V_{NO} are low in adults with PHN, and are negatively correlated with pulmonary artery (PA) pressures and with years since diagnosis of PHN [142–144]. Therapeutic interventions for PHN are associated with increased levels of FE_{NO} [144, 145]. Therefore, FE_{NO} may have a role in monitoring disease severity and response to therapy in children with PHN but further investigation is required.

Cystic Fibrosis (CF)

FE_{NO} is low in both children [40, 63, 146, 147] and infants [134, 148] with CF despite chronic airway inflammation, although FE_{NO} levels similar to or higher than control subjects are also reported in children and infants with CF [93, 139, 149]. FE_{NO} is negatively correlated with lung clearance index in CF [40] and FE_{NO} is lower in patients with severe CF lung disease than in those with mild disease [147, 150]. However, this association has not been shown in other trial [93]. FE_{NO} also has an inverse relationship with age, regardless of CF genotypes, and gradually decline throughout young childhood [149]. Several mechanisms for reduced FE_{NO} in CF [151] have been proposed including reduced iNOS or iNOS expression in CF [152–155], presence of NO reductase in *Pseudomonas aeruginosa* [156], trapping of NO metabolites in thick secretions [157], deficiency of L-arginine by increased sputum or systemic arginase activities [150, 158], and metabolism and consumptions of NO by reactive oxygen species present in the inflamed environment resulting in elevated nitrate and nitrotyrosine [159, 160].

After therapeutic interventions, the relationship between FE_{NO} and pulmonary function is not consistent. A significant increase in FE_{NO} following intravenous antibiotic treatment is noted in children with CF, but does not correlate with lung function [161]. On the other hand, inhaled L-arginine improves both FE_{NO} and pulmonary function [162]. FE_{NO} is also not associated with any marker of airway inflammation measured in bronchoalveolar lavage in infants with CF [149].

Decreased iNOS in bronchial epithelium and consequently decreased NO are associated with reduced bactericidal activity in the lung [152, 155], and with increased susceptibility of airway colonization with *P. aeruginosa* [163]. Interestingly, children with chronic *P. aeruginosa* infection demonstrated no significant increase in FE_{NO} after intravenous antibiotics [161, 164].

A study including both children and adult shows lower nasal NO concentration in CF than in controls and asthmatics [93]. However, no relationship between nasal NO and pulmonary function is noted in patients with CF.

C_{alv} and J_{NO} have been evaluated in children with CF [40, 43, 44]. J_{NO} can be similar to or lower than healthy children without CF but variable results were noted for C_{alv}. C_{alv} correlates negatively with other systemic inflammatory markers in CF [40]. Children with chronic *P. aeruginosa* colonization have higher levels of systemic inflammatory markers than those not colonized and also lower levels of C_{alv} [40].

Although FE_{NO} may have some utility as a biomarker of CF severity in children, roles of FE_{NO} in CF-related lung disease need further study and the use of FE_{NO} is currently very limited in CF.

Primary Ciliary Dyskinesia (PCD)

Children with PCD have lower FE_{NO} than healthy children. However, some overlap in FE_{NO} has been shown [165]; thereby, FE_{NO} cannot be used to differentiate patients with PCD from healthy controls. On the other hand, extremely low levels of nasal

NO occur in children with PCD, and can effectively discriminate those with PCD from children with other causes of bronchiectasis, CF, asthma, and healthy controls [104, 166–169]. A detailed description of the utility of nasal NO as a screening tool in PCD is explained further in Chap. 4.

Transplantation

Increased FE_{NO} has been noted with acute rejection [170], pulmonary infection [171], and development of bronchiolitis obliterans syndrome (BOS) [172, 173] in adult lung transplant recipients. However, no elevated FE_{NO} is also reported in pulmonary infection or BOS in human lung transplantation [170]. The data on pediatric lung and cardiac transplant recipients demonstrated that C_{alv} was significantly elevated in cardiac transplant recipients when compared to controls; lung transplant recipients had higher levels of C_{alv} than controls; however this difference did not reach statistical significance [174]. Nasal NO is significantly lower in pediatric lung transplant recipients when compared to other solid-organ recipients or healthy controls, and was negatively correlated with tacrolimus levels [175]. Higher FE_{NO} was also observed in children with pulmonary complications after hematopoietic stem cell transplantation [176].

Conclusion

NO is a molecule generated from various resident and inflammatory cells in the airway, and can be measured in exhaled air as FE_{NO} by a stationary chemiluminescence analyzer or a portable handheld device. ATS/ERS published recommendations to standardize the procedures to measure FE_{NO}, and official ATS clinical practice guidelines has also been published for interpretation of FE_{NO}. In the clinical setting, FE_{NO} can provide information on airway inflammation, and help the management of airway diseases, particularly asthma. In pediatric asthma, FE_{NO} can be complementary to lung function tests to guide asthma diagnosis, assessment of current asthma control, adjustment of anti-inflammatory medications, and future risk of exacerbation. In other pediatric respiratory diseases, there has been progress in clinical application of FE_{NO}, but further research is needed.

References

1. Barnes PJ, Dweik RA, Gelb AF, Gibson PG, George SC, Grasemann H, et al. Exhaled nitric oxide in pulmonary diseases: a comprehensive review. Chest. 2010;138(3):682–92. PubMed PMID: 20822990.
2. American Thoracic Society, European Respiratory Society. ATS/ERS recommendations for standardized procedures for the online and offline measurement of exhaled lower respiratory nitric oxide and nasal nitric oxide, 2005. Am J Respir Crit Care Med. 2005;171(8):912–30. PubMed PMID: 15817806.

3. Recommendations for standardized procedures for the on-line and off-line measurement of exhaled lower respiratory nitric oxide and nasal nitric oxide in adults and children-1999. This official statement of the American Thoracic Society was adopted by the ATS Board of Directors, July 1999. Am J Res Crit Care Med. 1999;160(6):2104–17. PubMed PMID: 10588636.

4. Silkoff PE, Erzurum SC, Lundberg JO, George SC, Marczin N, Hunt JF, et al. ATS workshop proceedings: exhaled nitric oxide and nitric oxide oxidative metabolism in exhaled breath condensate. Proc Am Thorac Soc. 2006;3(2):131–45. PubMed PMID: 16565422.

5. Dweik RA, Boggs PB, Erzurum SC, Irvin CG, Leigh MW, Lundberg JO, et al. An official ATS clinical practice guideline: interpretation of exhaled nitric oxide levels (FENO) for clinical applications. Am J Respir Crit Care Med. 2011;184(5):602–15. PubMed PMID: 21885636.

6. Baraldi E, de Jongste JC. European Respiratory Society/American Thoracic Society Task F. Measurement of exhaled nitric oxide in children, 2001. Eur Respir J. 2002;20(1):223–37.

7. Lane C, Knight D, Burgess S, Franklin P, Horak F, Legg J, et al. Epithelial inducible nitric oxide synthase activity is the major determinant of nitric oxide concentration in exhaled breath. Thorax. 2004;59(9):757–60. PubMed PMID: 15333851. Pubmed Central PMCID: 1747143.

8. Barreto M, Villa MP, Monti F, Bohmerova Z, Martella S, Montesano M, et al. Additive effect of eosinophilia and atopy on exhaled nitric oxide levels in children with or without a history of respiratory symptoms. Pediatr Allergy Immunol. 2005;16(1):52–8. PubMed PMID: 15693912.

9. Lex C, Ferreira F, Zacharasiewicz A, Nicholson AG, Haslam PL, Wilson NM, et al. Airway eosinophilia in children with severe asthma: predictive values of noninvasive tests. Am J Respir Crit Care Med. 2006;174(12):1286–91. PubMed PMID: 16973985.

10. Payne DN, Adcock IM, Wilson NM, Oates T, Scallan M, Bush A. Relationship between exhaled nitric oxide and mucosal eosinophilic inflammation in children with difficult asthma, after treatment with oral prednisolone. Am J Respir Crit Care Med. 2001;164(8 Pt 1):1376–81. PubMed PMID: 11704581.

11. Strunk RC, Szefler SJ, Phillips BR, Zeiger RS, Chinchilli VM, Larsen G, et al. Relationship of exhaled nitric oxide to clinical and inflammatory markers of persistent asthma in children. J Allergy Clin Immunol. 2003;112(5):883–92. PubMed PMID: 14610474.

12. van den Toorn LM, Overbeek SE, de Jongste JC, Leman K, Hoogsteden HC, Prins JB. Airway inflammation is present during clinical remission of atopic asthma. Am J Respir Crit Care Med. 2001;164(11):2107–13. PubMed PMID: 11739143.

13. Warke TJ, Fitch PS, Brown V, Taylor R, Lyons JD, Ennis M, et al. Exhaled nitric oxide correlates with airway eosinophils in childhood asthma. Thorax. 2002;57(5):383–7. PubMed PMID: 11978911. Pubmed Central PMCID: 1746317.

14. Thomas PS, Gibson PG, Wang H, Shah S, Henry RL. The relationship of exhaled nitric oxide to airway inflammation and responsiveness in children. J Asthma. 2005;42(4):291–5. PubMed PMID: 16032938.

15. Hemmingsson T, Linnarsson D, Gambert R. Novel hand-held device for exhaled nitric oxide-analysis in research and clinical applications. J Clin Monit Comput. 2004;18(5–6):379–87. PubMed PMID: 15957630.

16. Alving K, Janson C, Nordvall L. Performance of a new hand-held device for exhaled nitric oxide measurement in adults and children. Respir Res. 2006;7:67. PubMed PMID: 16626491. Pubmed Central PMCID: 1462993.

17. Pisi R, Aiello M, Tzani P, Marangio E, Olivieri D, Chetta A. Measurement of fractional exhaled nitric oxide by a new portable device: comparison with the standard technique. J Asthma. 2010;47(7):805–9. PubMed PMID: 20670207.

18. McGill C, Malik G, Turner SW. Validation of a hand-held exhaled nitric oxide analyzer for use in children. Pediatr Pulmonol. 2006;41(11):1053–7. PubMed PMID: 16871592.

19. Buchvald F, Baraldi E, Carraro S, Gaston B, De Jongste J, Pijnenburg MW, et al. Measurements of exhaled nitric oxide in healthy subjects age 4 to 17 years. J Allergy Clin Immunol. 2005;115(6):1130–6. PubMed PMID: 15940124.

20. Pijnenburg MW, Floor SE, Hop WC, De Jongste JC. Daily ambulatory exhaled nitric oxide measurements in asthma. Pediatr Allergy Immunol. 2006;17(3):189–93. PubMed PMID: 16672005.

21. Lundberg JO, Weitzberg E, Lundberg JM, Alving K. Nitric oxide in exhaled air. Eur Respir J. 1996;9(12):2671–80. PubMed PMID: 8980984.

22. Silkoff PE, McClean PA, Slutsky AS, Furlott HG, Hoffstein E, Wakita S, et al. Marked flow-dependence of exhaled nitric oxide using a new technique to exclude nasal nitric oxide. Am J Respir Crit Care Med. 1997;155(1):260–7. PubMed PMID: 9001322.

23. Pedroletti C, Zetterquist W, Nordvall L, Alving K. Evaluation of exhaled nitric oxide in schoolchildren at different exhalation flow rates. Pediatr Res. 2002;52(3):393–8. PubMed PMID: 12193674.

24. Silkoff PE, Sylvester JT, Zamel N, Permutt S. Airway nitric oxide diffusion in asthma: Role in pulmonary function and bronchial responsiveness. Am J Respir Crit Care Med. 2000;161 (4 Pt 1):1218–28. PubMed PMID: 10764315.

25. Lundberg JO, Farkas-Szallasi T, Weitzberg E, Rinder J, Lidholm J, Anggaard A, et al. High nitric oxide production in human paranasal sinuses. Nat Med. 1995;1(4):370–3. PubMed PMID: 7585069.

26. Baraldi E, Scollo M, Zaramella C, Zanconato S, Zacchello F. A simple flow-driven method for online measurement of exhaled NO starting at the age of 4 to 5 years. Am J Respir Crit Care Med. 2000;162(5):1828–32. PubMed PMID: 11069821.

27. Silkoff PE, Bates CA, Meiser JB, Bratton DL. Single-breath exhaled nitric oxide in preschool children facilitated by a servo-controlled device maintaining constant flow. Pediatr Pulmonol. 2004;37(6):554–8. PubMed PMID: 15114557.

28. Buchvald F, Bisgaard H. FeNO measured at fixed exhalation flow rate during controlled tidal breathing in children from the age of 2 yr. Am J Respir Crit Care Med. 2001;163(3 Pt 1):699–704. PubMed PMID: 11254527.

29. Debley JS, Stamey DC, Cochrane ES, Gama KL, Redding GJ. Exhaled nitric oxide, lung function, and exacerbations in wheezy infants and toddlers. J Allergy Clin Immunol. 2010;125(6):1228–34 e13. PubMed PMID: 20462633. Pubmed Central PMCID: 2879468.

30. Tepper RS, Llapur CJ, Jones MH, Tiller C, Coates C, Kimmel R, et al. Expired nitric oxide and airway reactivity in infants at risk for asthma. J Allergy Clin Immunol. 2008;122(4):760–5. PubMed PMID: 18760452.

31. Wildhaber JH, Hall GL, Stick SM. Measurements of exhaled nitric oxide with the single-breath technique and positive expiratory pressure in infants. Am J Respir Crit Care Med. 1999;159(1):74–8. PubMed PMID: 9872821.

32. Baraldi E, Dario C, Ongaro R, Scollo M, Azzolin NM, Panza N, et al. Exhaled nitric oxide concentrations during treatment of wheezing exacerbation in infants and young children. Am J Respir Crit Care Med. 1999;159(4 Pt 1):1284–8. PubMed PMID: 10194178.

33. Franklin PJ, Turner SW, Mutch RC, Stick SM. Measuring exhaled nitric oxide in infants during tidal breathing: methodological issues. Pediatr Pulmonol. 2004;37(1):24–30. PubMed PMID: 14679485.

34. Hall GL, Reinmann B, Wildhaber JH, Frey U. Tidal exhaled nitric oxide in healthy, unsedated newborn infants with prenatal tobacco exposure. J Appl Physiol. 2002;92(1):59–66. PubMed PMID: 11744643.

35. Franklin PJ, Turner SW, Mutch RC, Stick SM. Comparison of single-breath and tidal breathing exhaled nitric oxide levels in infants. Eur Respir J. 2004;23(3):369–72. PubMed PMID: 15065823.

36. Tsoukias NM, George SC. A two-compartment model of pulmonary nitric oxide exchange dynamics. J Appl Physiol. 1998;85(2):653–66. PubMed PMID: 9688744.

37. Lehtimaki L, Kankaanranta H, Saarelainen S, Hahtola P, Jarvenpaa R, Koivula T, et al. Extended exhaled NO measurement differentiates between alveolar and bronchial inflammation. Am J Respir Crit Care Med. 2001;163(7):1557–61. PubMed PMID: 11401873.

38. Lehtimaki L, Turjanmaa V, Kankaanranta H, Saarelainen S, Hahtola P, Moilanen E. Increased bronchial nitric oxide production in patients with asthma measured with a novel method of different exhalation flow rates. Ann Med. 2000;32(6):417–23. PubMed PMID: 11028690.

39. Lehtimaki L, Kankaanranta H, Saarelainen S, Turjanmaa V, Moilanen E. Increased alveolar nitric oxide concentration in asthmatic patients with nocturnal symptoms. Eur Respir J. 2002;20(4):841–5. PubMed PMID: 12412673.

40. Keen C, Gustafsson P, Lindblad A, Wennergren G, Olin AC. Low levels of exhaled nitric oxide are associated with impaired lung function in cystic fibrosis. Pediatr Pulmonol. 2010;45(3):241–8. PubMed PMID: 20146368.
41. Paraskakis E, Brindicci C, Fleming L, Krol R, Kharitonov SA, Wilson NM, et al. Measurement of bronchial and alveolar nitric oxide production in normal children and children with asthma. Am J Respir Crit Care Med. 2006;174(3):260–7. PubMed PMID: 16627868.
42. Sepponen A, Lehtimaki L, Huhtala H, Kaila M, Kankaanranta H, Moilanen E. Alveolar and bronchial nitric oxide output in healthy children. Pediatr Pulmonol. 2008;43(12):1242–8. PubMed PMID: 19009623.
43. Shin HW, Rose-Gottron CM, Sufi RS, Perez F, Cooper DM, Wilson AF, et al. Flow-independent nitric oxide exchange parameters in cystic fibrosis. Am J Respir Crit Care Med. 2002;165(3):349–57. PubMed PMID: 11818320.
44. Suri R, Paraskakis E, Bush A. Alveolar, but not bronchial nitric oxide production is elevated in cystic fibrosis. Pediatr Pulmonol. 2007;42(12):1215–21. PubMed PMID: 17969001.
45. See KC, Christiani DC. Normal values and thresholds for the clinical interpretation of exhaled nitric oxide levels in the US general population: results from the National Health and Nutrition Examination Survey 2007–2010. Chest. 2013;143(1):107–16. PubMed PMID: 22628492.
46. Malmberg LP, Petays T, Haahtela T, Laatikainen T, Jousilahti P, Vartiainen E, et al. Exhaled nitric oxide in healthy nonatopic school-age children: determinants and height-adjusted reference values. Pediatr Pulmonol. 2006;41(7):635–42. PubMed PMID: 16703576.
47. Kovesi T, Dales R. Exhaled nitric oxide and respiratory symptoms in a community sample of school aged children. Pediatr Pulmonol. 2008;43(12):1198–205. PubMed PMID: 19003883.
48. Kovesi T, Kulka R, Dales R. Exhaled nitric oxide concentration is affected by age, height, and race in healthy 9- to 12-year-old children. Chest. 2008;133(1):169–75. PubMed PMID: 17925422.
49. Saito J, Inoue K, Sugawara A, Yoshikawa M, Watanabe K, Ishida T, et al. Exhaled nitric oxide as a marker of airway inflammation for an epidemiologic study in schoolchildren. J Allergy Clin Immunol. 2004;114(3):512–6. PubMed PMID: 15356549.
50. Wong GW, Liu EK, Leung TF, Yung E, Ko FW, Hui DS, et al. High levels and gender difference of exhaled nitric oxide in Chinese schoolchildren. Clin Exp Allergy. 2005;35(7):889–93. PubMed PMID: 16008675.
51. Ekroos H, Karjalainen J, Sarna S, Laitinen LA, Sovijarvi AR. Short-term variability of exhaled nitric oxide in young male patients with mild asthma and in healthy subjects. Respir Med. 2002;96(11):895–900. PubMed PMID: 12418587.
52. Kharitonov SA, Gonio F, Kelly C, Meah S, Barnes PJ. Reproducibility of exhaled nitric oxide measurements in healthy and asthmatic adults and children. Eur Respir J. 2003;21(3):433–8. PubMed PMID: 12661997.
53. Santamaria F, Montella S, De Stefano S, Sperli F, Barbarano F, Valerio G. Relationship between exhaled nitric oxide and body mass index in children and adolescents. J Allergy Clin Immunol. 2005;116(5):1163–4. author reply 4–5. PubMed PMID: 16275394.
54. Olin AC, Aldenbratt A, Ekman A, Ljungkvist G, Jungersten L, Alving K, et al. Increased nitric oxide in exhaled air after intake of a nitrate-rich meal. Respir Med. 2001;95(2):153–8. PubMed PMID: 11217912.
55. Zetterquist W, Pedroletti C, Lundberg JO, Alving K. Salivary contribution to exhaled nitric oxide. Eur Respir J. 1999;13(2):327–33. PubMed PMID: 10065676.
56. Cardinale F, Tesse R, Fucilli C, Loffredo MS, Iacoviello G, Chinellato I, et al. Correlation between exhaled nitric oxide and dietary consumption of fats and antioxidants in children with asthma. J Allergy Clin Immunol. 2007;119(5):1268–70. PubMed PMID: 17321576.
57. Byrnes CA, Dinarevic S, Busst CA, Shinebourne EA, Bush A. Effect of measurement conditions on measured levels of peak exhaled nitric oxide. Thorax. 1997;52(8):697–701. PubMed PMID: 9337828. Pubmed Central PMCID: 1758633.
58. Bruce C, Yates DH, Thomas PS. Caffeine decreases exhaled nitric oxide. Thorax. 2002;57(4):361–3. PubMed PMID: 11923558. Pubmed Central PMCID: 1746303.
59. Yates DH, Kharitonov SA, Robbins RA, Thomas PS, Barnes PJ. The effect of alcohol ingestion on exhaled nitric oxide. Eur Respir J. 1996;9(6):1130–3. PubMed PMID: 8804927.

60. Kharitonov SA, Lubec G, Lubec B, Hjelm M, Barnes PJ. L-arginine increases exhaled nitric oxide in normal human subjects. Clin Sci. 1995;88(2):135–9. PubMed PMID: 7720336.

61. Mehta S, Stewart DJ, Levy RD. The hypotensive effect of L-arginine is associated with increased expired nitric oxide in humans. Chest. 1996;109(6):1550–5. PubMed PMID: 8769510.

62. Ogata H, Yatabe M, Misaka S, Shikama Y, Sato S, Munakata M, et al. Effect of oral L-arginine administration on exhaled nitric oxide (no) concentration in healthy volunteers. Fukushima J Med Sci. 2013;59(1):43–8. PubMed PMID: 23842514.

63. Zetterquist W, Marteus H, Kalm-Stephens P, Nas E, Nordvall L, Johannesson M, et al. Oral bacteria—the missing link to ambiguous findings of exhaled nitrogen oxides in cystic fibrosis. Respir Med. 2009;103(2):187–93. PubMed PMID: 19006660.

64. Baraldi E, Azzolin NM, Zanconato S, Dario C, Zacchello F. Corticosteroids decrease exhaled nitric oxide in children with acute asthma. J Pediatr. 1997;131(3):381–5. PubMed PMID: 9329413.

65. Kharitonov SA, Yates DH, Barnes PJ. Inhaled glucocorticoids decrease nitric oxide in exhaled air of asthmatic patients. Am J Respir Crit Care Med. 1996;153(1):454–7. PubMed PMID: 8542158.

66. Carra S, Gagliardi L, Zanconato S, Scollo M, Azzolin N, Zacchello F, et al. Budesonide but not nedocromil sodium reduces exhaled nitric oxide levels in asthmatic children. Respir Med. 2001;95(9):734–9. PubMed PMID: 11575894.

67. Bisgaard H, Loland L, Oj JA. NO in exhaled air of asthmatic children is reduced by the leukotriene receptor antagonist montelukast. Am J Respir Crit Care Med. 1999;160(4):1227–31. PubMed PMID: 10508811.

68. Silkoff PE, Romero FA, Gupta N, Townley RG, Milgrom H. Exhaled nitric oxide in children with asthma receiving Xolair (omalizumab), a monoclonal anti-immunoglobulin E antibody. Pediatrics. 2004;113(4):e308–12. PubMed PMID: 15060258.

69. Silkoff PE, Wakita S, Chatkin J, Ansarin K, Gutierrez C, Caramori M, et al. Exhaled nitric oxide after beta2-agonist inhalation and spirometry in asthma. Am J Respir Crit Care Med. 1999;159(3):940–4. PubMed PMID: 10051277.

70. Mitsufuji H, Kobayashi H, Imasaki T, Ichikawa T, Kawakami T, Tomita T. Acute changes in bronchoconstriction influences exhaled nitric oxide level. Jpn J Physiol. 2001;51(2):151–7. PubMed PMID: 11405907.

71. Kissoon N, Duckworth LJ, Blake KV, Murphy SP, Lima JJ. Effect of beta2-agonist treatment and spirometry on exhaled nitric oxide in healthy children and children with asthma. Pediatr Pulmonol. 2002;34(3):203–8. PubMed PMID: 12203849.

72. Lim S, Tomita K, Caramori G, Jatakanon A, Oliver B, Keller A, et al. Low-dose theophylline reduces eosinophilic inflammation but not exhaled nitric oxide in mild asthma. Am J Respir Crit Care Med. 2001;164(2):273–6. PubMed PMID: 11463600.

73. Deykin A, Halpern O, Massaro AF, Drazen JM, Israel E. Expired nitric oxide after bronchoprovocation and repeated spirometry in patients with asthma. Am J Respir Crit Care Med. 1998;157(3 Pt 1):769–75. PubMed PMID: 9517589.

74. Kharitonov SA, Robbins RA, Yates D, Keatings V, Barnes PJ. Acute and chronic effects of cigarette smoking on exhaled nitric oxide. Am J Respir Crit Care Med. 1995;152(2):609–12. PubMed PMID: 7543345.

75. Schilling J, Holzer P, Guggenbach M, Gyurech D, Marathia K, Geroulanos S. Reduced endogenous nitric oxide in the exhaled air of smokers and hypertensives. Eur Respir J. 1994;7(3):467–71. PubMed PMID: 8013603.

76. Yates DH, Breen H, Thomas PS. Passive smoke inhalation decreases exhaled nitric oxide in normal subjects. Am J Respir Crit Care Med. 2001;164(6):1043–6. PubMed PMID: 11587994.

77. Gabriele C, Asgarali R, Jaddoe VW, Hofman A, Moll HA, de Jongste JC. Smoke exposure, airway symptoms and exhaled nitric oxide in infants: the Generation R study. Eur Respir J. 2008;32(2):307–13. PubMed PMID: 18417508.

78. Frey U, Kuehni C, Roiha H, Cernelc M, Reinmann B, Wildhaber JH, et al. Maternal atopic disease modifies effects of prenatal risk factors on exhaled nitric oxide in infants. Am J Respir Crit Care Med. 2004;170(3):260–5. PubMed PMID: 15059789.

79. Franklin PJ, Turner S, Mutch R, Stick SM. Parental smoking increases exhaled nitric oxide in young children. Eur Respir J. 2006;28(4):730–3. PubMed PMID: 17012629.
80. Gabriele C, Pijnenburg MW, Monti F, Hop W, Bakker ME, de Jongste JC. The effect of spirometry and exercise on exhaled nitric oxide in asthmatic children. Pediatr Allergy Immunol. 2005;16(3):243–7. PubMed PMID: 15853954.
81. Deykin A, Massaro AF, Coulston E, Drazen JM, Israel E. Exhaled nitric oxide following repeated spirometry or repeated plethysmography in healthy individuals. Am J Respir Crit Care Med. 2000;161(4 Pt 1):1237–40. PubMed PMID: 10764317.
82. Piacentini GL, Bodini A, Costella S, Vicentini L, Suzuki Y, Boner AL. Exhaled nitric oxide is reduced after sputum induction in asthmatic children. Pediatr Pulmonol. 2000;29(6):430–3. PubMed PMID: 10821723.
83. Beier J, Beeh KM, Kornmann O, Buhl R. Sputum induction leads to a decrease of exhaled nitric oxide unrelated to airflow. Eur Respir J. 2003;22(2):354–7. PubMed PMID: 12952273.
84. ten Hacken NH, van der Vaart H, van der Mark TW, Koeter GH, Postma DS. Exhaled nitric oxide is higher both at day and night in subjects with nocturnal asthma. Am J Respir Crit Care Med. 1998;158(3):902–7. PubMed PMID: 9731024.
85. Ratjen F, Kavuk I, Gartig S, Wiesemann HG, Grasemann H. Airway nitric oxide in infants with acute wheezy bronchitis. Pediatr Allergy Immunol. 2000;11(4):230–5. PubMed PMID: 11110577.
86. Georges G, Bartelson BB, Martin RJ, Silkoff PE. Circadian variation in exhaled nitric oxide in nocturnal asthma. J Asthma. 1999;36(5):467–73. PubMed PMID: 10461936.
87. Mattes J, Storm van's Gravesande K, Moeller C, Moseler M, Brandis M, Kuehr J. Circadian variation of exhaled nitric oxide and urinary eosinophil protein X in asthmatic and healthy children. Pediatr Res. 2002;51(2):190–4. PubMed PMID: 11809913.
88. Vahlkvist S, Sinding M, Skamstrup K, Bisgaard H. Daily home measurements of exhaled nitric oxide in asthmatic children during natural birch pollen exposure. J Allergy Clin Immunol. 2006;117(6):1272–6. PubMed PMID: 16750986.
89. Morris NH, Carroll S, Nicolaides KH, Steer PJ, Warren JB. Exhaled nitric oxide concentration and amniotic fluid nitrite concentration during pregnancy. Eur J Clin Invest. 1995;25(2):138–41. PubMed PMID: 7737264.
90. Oguzulgen IK, Turktas H, Erbas D. Airway inflammation in premenstrual asthma. J Asthma. 2002;39(6):517–22. PubMed PMID: 12375711.
91. Morris NH, Sooranna SR, Steer PJ, Warren JB. The effect of the menstrual cycle on exhaled nitric oxide and urinary nitrate concentration. Eur J Clin Invest. 1996;26(6):481–4. PubMed PMID: 8817162.
92. Jilma B, Kastner J, Mensik C, Vondrovec B, Hildebrandt J, Krejcy K, et al. Sex differences in concentrations of exhaled nitric oxide and plasma nitrate. Life Sci. 1996;58(6):469–76. PubMed PMID: 8569419.
93. Dotsch J, Demirakca S, Terbrack HG, Huls G, Rascher W, Kuhl PG. Airway nitric oxide in asthmatic children and patients with cystic fibrosis. Eur Respir J. 1996;9(12):2537–40. PubMed PMID: 8980966.
94. Carlin RE, Ferrario L, Boyd JT, Camporesi EM, McGraw DJ, Hakim TS. Determinants of nitric oxide in exhaled gas in the isolated rabbit lung. Am J Respir Crit Care Med. 1997;155(3):922–7. PubMed PMID: 9117027.
95. Stromberg S, Lonnqvist PA, Persson MG, Gustafsson LE. Lung distension and carbon dioxide affect pulmonary nitric oxide formation in the anaesthetized rabbit. Acta Physiol Scand. 1997;159(1):59–67. PubMed PMID: 9124071.
96. Persson MG, Lonnqvist PA, Gustafsson LE. Positive end-expiratory pressure ventilation elicits increases in endogenously formed nitric oxide as detected in air exhaled by rabbits. Anesthesiology. 1995;82(4):969–74. PubMed PMID: 7717570.
97. Dweik RA, Laskowski D, Abu-Soud HM, Kaneko F, Hutte R, Stuehr DJ, et al. Nitric oxide synthesis in the lung. Regulation by oxygen through a kinetic mechanism. J Clin Invest. 1998;101(3):660–6. PubMed PMID: 9449700. Pubmed Central PMCID: 508610.

98. Schmetterer L, Strenn K, Kastner J, Eichler HG, Wolzt M. Exhaled NO during graded changes in inhaled oxygen in man. Thorax. 1997;52(8):736–8. PubMed PMID: 9337835. Pubmed Central PMCID: 1758631.

99. Brussee JE, Smit HA, Kerkhof M, Koopman LP, Wijga AH, Postma DS, et al. Exhaled nitric oxide in 4-year-old children: relationship with asthma and atopy. Eur Respir J. 2005;25(3): 455–61. PubMed PMID: 15738288.

100. Prasad A, Langford B, Stradling JR, Ho LP. Exhaled nitric oxide as a screening tool for asthma in school children. Respir Med. 2006;100(1):167–73. PubMed PMID: 15885997.

101. Malmberg LP, Pelkonen AS, Haahtela T, Turpeinen M. Exhaled nitric oxide rather than lung function distinguishes preschool children with probable asthma. Thorax. 2003;58(6):494–9. PubMed PMID: 12775859. Pubmed Central PMCID: 1746693.

102. Sivan Y, Gadish T, Fireman E, Soferman R. The use of exhaled nitric oxide in the diagnosis of asthma in school children. J Pediatr. 2009;155(2):211–6. PubMed PMID: 19394049.

103. Henriksen AH, Lingaas-Holmen T, Sue-Chu M, Bjermer L. Combined use of exhaled nitric oxide and airway hyperresponsiveness in characterizing asthma in a large population survey. Eur Respir J. 2000;15(5):849–55. PubMed PMID: 10853848.

104. Narang I, Ersu R, Wilson NM, Bush A. Nitric oxide in chronic airway inflammation in children: diagnostic use and pathophysiological significance. Thorax. 2002;57(7):586–9. PubMed PMID: 12096200. Pubmed Central PMCID: 1746369.

105. Nordvall SL, Janson C, Kalm-Stephens P, Foucard T, Toren K, Alving K. Exhaled nitric oxide in a population-based study of asthma and allergy in schoolchildren. Allergy. 2005;60(4):469–75. PubMed PMID: 15727578.

106. Hahn PY, Morgenthaler TY, Lim KG. Use of exhaled nitric oxide in predicting response to inhaled corticosteroids for chronic cough. Mayo Clin Proc. 2007;82(11):1350–5. PubMed PMID: 17976354.

107. Szefler SJ, Martin RJ, King TS, Boushey HA, Cherniack RM, Chinchilli VM, et al. Significant variability in response to inhaled corticosteroids for persistent asthma. J Allergy Clin Immunol. 2002;109(3):410–8. PubMed PMID: 11897984.

108. Szefler SJ, Phillips BR, Martinez FD, Chinchilli VM, Lemanske RF, Strunk RC, et al. Characterization of within-subject responses to fluticasone and montelukast in childhood asthma. J Allergy Clin Immunol. 2005;115(2):233–42. PubMed PMID: 15696076.

109. Zeiger RS, Szefler SJ, Phillips BR, Schatz M, Martinez FD, Chinchilli VM, et al. Response profiles to fluticasone and montelukast in mild-to-moderate persistent childhood asthma. J Allergy Clin Immunol. 2006;117(1):45–52. PubMed PMID: 16387583.

110. Knuffman JE, Sorkness CA, Lemanske Jr RF, Mauger DT, Boehmer SJ, Martinez FD, et al. Phenotypic predictors of long-term response to inhaled corticosteroid and leukotriene modifier therapies in pediatric asthma. J Allergy Clin Immunol. 2009;123(2):411–6. PubMed PMID: 19121860. Pubmed Central PMCID: 2662352.

111. Smith AD, Cowan JO, Brassett KP, Filsell S, McLachlan C, Monti-Sheehan G, et al. Exhaled nitric oxide: a predictor of steroid response. Am J Respir Crit Care Med. 2005;172(4):453–9. PubMed PMID: 15901605.

112. Silkoff PE, McClean P, Spino M, Erlich L, Slutsky AS, Zamel N. Dose-response relationship and reproducibility of the fall in exhaled nitric oxide after inhaled beclomethasone dipropionate therapy in asthma patients. Chest. 2001;119(5):1322–8. PubMed PMID: 11348935.

113. Cowan DC, Cowan JO, Palmay R, Williamson A, Taylor DR. Effects of steroid therapy on inflammatory cell subtypes in asthma. Thorax. 2010;65(5):384–90. PubMed PMID: 19996343.

114. Jones SL, Herbison P, Cowan JO, Flannery EM, Hancox RJ, McLachlan CR, et al. Exhaled NO and assessment of anti-inflammatory effects of inhaled steroid: dose-response relationship. Eur Respir J. 2002;20(3):601–8. PubMed PMID: 12358335.

115. Kharitonov SA, Donnelly LE, Montuschi P, Corradi M, Collins JV, Barnes PJ. Dose-dependent onset and cessation of action of inhaled budesonide on exhaled nitric oxide and symptoms in mild asthma. Thorax. 2002;57(10):889–96. PubMed PMID: 12324677. Pubmed Central PMCID: 1746196.

116. Pijnenburg MW, Hofhuis W, Hop WC, De Jongste JC. Exhaled nitric oxide predicts asthma relapse in children with clinical asthma remission. Thorax. 2005;60(3):215–8. PubMed PMID: 15741438. Pubmed Central PMCID: 1747332.

117. Li AM, Tsang TW, Lam HS, Sung RY, Chang AB. Predictors for failed dose reduction of inhaled corticosteroids in childhood asthma. Respirology. 2008;13(3):400–7. PubMed PMID: 18399863.

118. Zacharasiewicz A, Wilson N, Lex C, Erin EM, Li AM, Hansel T, et al. Clinical use of noninvasive measurements of airway inflammation in steroid reduction in children. Am J Respir Crit Care Med. 2005;171(10):1077–82. PubMed PMID: 15709050.

119. de Jongste JC, Carraro S, Hop WC, Group CS, Baraldi E. Daily telemonitoring of exhaled nitric oxide and symptoms in the treatment of childhood asthma. Am J Respir Crit Care Med. 2009;179(2):93–7. PubMed PMID: 18931330.

120. Fritsch M, Uxa S, Horak Jr F, Putschoegl B, Dehlink E, Szepfalusi Z, et al. Exhaled nitric oxide in the management of childhood asthma: a prospective 6-months study. Pediatr Pulmonol. 2006;41(9):855–62. PubMed PMID: 16850457.

121. Pijnenburg MW, Bakker EM, Hop WC, De Jongste JC. Titrating steroids on exhaled nitric oxide in children with asthma: a randomized controlled trial. Am J Respir Crit Care Med. 2005;172(7):831–6. PubMed PMID: 15976380.

122. Smith AD, Cowan JO, Brassett KP, Herbison GP, Taylor DR. Use of exhaled nitric oxide measurements to guide treatment in chronic asthma. N Engl J Med. 2005;352(21):2163–73. PubMed PMID: 15914548.

123. Szefler SJ, Mitchell H, Sorkness CA, Gergen PJ, O'Connor GT, Morgan WJ, et al. Management of asthma based on exhaled nitric oxide in addition to guideline-based treatment for inner-city adolescents and young adults: a randomised controlled trial. Lancet. 2008;372(9643):1065–72. PubMed PMID: 18805335. Pubmed Central PMCID: 2610850.

124. Petsky HL, Cates CJ, Lasserson TJ, Li AM, Turner C, Kynaston JA, et al. A systematic review and meta-analysis: tailoring asthma treatment on eosinophilic markers (exhaled nitric oxide or sputum eosinophils). Thorax. 2012;67(3):199–208. PubMed PMID: 20937641.

125. Powell H, Murphy VE, Taylor DR, Hensley MJ, McCaffery K, Giles W, et al. Management of asthma in pregnancy guided by measurement of fraction of exhaled nitric oxide: a double-blind, randomised controlled trial. Lancet. 2011;378(9795):983–90. PubMed PMID: 21907861.

126. Beck-Ripp J, Griese M, Arenz S, Koring C, Pasqualoni B, Bufler P. Changes of exhaled nitric oxide during steroid treatment of childhood asthma. Eur Respir J. 2002;19(6):1015–9. PubMed PMID: 12108850.

127. van Veen IH, Ten Brinke A, Sterk PJ, Sont JK, Gauw SA, Rabe KF, et al. Exhaled nitric oxide predicts lung function decline in difficult-to-treat asthma. Eur Respir J. 2008;32(2):344–9. PubMed PMID: 18508818.

128. de Gouw HW, Grunberg K, Schot R, Kroes AC, Dick EC, Sterk PJ. Relationship between exhaled nitric oxide and airway hyperresponsiveness following experimental rhinovirus infection in asthmatic subjects. Eur Respir J. 1998;11(1):126–32. PubMed PMID: 9543281.

129. Murphy AW, Platts-Mills TA, Lobo M, Hayden F. Respiratory nitric oxide levels in experimental human influenza. Chest. 1998;114(2):452–6. PubMed PMID: 9726729.

130. Kharitonov SA, Yates D, Barnes PJ. Increased nitric oxide in exhaled air of normal human subjects with upper respiratory tract infections. Eur Respir J. 1995;8(2):295–7. PubMed PMID: 7538934.

131. Franklin PJ, Turner SW, Hall GL, Moeller A, Stick SM. Exhaled nitric oxide is reduced in infants with rhinorrhea. Pediatr Pulmonol. 2005;39(2):117–9. PubMed PMID: 15573394.

132. Pena Zarza JA, Osona B, Gil-Sanchez JA, Figuerola J. Exhaled nitric oxide in acute phase of bronchiolitis and its relation with episodes of subsequent wheezing in children of preschool age. Pediatr Allergy Immunol Pulmonol. 2012;25(2):92–6. PubMed PMID: 22768386. Pubmed Central PMCID: 3377953.

133. Moeller A, Diefenbacher C, Lehmann A, Rochat M, Brooks-Wildhaber J, Hall GL, et al. Exhaled nitric oxide distinguishes between subgroups of preschool children with respiratory symptoms. J Allergy Clin Immunol. 2008;121(3):705–9. PubMed PMID: 18177695.

134. Gabriele C, Nieuwhof EM, Van Der Wiel EC, Hofhuis W, Moll HA, Merkus PJ, et al. Exhaled nitric oxide differentiates airway diseases in the first two years of life. Pediatr Res. 2006;60(4):461–5. PubMed PMID: 16940253.

135. Roiha HL, Kuehni CE, Zanolari M, Zwahlen M, Baldwin DN, Casaulta C, et al. Alterations of exhaled nitric oxide in pre-term infants with chronic lung disease. Eur Respir J. 2007;29(2):251–8. PubMed PMID: 17050555.

136. Williams O, Dimitriou G, Hannam S, Rafferty GF, Greenough A. Lung function and exhaled nitric oxide levels in infants developing chronic lung disease. Pediatr Pulmonol. 2007;42(2):107–13. PubMed PMID: 17186509.

137. Leipala JA, Williams O, Sreekumar S, Cheeseman P, Rafferty GF, Hannam S, et al. Exhaled nitric oxide levels in infants with chronic lung disease. Eur J Pediatr. 2004;163(9):555–8. PubMed PMID: 15205950.

138. May C, Williams O, Milner AD, Peacock J, Rafferty GF, Hannam S, et al. Relation of exhaled nitric oxide levels to development of bronchopulmonary dysplasia. Arch Dis Child Fetal Neonatal Ed. 2009;94(3):F205–9. PubMed PMID: 19383857.

139. Storme L, Riou Y, Leclerc F, Dubois A, Deschildre A, Pierre MH, et al. Exhale nitric oxide (NO) and respiratory function measured with body plethysmography in children. Arch Pediatr. 1998;5(4):389–96. PubMed PMID: 9759158. Monoxyde d'azote (NO) exhale et fonction ventilatoire mesuree par plethysmographie corporelle chez l'enfant.

140. Mieskonen ST, Malmberg LP, Kari MA, Pelkonen AS, Turpeinen MT, Hallman NM, et al. Exhaled nitric oxide at school age in prematurely born infants with neonatal chronic lung disease. Pediatr Pulmonol. 2002;33(5):347–55. PubMed PMID: 11948979.

141. Baraldi E, Bonetto G, Zacchello F, Filippone M. Low exhaled nitric oxide in school-age children with bronchopulmonary dysplasia and airflow limitation. Am J Respir Crit Care Med. 2005;171(1):68–72. PubMed PMID: 15477497.

142. Kaneko FT, Arroliga AC, Dweik RA, Comhair SA, Laskowski D, Oppedisano R, et al. Biochemical reaction products of nitric oxide as quantitative markers of primary pulmonary hypertension. Am J Respir Crit Care Med. 1998;158(3):917–23. PubMed PMID: 9731026.

143. Clini E, Cremona G, Campana M, Scotti C, Pagani M, Bianchi L, et al. Production of endogenous nitric oxide in chronic obstructive pulmonary disease and patients with cor pulmonale. Correlates with echo-Doppler assessment. Am J Respir Crit Care Med. 2000;162(2 Pt 1): 446–50. PubMed PMID: 10934068.

144. Machado RF, Londhe Nerkar MV, Dweik RA, Hammel J, Janocha A, Pyle J, et al. Nitric oxide and pulmonary arterial pressures in pulmonary hypertension. Free Radic Biol Med. 2004;37(7):1010–7. PubMed PMID: 15336317.

145. Ozkan M, Dweik RA, Laskowski D, Arroliga AC, Erzurum SC. High levels of nitric oxide in individuals with pulmonary hypertension receiving epoprostenol therapy. Lung. 2001;179(4):233–43. PubMed PMID: 11891614.

146. Robroeks CM, Rosias PP, van Vliet D, Jobsis Q, Yntema JB, Brackel HJ, et al. Biomarkers in exhaled breath condensate indicate presence and severity of cystic fibrosis in children. Pediatr Allergy Immunol. 2008;19(7):652–9. PubMed PMID: 18312532.

147. Grasemann H, Michler E, Wallot M, Ratjen F. Decreased concentration of exhaled nitric oxide (NO) in patients with cystic fibrosis. Pediatr Pulmonol. 1997;24(3):173–7. PubMed PMID: 9330413.

148. Elphick HE, Demoncheaux EA, Ritson S, Higenbottam TW, Everard ML. Exhaled nitric oxide is reduced in infants with cystic fibrosis. Thorax. 2001;56(2):151–2. PubMed PMID: 11209106. Pubmed Central PMCID: 1746000.

149. Franklin PJ, Hall GL, Moeller A, Horak Jr F, Brennan S, Stick SM. Exhaled nitric oxide is not reduced in infants with cystic fibrosis. Eur Respir J. 2006;27(2):350–3. PubMed PMID: 16452591.

150. Grasemann H, Schwiertz R, Matthiesen S, Racke K, Ratjen F. Increased arginase activity in cystic fibrosis airways. Am J Respir Crit Care Med. 2005;172(12):1523–8. PubMed PMID: 16166623.

151. de Winter-de Groot KM, van der Ent CK. Nitric oxide in cystic fibrosis. J Cyst Fibros. 2005;4 Suppl 2:25–9. PubMed PMID: 15982933.

152. Kelley TJ, Drumm ML. Inducible nitric oxide synthase expression is reduced in cystic fibrosis murine and human airway epithelial cells. J Clin Invest. 1998;102(6):1200–7. PubMed PMID: 9739054. Pubmed Central PMCID: 509103.
153. Moeller A, Horak Jr F, Lane C, Knight D, Kicic A, Brennan S, et al. Inducible NO synthase expression is low in airway epithelium from young children with cystic fibrosis. Thorax. 2006;61(6):514–20. PubMed PMID: 16517573. Pubmed Central PMCID: 2111217.
154. Zheng S, Xu W, Bose S, Banerjee AK, Haque SJ, Erzurum SC. Impaired nitric oxide synthase-2 signaling pathway in cystic fibrosis airway epithelium. Am J Physiol Lung Cell Mol Physiol. 2004;287(2):L374–81. PubMed PMID: 15107292.
155. Meng QH, Springall DR, Bishop AE, Morgan K, Evans TJ, Habib S, et al. Lack of inducible nitric oxide synthase in bronchial epithelium: a possible mechanism of susceptibility to infection in cystic fibrosis. J Pathol. 1998;184(3):323–31. PubMed PMID: 9614386.
156. Gaston B, Ratjen F, Vaughan JW, Malhotra NR, Canady RG, Snyder AH, et al. Nitrogen redox balance in the cystic fibrosis airway: effects of antipseudomonal therapy. Am J Respir Crit Care Med. 2002;165(3):387–90. PubMed PMID: 11818326.
157. Grasemann H, Ioannidis I, Tomkiewicz RP, de Groot H, Rubin BK, Ratjen F. Nitric oxide metabolites in cystic fibrosis lung disease. Arch Dis Child. 1998;78(1):49–53. PubMed PMID: 9534676. Pubmed Central PMCID: 1717443.
158. Grasemann H, Schwiertz R, Grasemann C, Vester U, Racke K, Ratjen F. Decreased systemic bioavailability of L-arginine in patients with cystic fibrosis. Respir Res. 2006;7:87. PubMed PMID: 16764721. Pubmed Central PMCID: 1526723.
159. Jones KL, Hegab AH, Hillman BC, Simpson KL, Jinkins PA, Grisham MB, et al. Elevation of nitrotyrosine and nitrate concentrations in cystic fibrosis sputum. Pediatr Pulmonol. 2000;30(2):79–85. PubMed PMID: 10922128.
160. Morrissey BM, Schilling K, Weil JV, Silkoff PE, Rodman DM. Nitric oxide and protein nitration in the cystic fibrosis airway. Arch Biochem Biophys. 2002;406(1):33–9. PubMed PMID: 12234487.
161. Jaffe A, Slade G, Rae J, Laverty A. Exhaled nitric oxide increases following admission for intravenous antibiotics in children with cystic fibrosis. J Cyst Fibros. 2003;2(3):143–7. PubMed PMID: 15463863.
162. Grasemann H, Kurtz F, Ratjen F. Inhaled L-arginine improves exhaled nitric oxide and pulmonary function in patients with cystic fibrosis. Am J Respir Crit Care Med. 2006;174(2):208–12. PubMed PMID: 16627863.
163. Grasemann H, Knauer N, Buscher R, Hubner K, Drazen JM, Ratjen F. Airway nitric oxide levels in cystic fibrosis patients are related to a polymorphism in the neuronal nitric oxide synthase gene. Am J Respir Crit Care Med. 2000;162(6):2172–6. PubMed PMID: 11112133.
164. Jobsis Q, Raatgeep HC, Schellekens SL, Kroesbergen A, Hop WC, de Jongste JC. Hydrogen peroxide and nitric oxide in exhaled air of children with cystic fibrosis during antibiotic treatment. Eur Respir J. 2000;16(1):95–100. PubMed PMID: 10933092.
165. Karadag B, James AJ, Gultekin E, Wilson NM, Bush A. Nasal and lower airway level of nitric oxide in children with primary ciliary dyskinesia. Eur Respir J. 1999;13(6):1402–5. PubMed PMID: 10445619.
166. Baraldi E, Pasquale MF, Cangiotti AM, Zanconato S, Zacchello F. Nasal nitric oxide is low early in life: case study of two infants with primary ciliary dyskinesia. Eur Respir J. 2004;24(5):881–3. PubMed PMID: 15516684.
167. Corbelli R, Bringolf-Isler B, Amacher A, Sasse B, Spycher M, Hammer J. Nasal nitric oxide measurements to screen children for primary ciliary dyskinesia. Chest. 2004;126(4):1054–9. PubMed PMID: 15486363.
168. Horvath I, Loukides S, Wodehouse T, Csiszer E, Cole PJ, Kharitonov SA, et al. Comparison of exhaled and nasal nitric oxide and exhaled carbon monoxide levels in bronchiectatic patients with and without primary ciliary dyskinesia. Thorax. 2003;58(1):68–72. PubMed PMID: 12511725. Pubmed Central PMCID: 1746449.
169. Lundberg JO, Weitzberg E, Nordvall SL, Kuylenstierna R, Lundberg JM, Alving K. Primarily nasal origin of exhaled nitric oxide and absence in Kartagener's syndrome. Eur Respir J. 1994;7(8):1501–4. PubMed PMID: 7957837.

170. Silkoff PE, Caramori M, Tremblay L, McClean P, Chaparro C, Kesten S, et al. Exhaled nitric oxide in human lung transplantation. A noninvasive marker of acute rejection. Am J Respir Crit Care Med. 1998;157(6 Pt 1):1822–8. PubMed PMID: 9620912.

171. Antus B, Csiszer E, Czebe K, Horvath I. Pulmonary infections increase exhaled nitric oxide in lung transplant recipients: a longitudinal study. Clin Transplant. 2005;19(3):377–82. PubMed PMID: 15877802.

172. Gabbay E, Walters EH, Orsida B, Whitford H, Ward C, Kotsimbos TC, et al. Post-lung transplant bronchiolitis obliterans syndrome (BOS) is characterized by increased exhaled nitric oxide levels and epithelial inducible nitric oxide synthase. Am J Respir Crit Care Med. 2000;162(6):2182–7. PubMed PMID: 11112135.

173. Neurohr C, Huppmann P, Leuschner S, von Wulffen W, Meis T, Leuchte H, et al. Usefulness of exhaled nitric oxide to guide risk stratification for bronchiolitis obliterans syndrome after lung transplantation. Am J Transplant. 2011;11(1):129–37. PubMed PMID: 21087415.

174. Bendiak GN, Kritzinger F, Dipchand AI, Ng VL, Solomon M, Grasemann H. Flow-independent exhaled nitric oxide parameters in pediatric lung and cardiac transplant recipients. Transplantation. 2011;91(10):e75–7. PubMed PMID: 21540720.

175. Grasemann H, Kritzinger F, Dipchand A, Hebert D, Solomon M. Nasal nitric oxide is reduced in children after solid-organ transplantation. J Heart Lung Transplant. 2011;30(1):108–9. PubMed PMID: 20934886.

176. Fazekas T, Eickhoff P, Lawitschka A, Knotek B, Potschger U, Peters C. Exhaled nitric oxide and pulmonary complications after paediatric stem cell transplantation. Eur J Pediatr. 2012;171(7):1095–101. PubMed PMID: 22350283.

Index

© Springer Science+Business Media New York 2015

309

S.D. Davis et al. (eds.), *Diagnostic Tests in Pediatric Pulmonology*,
Respiratory Medicine, DOI 10.1007/978-1-4939-1801-0